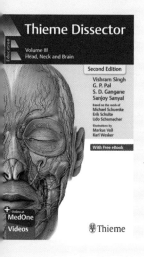

Thieme Dissector

Volume III
Head, Neck and Brain

Second Edition

Vishram Singh
G. P. Pal
S. D. Gangane
Sanjoy Sanyal

Based on the work of
Michael Schuenke
Erik Schulte
Udo Schumacher

Illustrations by
Markus Voll
Karl Wesker

With Free eBook

Online at
MedOne
Videos

Thieme

Access your free e-book now!

With three easy steps, unlock free access to your e-book on MedOne, Thieme's online platform.

1. Note your personal access code below. Once this code is activated, your printed book can no longer be returned.

T0329757

2. Scan this QR code or enter your access code at **medone.thieme.com/code**.

3. Set up a username on MedOne and sign in to activate your e-book on most phones, tablets, or PCs.

Quick Access

After you successfully register and activate your code, you can find your book and additional online media at **medone.thieme.com/9789392819254** or with this QR code.

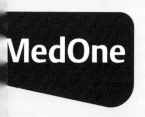

MedOne

...edical information how ...d when you need it.

Thieme
Dissector

Second Edition

Volume III

Head, Neck and Brain

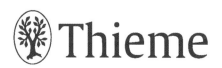

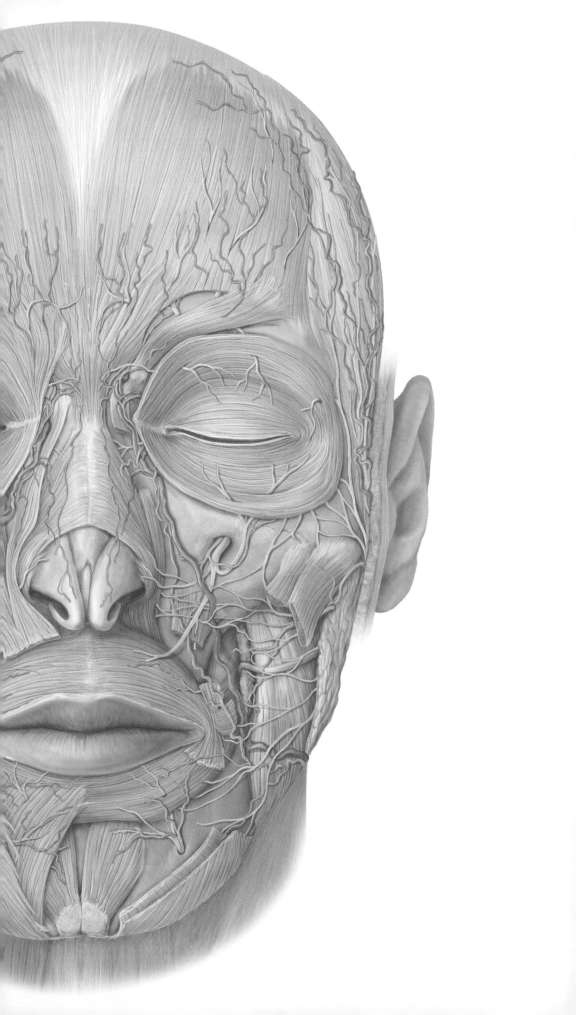

Thieme
Dissector

Second Edition

Volume III

Head, Neck and Brain

Vishram Singh, MBBS, MS, PhD (hc), MICPS, FASI, FIMSA
Adjunct Professor
Department of Anatomy
KMC, Manipal Academy of Higher Education
Mangalore, Karnataka, India;
Editor-in-Chief
Journal of the Anatomical Society of India;
Member, Federative International Committee for Scientific Publications (FICSP)
International Federation of Association on Anatomists (IFAA)
Geneva, Switzerland

G. P. Pal, MBBS, MS, DSc, FASI, FAMS, FNASc, FASc, Bhatnagar Laureate
Director Professor
Department of Anatomy
Index Medical College;
Emeritus Professor
MGM Medical College
Indore, Madhya Pradesh, India

S. D. Gangane, MBBS, MS, FAIMS
Professor and Head
Department of Anatomy
Terna Medical College
Navi Mumbai, Maharashtra, India

Sanjoy Sanyal MBBS, MS, MSc, ADPHA
Provost and Dean
Professor and Department Chair Anatomical Sciences
Richmond Gabriel University College of Medicine
St. Vincent and the Grenadines
Canada

Based on the work of
Michael Schuenke
Erik Schulte
Udo Schumacher

Illustrations by
Markus Voll
Karl Wesker

Thieme
Delhi • Stuttgart • New York • Rio de Janeiro

Publishing Director: Ritu Sharma
Senior Development Editor: Dr. Gurvinder Kaur
Director-Editorial Services: Rachna Sinha
Project Manager: Snehil Sharma
National Sales Manager: Bishwajit Kumar Mishra
Managing Director & CEO: Ajit Kohli

Thieme Medical and Scientific Publishers Private Limited.
A - 12, Second Floor, Sector - 2, Noida - 201 301,
Uttar Pradesh, India, +911204556600
Email: customerservice@thieme.in
www.thieme.in

Cover design: Thieme Publishing Group
Cover image source: Voll M and Wesker K

Illustrations by Voll M and Wesker K. From: Schuenke M,
Schulte E, Schumacher U, THIEME Atlas of Anatomy.

Page make-up by RECTO Graphics, India

Printed in India

First Reprint, 2022
Second Reprint, 2023
Third Reprint, 2023

ISBN: 978-93-92819-25-4
Also available as an e-book:
eISBN (PDF): 978-93-92819-30-8
eISBN (ePub): 978-93-92819-35-3

Important note: Medicine is an ever-changing science undergoing continual development. Research and clinical experience are continually expanding our knowledge, in particular, our knowledge of proper treatment and drug therapy. Insofar as this book mentions any dosage or application, readers may rest assured that the authors, editors, and publishers have made every effort to ensure that such references are in accordance with **the state of knowledge at the time of production of the book**.

Nevertheless, this does not involve, imply, or express any guarantee or responsibility on the part of the publishers in respect to any dosage instructions and forms of applications stated in the book. **Every user is requested to examine carefully** the manufacturers' leaflets accompanying each drug and to check, if necessary, in consultation with a physician or specialist, whether the dosage schedules mentioned therein or the contraindications stated by the manufacturers differ from the statements made in the present book. Such examination is particularly important with drugs that are either rarely used or have been newly released in the market. Every dosage schedule or every form of application used is entirely at the user's own risk and responsibility. The authors and publishers request every user to report to the publishers any discrepancies or inaccuracies noticed. If errors in this work are found after publication, errata will be posted at www.thieme.com on the product description page.

Some of the product names, patents, and registered designs referred to in this book are in fact registered trademarks or proprietary names even though specific reference to this fact is not always made in the text. Therefore, the appearance of a name without designation as proprietary is not to be construed as a representation by the publisher that it is in the public domain.

Thieme addresses people of all gender identities equally. We encourage our authors to use gender-neutral or gender-equal expressions wherever the context allows.

To my students, past and present.
Vishram Singh

To my grandson, Yatharth.
G. P. Pal

To my family and colleagues, for their support;
my patients and students, for teaching me to learn from them;
the willed body-donors, for their silent altruism to medical science.
Sanjoy Sanyal

Contents

Video Contents   ix

Note from the Authors   xi

About the Authors   xv

1. Introduction and Osteology of the Head and Neck   1

2. Scalp and Superficial Temporal Region   21

3. Face   31

4. Eyelids and Lacrimal Apparatus   43

5. Posterior Triangle   49

6. Back of the Neck and Suboccipital Triangle   57

7. Anterior Triangle of the Neck   65

8. Parotid Region   75

9. Temporal and Infratemporal Regions   85

10. Temporomandibular Joint   95

11. Submandibular Region and Submandibular Gland   103

12. Removal of the Brain from the Cranial Cavity, Cranial Meninges,
    and Dural Venous Sinuses   113

13. Cranial Fossae   123

14. Orbit   133

15. Deep Dissection of the Neck—I: Thyroid Gland   147

16. Deep Dissection of the Neck—II: Structures under Cover of the
    Sternocleidomastoid and Posterior Belly of Digastric   157

17. Deep Dissection of the Neck—III: Root of the Neck   165

18. Deep Dissection of the Neck—IV: Upper Part of the Cervical Vessels
    and Nerves   177

19. Dissection of the Prevertebral Region and Cervical Plexus   191

20. Pharynx, Palatine Tonsil, and Soft Palate   197

21. Tongue   209

22. Nasal Cavity and Paranasal Air Sinuses   219

23. Larynx   231

24. Eyeball   241

25. Ear 249

26. Joints of the Neck Region 261

27. Brain—Introduction and its Blood Vessels 269

28. Brainstem 283

29. Cerebellum 295

30. Fourth Ventricle 303

31. Cerebrum: External Features 307

32. Structures Seen on the Midsagittal Section of the Forebrain 317

33. White Matter of the Cerebrum 321

34. Dissection of the Lateral Ventricle 329

35. Dissection of Basal Nuclei 337

36. Sections of the Brain 341

Index 355

Video Contents

Video 2.1	Layers of scalp	24
Video 2.2	Dissection of superficial temporal region	28
Video 3.1	External nose	32
Video 4.1	Layers of eyelid, orbicularis oculi muscle, and lacrimal gland	47
Video 5.1	Posterior triangle of neck	55
Video 5.2	Lateral aspect of neck, external jugular vein variant, cervical plexus, CN XI, and scalene triangle	55
Video 7.1	Anterior triangle of neck	67
Video 7.2	Submental, submandibular, carotid and muscular triangles	68
Video 7.3	Carotid triangle	68
Video 8.1	Parotid gland and Parotid duct/Stensen duct	76
Video 9.1	Infratemporal fossa and pterygomaxillary fissure	86
Video 9.2	Infratemporal fossa: Part I	89
Video 9.3	Infratemporal fossa: Part II	89
Video 11.1	Submandibular region	107
Video 12.1	Intracranial dural venous sinuses	115
Video 13.1	Cranial venous sinus, superior sagittal sinus (SSS), cavernous sigmoid petrosal dural folds, clinicals	124
Video 13.2	Cavernous petrosal sinus, origin, tributaries, cavernous sinus (CS) syndrome, carotid-cavernous fistula (CCF), clinicals	124
Video 14.1	Salient features of bony orbit	134
Video 14.2	Ocular muscles, lacrimal gland, and optic nerve	134
Video 14.3	Orbit extraocular eye muscles and neurovascular structures	136
Video 15.1	Thyroid gland and its relations	149
Video 15.2	Larynx and trachea	149
Video 16.1	Cranial nerves X, XI, XII and ansa cervicalis in neck	159
Video 17.1	Carotid, jugular, vagus, recurrent laryngeal nerve	168
Video 17.2	Scalene triangle	168
Video 17.3	Subclavian vessels, brachial plexus, and scalene triangle	169

Video 18.1   Last four cranial nerves: Glosso-Pharyngeal vagus, hypoglossal,
             and accessory nerves in neck   179

Video 18.2   Carotid arteries   180

Video 19.1   Cervical plexus   192

Video 20.1   Laryngopharynx and piriform fossa   200

Video 21.1   Floor of the mouth   212

Video 23.1   Larynx–Part 1: external structure   232

Video 23.2   Larynx–Part 2: internal structure   236

Video 23.3   Interior of larynx, trachea, laryngopharynx, and piriform fossa   238

Video 24.1   Exenterated eyeball showing ocular muscles, lacrimal gland,
             and optic nerve   242

Video 27.1   Human brain: vertebrobasilar circulation of brain   273

Video 27.2   Human brain: carotid middle cerebral, and anterior cerebral arteries   273

Video 27.3   Tracking brain circulation via 2D time of flight angiography (TOF)
             serial MRI axial slices with narration   281

Video 29.1   Cerebellar dissection: Part I   296

Video 29.2   Cerebellar dissection: Part II   296

Video 29.3   Deep nuclei of cerebellum   297

Video 30.1   Ventricles of brain   304

Video 31.1   Hippocampus and fornix   311

Video 31.2   Papez circuit   311

Video 32.1   Circumventricular organs, location, cytoarchitecture description   320

Video 33.1   Caudate nucleus, lentiform nucleus, thalamus, and internal capsule   323

Video 34.1   Lateral ventricle   330

Video 35.1   Basal ganglia: Part I   340

Video 35.2   Basal ganglia: Part II   340

Note from the Authors

There was a long-felt need of a good dissection manual for first-year undergraduate medical students undertaking the anatomy course. Anatomy is the foundation of all medical subjects, and hence, its thorough knowledge is essential for all students aspiring to become good doctors, especially in surgical fields.

The best *modus operandi* to learn anatomy is through dissection. Recently, due to information explosion in the medical field, the health sciences curricula have markedly reduced the time allocation for studying and teaching anatomy; yet it is realized by all that the gross structure of the human body, including its three-dimensional conceptualization, must be understood thoroughly before proceeding further to learn medicine.

Therefore, we have made a sincere effort to meet all the needs of the students in creating this three-volume set of dissection manuals. They not only delineate instructions for students to perform perfect dissection but also provide gross anatomy descriptions, supplemented by clinical correlations of gross structures studied during dissection. The textual descriptions are complemented by numerous colored illustrations that will help students recognize significant structures with more precision. To further enhance understanding, the content of the volumes is organized in sections like (a) Learning Objectives, (b) Surface Landmarks, (c) Dissection and Identification, (d) Description of Gross Anatomy, and (e) Clinical Notes. Laced with all these features, we hope that these volumes will be useful not only for medical and dental students but also for teachers of anatomy. The value of these volumes is further enhanced by providing videos at relevant places.

As educators of anatomy, we have tried our best to make these manuals easy for learning. We highly appreciate the contribution of Prof. Poonam Kharb and Mr. D. Krishna Chaitanya in Volume II and Prof. Shabana M. Borate in Volume I. For further improvements, we would sincerely welcome comments and suggestions from all students and teachers.

The second edition of this dissection manual is thoroughly updated with new line diagrams, X-ray pictures, and CT and MRI scans.

All dissection steps are supplemented by dissection videos in all the three volumes for easy understanding of gross and clinical anatomy by the students.

Vishram Singh, MBBS, MS, PhD (hc), MICPS, FASI, FIMSA

The medical curriculum in India requires basic anatomy, along with some other basic subjects, to be taught to students in the first year of the course. This often leads to an information overload for them. For some students, the situation is made even more difficult due to linguistic limitations and late admissions. As a result, there has long been a pressing need for comprehensive teaching resources that create thorough understanding of these courses in a short time span. Specifically for anatomy, one cannot stress enough on the value of a complete and detailed dissection manual that explains basic concepts in a simple and lucid manner, without duplication of facts or unnecessary complexities.

In Volume III, every care has been taken to describe all steps involved in the dissection of the head, neck, and brain in a stepwise manner that is easy to understand for the beginners. Several high-quality illustrations have been used to explain each step. They help show the dissections with a great amount of detailing and clarity. To make the discourse interesting, relevant clinical conditions have also been presented under separate sections called "Clinical Notes."

Producing a book with hundreds of illustrations is a joint effort by the author and the publisher in a true sense.

I strongly believe that this book will be an invaluable learning resource for students and teachers of anatomy in medical and dental courses.

G. P. Pal, MBBS, MS, DSc, FASI, FAMS, FNASc, FASc, Bhatnagar Laureate

Cadaveric dissection is an integral part of teaching anatomy in medical schools. It offers an unmatched firsthand experience of exploring the structure of organs and their relationship with each other. *Thieme Dissector* provides a complete account of dissection of human body through a set of three volumes.

The first volume deals with the upper limb and thorax. The introduction of this volume gives general information about preservation of cadaver, instruments required for dissection, and anatomical terms, followed by a discussion on basic tissues of the body. This is followed by 10 chapters on upper limb and 5 chapters on thorax. Each chapter begins with "Learning Objectives," followed by an introduction to the topic, dissection steps with description of the relevant structures, and clinical notes.

To facilitate understanding of the subject, photographs of actual dissected parts and real dissection videos have been provided. Access to these videos will help and enrich students' learning process.

My heartfelt gratitude to Dr. Shabana M. Borate, Associate Professor, Department of Anatomy, at Grant Government Medical College and Sir J. J. Group of Hospitals, Mumbai, Maharashtra, India, Dr. Sachin Yadav, Assistant Professor at Grant Government Medical College and Sir J. J. Group of Hospitals, Mumbai, Maharashtra, India, and Dr. Shilpa Domkundwar, Professor and Head, Department of Radiodiagnosis, Grant Government Medical College and Sir J. J. Group of Hospitals, Mumbai, Maharashtra, India, for their untiring efforts in preparation of this volume. I am grateful to the entire team of Thieme Publishers for their constant support, and special thanks to Dr. Vishram Singh sir, who has been the guiding force for all of us in preparation of the *Thieme Dissector*.

S. D. Gangane, MBBS, MS, FAIMS

Thieme has taken a positive step by introducing this book for imparting anatomy education to medical students worldwide. The process of depicting videos and pictures of actual cadaver dissections in a textbook is indeed a monumental task. It starts with planning of the region to be dissected. This is followed by meticulous dissection of the region itself, which can take hours if not days. Then comes the process of accurate live narration of the dissection of the region on camera, while the video recording is in progress. The back-breaking task of editing and captioning the video frames and clips follows next, because many anatomical and medical terms used in the narration may otherwise be incomprehensible to the student. Since clinical students like content related to radiology, some videos have radiological images embedded within the frames. The relevant still shots from the dissections are then edited and labeled. Finally, of course, comes the task of publishing the finished product.

There are many digital anatomy tools available to the medical academia, ranging in size and versatility from usage in classrooms and digital labs to those used in individual laptops and tablets. Some have virtual reality–like, immersive three-dimensional, or augmented reality applications. They vary in accuracy, comprehensiveness, and versatility. They are good study tools, which are interactive and interesting to use in teaching and learning anatomy. They show body parts and spatial relationships. They are available offline, accessible anytime, anywhere, and can even show rare pathology. They present consolidated anatomy information to suit users' learning styles. They do not have the legal, ethical, religious, social, regional, and logistical constraints of human cadaver procurement. These factors are weaning away institutions from the hoary art of cadaver dissection.

However, cadaver dissection is still the gold standard for learning human anatomy and surgery. It is the benchmark for measuring the success of newer learning technologies. Cadavers are medical students' first "patients." Digital resources are to be considered as supplements to the armamentarium of learning methods in human anatomy. Digital technologies lack haptic qualities of human tissue, which are essential for a surgeon. Therefore, they can never completely replace cadaver dissection for anatomy students and surgical residents under training. Nobody would want to be treated by surgeons who acquired their entire quantum of expertise in operating on the human body through virtual reality alone, just like nobody would want to be flown by an airline pilot whose only flying experience was in the digital flight simulator.

The author is truly gratified knowing that students have learned the subject of anatomy and mastered the intricacies of the human body by watching *Thieme Dissector* videos and illustrations.

Sanjoy Sanyal, MBBS, MS, MSc, ADPHA

About the Authors

Vishram Singh
(Editor-in-Chief and Author, Volume II, Abdomen and Lower Limb)
Vishram Singh, MBBS, MS, PhD (hc), MICPS, FASI, FIMSA, is currently the Adjunct Professor, Department of Anatomy, KMC, Manipal Academy of Higher Education, Mangalore, Karnataka, India; Editor-in-Chief, *Journal of the Anatomical Society of India*; and Member, Federative International Committee for Scientific Publications (FICSP), International Federation of Association on Anatomists (IFAA), Geneva, Switzerland.

A renowned anatomist, Prof. Singh has taught undergraduate and postgraduate students at several colleges and institutes, such as GSVM Medical College, Kanpur; King George Medical College, Lucknow; All India Institute of Medical Sciences, New Delhi; and Al Arab Medical University, Benghazi, Libya. He has more than 50 years of experience in teaching, research, and clinical practice. He has various bestselling titles to his credit, such as *Textbook of Clinical Neuroanatomy, Textbook of Anatomy*—three volumes, and *Textbook of Clinical Embryology*. He has published more than 20 books and more than 100 research articles in reputed national and international journals.

Prof. Singh has received various recognitions and awards for his contributions in the field of gross anatomy, neuroanatomy, and embryology.

He has been elected Vice President of the Anatomical Society of India many times. He is currently Editor-in-Chief, *Journal of Anatomical Society of India* (JASI).

G. P. Pal
(Author, Volume III, Head, Neck, and Brain)
G. P. Pal, MBBS, MS, DSc, FASI, FAMS, FNASc, FASc, Bhatnagar Laureate, is currently the Director Professor of Anatomy at the Index Medical College; Emeritus Professor at MGM Medical College, Indore, Madhya Pradesh, India. Dr. Pal is an eminent teacher with almost five decades of teaching experience in various medical colleges of India and the United States.

He has to his credit numerous publications in journals of international repute. He has received several national awards and honors for his research works, which includes Shakuntala Amir Chand Prize of Indian Council of Medical Research (ICMR), Shanti Swarup Bhatnagar Prize of Council of Scientific and Industrial Research (CSIR), and several gold medals, oration awards, and Lifetime Achievement Award by the Anatomical Society of India. He has been elected Fellow at various leading academies of sciences in India—Anatomical Society of India; National Academy of Medical Sciences (New Delhi), National Academy of Sciences (Allahabad), and Indian Academy of Sciences (Bengaluru). His research work is cited in more than 100 standard medical textbooks throughout the world. Recently, his name featured in the list of top 2% scientists of the world. As per a survey conducted by the Stanford University, USA, in 2020, he is ranked as no. 1 Anatomy Scientist in India and 102 in the world.

Dr. Pal has authored many well-received books such as *Textbook of Histology, Illustrated Textbook of Neuroanatomy, Medical Genetics, Genetics in Dentistry, General Anatomy, Basics of Medical Genetics, Human Osteology, Genetics for Dental Student, Neuroanatomy for Medical Students,* and *Thieme Dissector*. He has edited First South Asian edition of *Grant's Atlas of Anatomy*. He has also coauthored Prof. Inderbir Singh's *Human Embryology* from the 7th to 9th editions. For more information about the author and his works, Google "Indian Anatomists - Wikipedia" or "Gaya Prasad Pal - Wikipedia."

S. D. Gangane
(Author, Volume I, Upper Limb and Thorax)

S. D. Gangane, MBBS, MS, FAIMS, is currently serving as Professor and Head, Department of Anatomy at Terna Medical College, Navi Mumbai, Maharashtra, India. He has been Professor and Head, Department of Anatomy and Genetic Division at Grant Medical College, Mumbai and Sir J. J. Group of Hospitals, Mumbai. This is a unique Anatomy Department offering services to patients having genetic disorders. Prof. Gangane has authored a bestselling book titled *Human Genetics* which has been widely accepted by faculty and both undergraduate and postgraduate students.

Prof. Gangane has over four decades of teaching experience and has been guiding students for MD Anatomy, and MSc and PhD in Applied Biology courses at the Mumbai University. He has also been a guide for the MD Anatomy and PhD Genetics courses at Maharashtra University of Health Sciences (the State Health University). He has published several articles in national and international journals and is also a coauthor of the recently published *Textbook of Pathology and Genetics for Nurses*. In addition, he has been on the national advisory board and the executive editorial board for a few journals, including *Indian Journal of Anatomy* and *National Journal of Medical Sciences*.

Prof. Gangane has also worked as an Officer of Special Duty (OSD) for the Government of Maharashtra under the Directorate of Medical Education and Research. He is a member of the advisory panel for the South Asian region of the international publishing house, Lippincott Williams and Wilkins. He is the founder Trustee of "Sandnya Sanwardhan Sanstha", an organization that takes care of mentally challenged children by imparting vocational training and enabling them to lead better lives.

Sanjoy Sanyal
(Contributor of Videos, Volumes I, II, and III)

Sanjoy Sanyal, MBBS, MS, MSc, ADPHA, is the Provost and Dean of Richmond Gabriel University College of Medicine, St. Vincent and the Grenadines, Canada. He is also the Professor and Department Chair of Anatomical Sciences in the same university. With medical degrees from India and the United Kingdom, Dr. Sanyal has 39 years of clinical, surgical, and teaching experience as a surgeon, surgical anatomist, neuroscientist, and medical informatician.

A prolific medical and educational researcher, he has published 25 original research papers in peer-reviewed journals and presented 15 papers in many international conferences in 11 countries. He is the recipient of five Outstanding Professor Awards from several different universities and medical schools.

He is a surgical skills instructor to American Medical Students' Association (AMSA). He is a life-member of Indian Medical Association (IMA), and annual member of American Association for Anatomy (AAA) and American Association of Clinical Anatomists (AACA). He is a provisional patent holder (January 2014) of a computerized medical program from the United States Patent and Trademark Office (USPTO). He is peer reviewer of several medical journals.

Dr. Sanjoy Sanyal is honorary faculty of the Multimedia Educational Resource for Learning and Online Teaching (MERLOT), a program of the California State University (CSU), Long Beach, partnering with educational institutions, professional societies, and industry. He is Gold-level MERLOT contributor, having authored more than 350 learning materials. He is a member of Virtual Speaker's Bureau (VSB) of MERLOT. He is also the recipient of Innovative Use of MERLOT award.

With an underpinning philosophy of lifelong learning, his motto is to make each succeeding generation better than the previous.

Introduction and Osteology of the Head and Neck

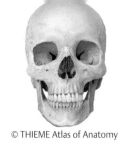

© THIEME Atlas of Anatomy

Introduction

The head is the upper globular part of the body which contains the brain. The neck is an elongated, cylindrical region of the body which connects the head to the trunk.

The bones of the head and neck region consist of *skull, cervical vertebrae,* and *hyoid bone.*

1. The skull forms the skeleton of the head region.

2. The cervical vertebrae form the skeleton of neck region.

3. The hyoid bone is present in the upper part of the neck in front of the third cervical vertebra.

Skull

The skull is formed by many paired and unpaired bones (**Table 1.1**), most of which unite with each other by sutures. A suture is narrow, linear gap filled with dense, fibrous tissue. Students are suggested to identify various bones of a dry skull and intervening sutures with the help of **Figs. 1.1** to **1.5**. We may study the dry skull by looking at it from various aspects, that is, from above (superior view), behind (posterior view), front (anterior view), side (lateral view), below (external view of the base), and inside (internal views of the base and the skull cap).

The skull consists of a brain box/cranium and facial skeleton. The facial skeleton is located beneath the anterior part of the cranium.

Table 1.1 Bones of skull

Part of skull	Paired	Unpaired
Cranium	Parietal bone, temporal bone	Frontal bone, ethmoid bone, occipital bone, sphenoid bone
Facial skeleton	Nasal bones, lacrimal bones, maxillae, zygomatic bones, palatine bones, inferior conchae	Frontal bone, vomer bone, mandible

Anatomical Position of the Skull

Anatomical position of the skull is obtained by keeping it in "Frankfurt horizontal plane." This plane is obtained by holding the skull in such a way that the inferior border of the orbit and superior border of external acoustic meatus of right and left sides lie in the same horizontal plane.

Superior Aspect of the Skull

Bones: On the superior aspect of the skull, the scalp covers the parts of the frontal bone, right and left parietal bones, and occipital bone.

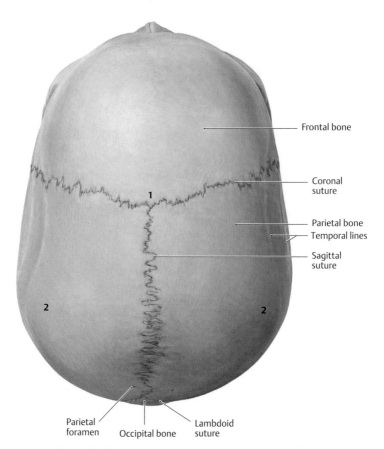

Frontal bone

Coronal
suture

Parietal bone
Temporal lines

Sagittal
suture

Parietal
foramen   Occipital bone   Lambdoid
suture

Fig. 1.1 Superior view of the skull. 1, Bregma; 2, parietal eminence. (From: Schuenke M, Schulte E, Schumacher U. THIEME Atlas of Anatomy. Head, Neck, and Neuroanatomy. Illustrations by Voll M and Wesker K. © Thieme 2020.)

Sutures: With the help of **Fig. 1.1**, identify the coronal, sagittal, and lambdoid sutures in this view. The bregma is the meeting point between the coronal and sagittal sutures, while lambda is the meeting point between the sagittal and lambdoid sutures.

Bony features: Identify the parietal eminence, parietal foramen, temporal lines (superior and inferior), and vertex (highest point of the skull).

Posterior Aspect of the Skull

Bones: With the help of **Fig. 1.2**, look for the following bones on the posterior aspect of the skull: posterior portions of the parietal bones, upper part of the occipital bone, and mastoid parts of the temporal bone.

Sutures: Look for the following sutures seen in this view: lambdoidal suture, occipitomastoid suture, and parietomastoid suture.

Bony features: With the help of **Fig. 1.2**, identify the following bony features on a dry skull: external occipital protuberance, external occipital crest, highest nuchal lines (supreme nuchal lines), superior nuchal lines, and inferior nuchal lines.

Anterior Aspect of the Skull

The anterior aspect of the skull forms the facial skeleton. It consists of forehead, orbits, nasal region, and upper and lower jaws.

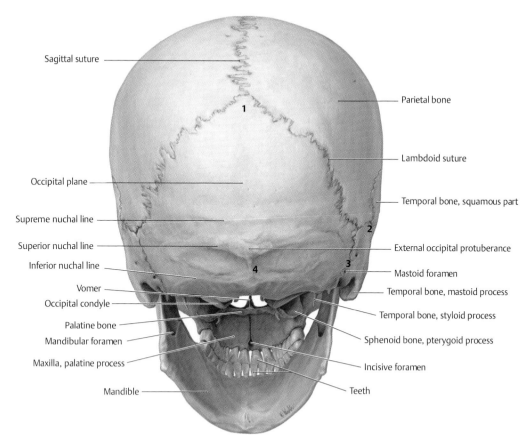

Fig. 1.2 Posterior view of the skull. 1, Lambda; 2, parietomastoid suture; 3, occipitomastoid suture; 4, external occipital crest. (From: Schuenke M, Schulte E, Schumacher U. THIEME Atlas of Anatomy. Head, Neck, and Neuroanatomy. Illustrations by Voll M and Wesker K. © Thieme 2020.)

Bones: Identify the bones of the facial skeleton with the help of **Fig. 1.3**. These bones are the frontal bone, right and left nasal bones, right and left zygomatic bones, and right and left maxilla and mandible.

Sutures: Look at **Fig. 1.3** for the following sutures present in this view: frontonasal suture, frontomaxillary suture, internasal suture, nasomaxillary suture, intermaxillary suture, frontozygomatic suture, and zygomaticomaxillary suture.

Bony features:

1. *Forehead*: Look for the following features on the forehead: glabella, superciliary arches, and frontal eminences.

2. *Orbital opening*: It is quadrilateral in shape and presents four margins: supraorbital, infraorbital, lateral, and medial.

3. *Malar prominence*: It is formed by the zygomatic bone and presents the zygomaticofacial foramen.

4. *Anterior nasal aperture*: It is piriform in shape. Note the presence of the median nasal septum, anterior nasal spine, and nasal notch of the right and left maxillae.

5. *Upper jaw (maxillae)*: It is formed by the right and left maxillae. Note the bony features, such as the alveolar process, canine eminence, incisive fossa, and canine fossa.

6. *Lower jaw (mandible)*: It is formed by the mandible. Note the features, such as alveolar process, mental foramen, symphysis menti, and mental protuberance.

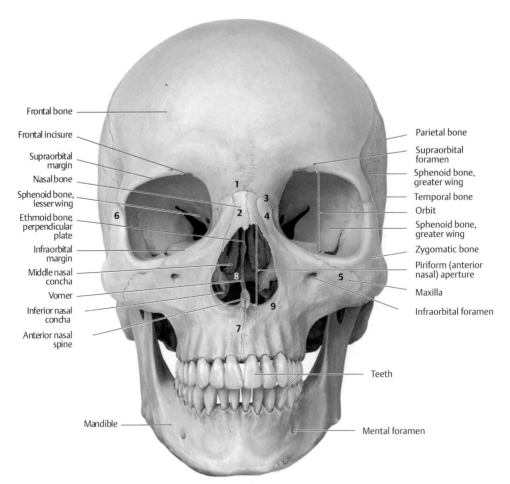

Fig. 1.3 Anterior view of the skull. 1, Frontonasal suture; 2, internasal suture; 3, frontomaxillary suture; 4, nasomaxillary suture; 5, zygomaticomaxillary suture; 6, frontozygomatic suture; 7, intermaxillary suture. Note the median nasal septum (8) formed by vomer and perpendicular plate of ethmoid. 9, Nasal notch. (From: Schuenke M, Schulte E, Schumacher U. THIEME Atlas of Anatomy. Head, Neck, and Neuroanatomy. Illustrations by Voll M and Wesker K. © Thieme 2020.)

Lateral Aspect of the Skull

Bones: This aspect of the skull is formed by the cranial and facial bones. Identify the following bones on the lateral aspect of the skull: frontal, parietal, occipital, nasal, maxilla, zygomatic, sphenoid, temporal, and mandible (**Fig. 1.4**).

Sutures: Many sutures, which are seen on this aspect, have already been observed while studying the superior, anterior, and lateral views of the dry skull. Hence, we shall study the sutures present in the central region of the lateral view (**Fig. 1.4**).

Identify an H-shaped suture present in the floor of the temporal fossa. This H-shaped suture is formed by the parietosphenoid, frontosphenoid, and temporosphenoid sutures. A small circular area enclosing this H-shaped suture is called a *pterion*. Also, identify the parietosquamous (squamous) and parietomastoid sutures, lambdoid suture, and occipitomastoid suture.

Bony features: Identify the superior and inferior temporal lines, zygomatic arch, supramastoid crest, external acoustic meatus, suprameatal triangle, mastoid process, and styloid process.

1. *Temporal fossa*: This fossa lies above the zygomatic arch. It is bounded above by the temporal lines. The temporal fossa communicates below with the infratemporal fossa.

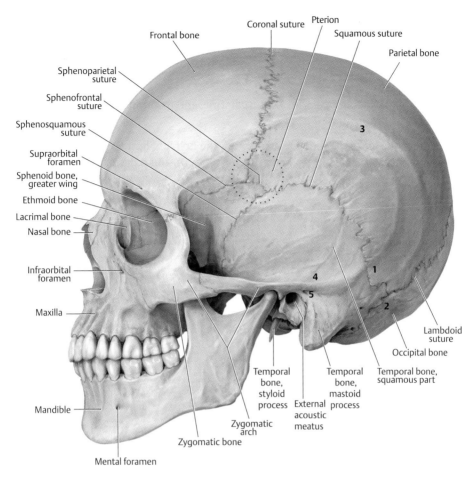

Fig. 1.4   Lateral view of the skull. 1, Parietomastoid suture; 2, occipitomastoid suture; 3, superior and inferior temporal lines; 4, supramastoid crest; 5, suprameatal triangle. (From: Schuenke M, Schulte E, Schumacher U. THIEME Atlas of Anatomy. Head, Neck, and Neuroanatomy. Illustrations by Voll M and Wesker K. © Thieme 2020.)

2. *Infratemporal fossa*: It is an irregular fossa below the zygomatic arch and behind the maxilla. It communicates above with the temporal fossa deep to the zygomatic arch. It consists of the roof, anterior, medial, and lateral walls, while the posterior wall and floor are open.

3. *Pterygopalatine fossa*: The junction of the anterior and medial walls shows a fissure called ptery-gomaxillary fissure. Deep to the fissure lies the pterygopalatine fossa.

(Students should note that infratemporal and pterygopalatine fossae are not properly visualized in these figures. They should study these fossae on a dry skull with the help of their teacher.)

Base of the Skull

You should note that to visualize the base of the skull, it is necessary to detach the mandible from the rest of the skull. The base of the skull is formed, from anterior to posterior, by the maxil-lae, palatine, vomer, sphenoid, temporal, and occipital bones (**Fig. 1.5**). For the convenience of description, the base of the skull is divided into anterior, middle, and posterior parts by two imagi-nary horizontal lines. The first imaginary horizontal line is drawn along the posterior border of the hard palate, and the second line passes through the anterior margin of the foramen magnum.

Anterior Part of the External Aspect of the Base of the Skull

Bones: It is formed by the alveolar arch of the maxilla and hard palate (**Fig. 1.5**). Hard palate is formed by the palatine processes of the right and left maxillae and horizontal plates of the palatine bones.

Sutures: Intermaxillary (median palatine), interpalatine, and palatomaxillary (transverse palatine) sutures form a cruciform suture.

Bony features: Note the following bony features with the help of **Fig. 1.5**: greater palatine foramen, lesser palatine foramen, incisive fossa, posterior nasal spine, and palatine crest.

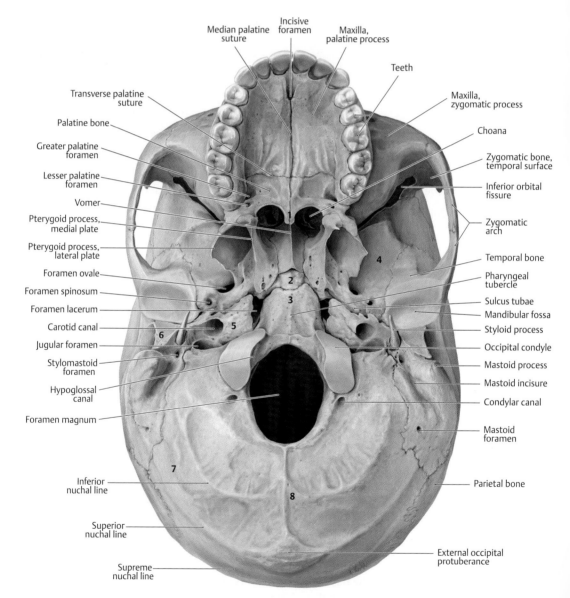

Fig. 1.5 Base of the skull. 1, Posterior nasal spine; 2, body of sphenoid; 3, basilar part of occipital bone; 4, greater wing of sphenoid; 5, petrous bone; 6, tympanic bone; 7, asterion; 8, external occipital crest. (From: Schuenke M, Schulte E, Schumacher U. THIEME Atlas of Anatomy. Head, Neck, and Neuroanatomy. Illustrations by Voll M and Wesker K. © Thieme 2020.)

Middle Part of the Base of the Skull

Bones: The bones present in the region are divided into median, right, and left areas. In the median area, bones are posterior border of vomer, body of sphenoid, and basilar part of the occipital bone. The bones in the lateral area are medial and lateral pterygoid plates, greater wing of the sphenoid, and temporal bone with its squamous, tympanic and petrous parts.

Sutures: The infratemporal surface of the greater wing of the sphenoid articulates with the squamous part of the temporal bone, posterolaterally, and with the petrous part of the temporal bone, posteromedially (sulcus tubae). Also, look for the squamotympanic fissure, petrosquamous fissure, and petrotympanic fissure.

Bony features: Note the posterior nasal apertures on either side of the vomer and pharyngeal tubercle in front of the foramen magnum. On the lateral side, look for the pterygoid fossa, scaphoid fossa, and hamulus. More laterally, note the tubercle of the root of the zygoma, articular tubercle, and mandibular fossa. Note the tympanic plate forming the posterior nonarticular part of the mandibular fossa.

Posterior Part of the Base of the Skull

Bones: The median area of the posterior part consists of the foramen magnum, which is bounded anteriorly by the basilar part, laterally by the condylar part and posteriorly by the squamous part of the occipital bone. In the lateral area of this part, look for the mastoid and styloid processes.

Sutures: Note the meeting point of the three sutures, that is, the occipitomastoid, lambdoid, and parietomastoid at the asterion.

Bony features: In the median part, identify the foramen magnum, jugular foramen, and occipital condyles. Posterior to the foramen magnum, look for the external occipital crest, protuberance, and nuchal lines with the help of **Fig. 1.5**. In the lateral part, note the presence of the styloid and mastoid processes.

Internal Aspect of the Skull

When the upper part of the vault of the skull (skull cap or calvaria) is removed, we may see the inner surface of the cranial vault and the interior of the base of the skull.

Inner Surface of the Cranial Vault

Bones and sutures: The various bones and the intervening sutures forming the cranial vault are the same as observed in the superior aspect of the skull (**Fig. 1.1**).

Bony features: In the midline, note the frontal crest and sagittal sulcus (groove). Many small depressions (*granular pits or foveolae*) are observed on each side of the sagittal sulcus. The inner aspect of the calvaria shows the presence of grooves for the meningeal vessels (**Fig. 1.6**).

Interior of the Base of the Skull

The internal aspect of the base of the skull can be divided into three fossae, that is, *anterior, middle,* and *posterior cranial fossae* (**Fig. 1.7**). The posterior border of the lesser wing of the sphenoid, anterior clinoid process and the anterior border of the sulcus chiasmaticus separates the anterior cranial fossa from the middle fossa. The middle and posterior fossae are separated from each other by the superior border of the petrous part of the temporal bone, posterior clinoid process, and dorsum sellae.

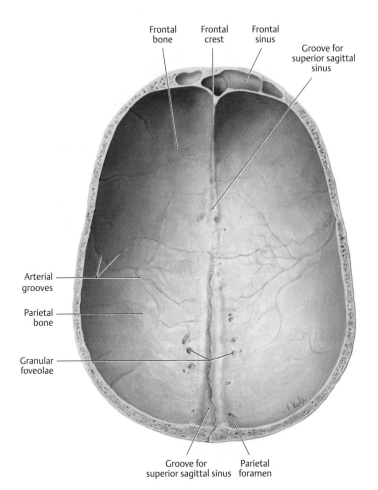

Frontal bone — Frontal crest — Frontal sinus — Groove for superior sagittal sinus

Arterial grooves

Parietal bone

Granular foveolae

Groove for superior sagittal sinus — Parietal foramen

Fig. 1.6 Inner surface of the cranial vault. (From: Schuenke M, Schulte E, Schumacher U. THIEME Atlas of Anatomy. Head, Neck, and Neuroanatomy. Illustrations by Voll M and Wesker K. © Thieme 2020.)

Anterior Cranial Fossa

Bones: The anterior cranial fossa is formed by the frontal bone, cribriform plate of the ethmoid, lesser wing of the sphenoid, and the anterior part of the superior surface of the body of the sphenoid (*jugum sphenoidale*).

Sutures: With the help of **Fig. 1.7a**, identify the frontoethmoidal, frontosphenoidal, and sphenoethmoidal sutures.

Bony features: In the median region of the floor of the anterior cranial fossa, note the frontal crest, crista galli, cribriform plate of the ethmoid, and jugum sphenoidale. The lateral region of the floor consists of the orbital plate and lesser wing of the sphenoid.

Middle Cranial Fossa

Bones: The median part is formed by the body of the sphenoid. Most anteriorly, the *sulcus chiasmaticus* is present. Behind the sulcus chiasmaticus, a saddle-shaped depression is present on the superior surface of the body of the sphenoid. It is known as *sella turcica*. The sella turcica consists of the *tuberculum sellae, hypophyseal fossa,* and *dorsum sellae* from anterior to posterior. Laterally, the floor of the middle cranial fossa is formed by three bones, that is, the cranial surface of the greater wing of the sphenoid, squamous, and petrous parts of the temporal bone.

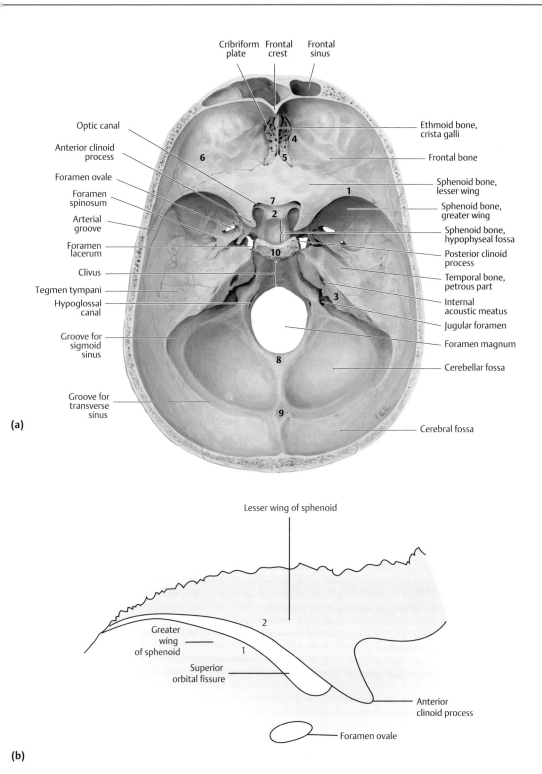

(a)

(b)

Fig. 1.7 **(a)** Interior of the base of the skull. 1, Posterior border of lesser wing of sphenoid; 2, sulcus chiasmaticus; 3, superior border of petrous temporal bone; 4, frontoethmoidal suture; 5, sphenoethmoidal suture; 6, frontosphenoidal; 7, jugum sphenoidale; 8, internal occipital crest; 9, internal occipital protuberance; 10, dorsum sellae. Superior orbital fissure is not seen as it is hidden below the free margin of lesser wing of sphenoid (refer to **b**). **(b)** Diagram of left superior orbital fissure as seen through middle cranial fossa. Superior orbital fissure is located between the 1. free margin of greater wing and 2. free margin of lesser wing of sphenoid bone. (Figure a: From: Schuenke M, Schulte E, Schumacher U. THIEME Atlas of Anatomy. Head, Neck, and Neuroanatomy. Illustrations by Voll M and Wesker K. © Thieme 2020.)

Sutures: At the base of the middle cranial fossa, look for a suture between the greater wing of the sphenoid and the squamous part of the temporal bone, and a suture between the petrous part and greater wing of the sphenoid.

Bony features: The *superior orbital fissure* (**Figs. 1.7b** and **1.8a**) is a triangular oblique cleft present most anteriorly in the middle cranial fossa. It connects the middle fossa with the orbit. Identify the foramen rotundum, foramen ovale, foramen spinosum, and foramen lacerum. In the median part, identify the hypophyseal fossa.

Posterior Cranial Fossa

Bones: The posterior part of the body of the sphenoid, occipital bone, posterior surface of the petrous temporal bone, mastoid part of the temporal bone, and posteroinferior angle of the parietal bone.

Sutures: The lower end of the lambdoid suture is present between the parietal and occipital bone, the parietomastoid suture, occipitomastoid suture, and petro-occipital suture.

Bony features: The median part of the floor presents the most striking structure, that is, the foramen magnum. The part anterior to the foramen magnum is called *clivus*. The parts posterior to the foramen magnum are internal occipital crest and internal occipital protuberance. In the lateral part of the floor, identify the *internal acoustic meatus,* jugular foramen, and transverse sulcus.

Orbital Cavity

The orbit is like a four-sided pyramid. It has a base, an apex, a roof, a floor, a medial wall, and a lateral wall (**Fig. 1.8a–c**).

The base: The base of the orbit is the orbital opening. It has four margins, that is, upper, lateral, medial, and inferior margins (**Fig. 1.3**).

The apex: The apex of the orbit lies posteriorly.

The medial wall: From anterior to posterior, the medial wall of the orbit is formed by the frontal process of the maxilla, lacrimal bone, orbital plate of the ethmoid, and body of the sphenoid.

The superior wall or roof: The superior wall is formed mainly by the orbital plate of the frontal bone and posteriorly by the lesser wing of the sphenoid.

The lateral wall: The lateral wall is formed anteriorly by the zygomatic bone and posteriorly by the greater wing of the sphenoid.

The inferior wall or floor: The inferior wall is mainly formed by the maxilla and a small part by the zygomatic bone.

Fissures, canal, and foramina of the orbital cavity: You should note that the orbital cavity communicates with the neighboring regions of the skull through the superior and inferior orbital fissures, optic and infraorbital canals, and various foramina.

Nasal Cavity

The nasal cavity is divided into right and left halves by the vertical median septum (i.e., the nasal septum). Each half of the cavity consists of an anterior opening, that is, the anterior nasal aperture, posterior nasal aperture, lateral wall, medial wall, roof, and floor.

The medial wall: The medial wall (median nasal septum) is formed by the perpendicular plate of the ethmoid, vomer bone, and septal cartilage (**Fig. 1.9a**).

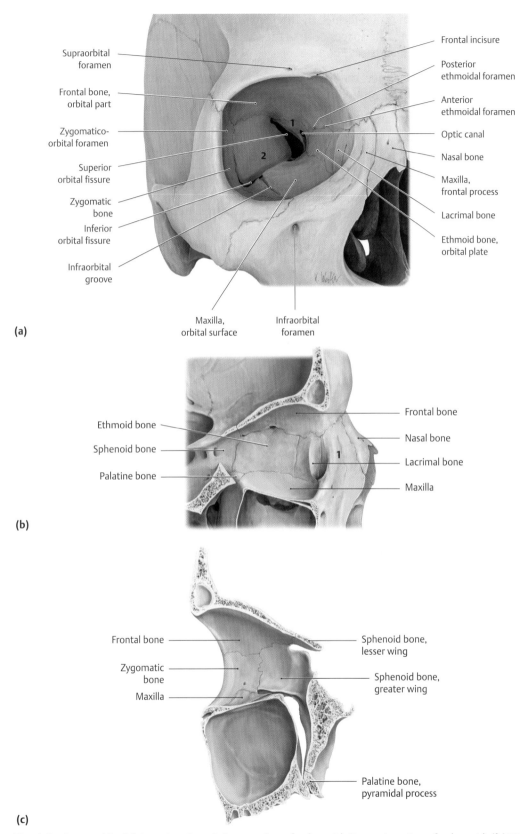

Fig. 1.8 Bony orbit: **(a)** Anterior view. 1, Lesser wing of sphenoid; 2, greater wing of sphenoid. **(b)** View of the medial wall with the lateral wall removed. 1, Frontal process of maxilla. **(c)** View of the lateral wall with the medial wall removed. (From: Schuenke M, Schulte E, Schumacher U. THIEME Atlas of Anatomy. Head, Neck, and Neuroanatomy. Illustrations by Voll M and Wesker K. © Thieme 2020.)

The lateral wall: The lateral wall is formed by three irregular bony projections, that is, the *superior, inferior,* and *middle conchae*. The spaces deep to the conchae are called *meatuses*, that is, the superior, middle, and inferior meatuses (**Fig. 1.9b, c**).

Roof: From anterior to posterior, the roof is formed by the nasal bone, frontal bone, cribriform plate of the ethmoid, anterior surface of the body of the sphenoid, and ala of vomer (**Fig. 1.9a**).

Floor: It is formed by the palatine process of the maxilla and horizontal plate of the palatine bone (**Fig. 1.9a–d**).

Bony features: Students are suggested to identify the following important features: sphenoethmoidal recess, superior, inferior, and middle conchae, bulla ethmoidal, uncinate process, and maxillary hiatus (**Fig. 1.9b, c**).

   The relative positions of the nasal cavity, orbit, maxillary air sinus, and ethmoidal air sinuses are shown in **Fig. 1.9d**.

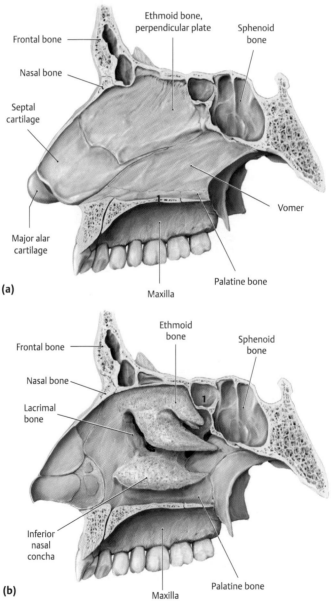

(a)

(b)

Fig. 1.9   Bony nose: **(a)** Bones of the nasal septum (left lateral view). 1, Palatine process of maxilla. **(b)** Bones of the lateral nasal wall (left lateral view). 1, Sphenoethmoidal recess.

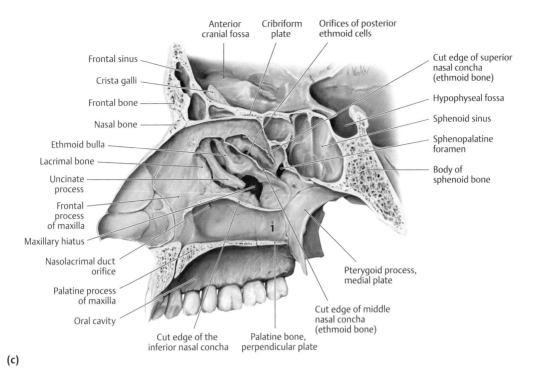

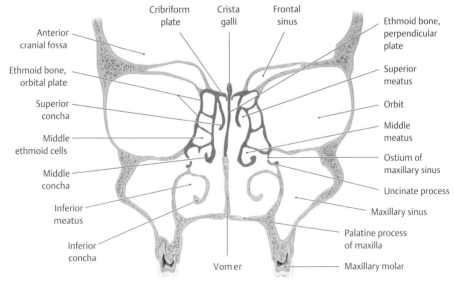

Fig. 1.9 Bony nose: **(c)** Lateral wall of the nose (left lateral view with nasal conchae removed). 1, Horizontal plate of palatine bone. **(d)** Coronal section through the skull to show the relative positions of the nasal cavity, orbit, maxillary air sinus, and ethmoidal air sinuses. (From: Schuenke M, Schulte E, Schumacher U. THIEME Atlas of Anatomy. Head, Neck, and Neuroanatomy. Illustrations by Voll M and Wesker K. © Thieme 2020.)

Mandible

The mandible is the bone of the lower jaw. It has a horseshoe-shaped body and two vertical broad rami.

Body: The body is U-shaped and has two surfaces and two borders. It consists of right and left halves united in the median plane at the symphysis menti. The upper border of the mandible is also known as the alveolar border. It bears sockets for the teeth. The lower border is also known as the base of the mandible (**Fig. 1.10a–c**).

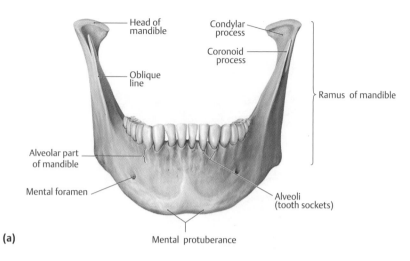

(a)

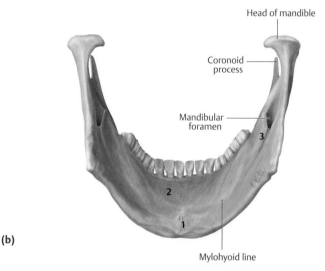

(b)

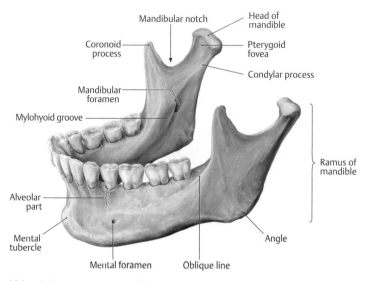

(c)

Fig. 1.10 Mandible: **(a)** Anterior view. **(b)** Posterior view. 1, Genial tubercles; 2, sublingual fossa; 3, mylohyoid groove. **(c)** Oblique left lateral view. (From: Schuenke M, Schulte E, Schumacher U. THIEME Atlas of Anatomy. Head, Neck, and Neuroanatomy. Illustrations by Voll M and Wesker K. © Thieme 2020.)

Ramus: The ramus of the mandible projects upward from the posterior part of the body. It has four borders (anterior, posterior, upper, and lower), two surfaces (lateral and medial), and two processes (coronoid and condylar).

Bony features: Identify the following bony features of the body of the mandible with the help of **Fig. 1.10a–c**: mental foramen, oblique line, mylohyoid line, sublingual fossa, and genial tubercles. In the ramus of the mandible, identify the mandibular notch, pterygoid fovea, mandibular foramen, and mylohyoid groove.

Hyoid Bone

Hyoid is a small U-shaped bone present in the upper part of the neck. The hyoid bone consists of a central body and greater and lesser cornua (horn) (**Fig. 1.11a–c**). It is not attached to any other bone but hangs at the level of third cervical vertebra with the help of the muscles and ligaments. The body has an anterior and posterior surface. Each end of the body is continuous posterolaterally as greater cornua. The lesser cornua are small conical projections attached to the bone at the junction of the body and greater cornu on each side.

Cervical Vertebrae

The cervical part of the vertebral column is highly mobile, and its curvature is convex anteriorly. It is made up of seven cervical vertebrae (**Fig. 1.12**). A cervical vertebra is characterized by the presence of a foramen in each transverse process (foramen transversarium). The first, second, and seventh vertebrae are atypical, while the third, fourth, fifth, and sixth vertebrae are typical.

Typical Cervical Vertebrae (C3–C6)

A typical cervical vertebra consists of a body and vertebral arch (**Fig. 1.13a**). The body is relatively small and rectangular shaped. The vertebral arch consists of the pedicle and lamina. The body and

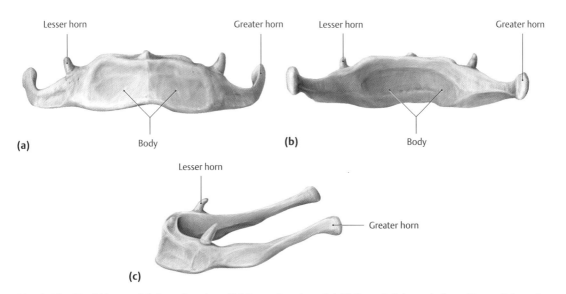

Fig. 1.11 Hyoid bone: **(a)** Anterior view. **(b)** Posterior view. **(c)** Oblique left lateral view. (From: Schuenke M, Schulte E, Schumacher U. THIEME Atlas of Anatomy. Head, Neck, and Neuroanatomy. Illustrations by Voll M and Wesker K. © Thieme 2020.)

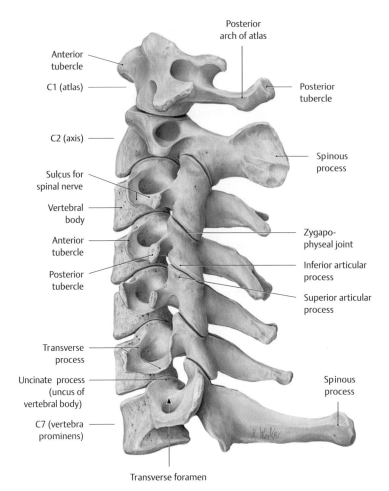

Fig. 1.12   Cervical spine (left lateral view).* (From: Schuenke M, Schulte E, Schumacher U. THIEME Atlas of Anatomy. Head, Neck, and Neuroanatomy. Illustrations by Voll M and Wesker K. © Thieme 2020.)

vertebral arch enclose a vertebral foramen, which is large and triangular in shape. The vertebral foramen lodges the spinal cord and its meninges. The vertebral arch consists of various processes, that is, the superior and inferior articular processes, transverse processes, and spine. The superior and inferior articular processes are broad and flat (**Fig. 1.13b**). The transverse processes bear foramen transversarium, which give passage to the vertebral artery. The spinous processes in the typical cervical vertebrae are short and bifid.

First Cervical Vertebra (Atlas)

The first cervical vertebra is also known as *atlas*. It is easily identified from the rest of the cervical vertebrae because it is ring shaped, has no body, is the widest of all the other cervical vertebrae, and has no spinous process (**Fig. 1.14a**). It has two lateral masses joined anteriorly by the anterior arch and posteriorly by the posterior arch. Each lateral mass has a superior articular facet and an inferior articular facet (**Fig. 1.14b**). The superior facets form the atlanto-occipital joints, whereas the inferior facets form the atlantoaxial joints. The transverse process projects laterally from the lateral mass. It has foramen transversarium which transmits the vertebral artery, vein, and sympathetic nerve.

*Illustrations in this volume variably depict the artery, nerve, vein either by their full name or through the shortened version, i.e., a., n., v.

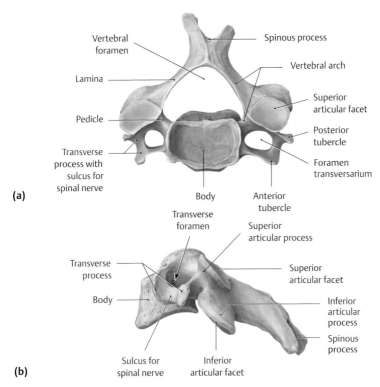

Fig. 1.13 Typical cervical vertebra: **(a)** Superior view. **(b)** Left lateral view. (From: Schuenke M, Schulte E, Schumacher U. THIEME Atlas of Anatomy. Head, Neck, and Neuroanatomy. Illustrations by Voll M and Wesker K. © Thieme 2020.)

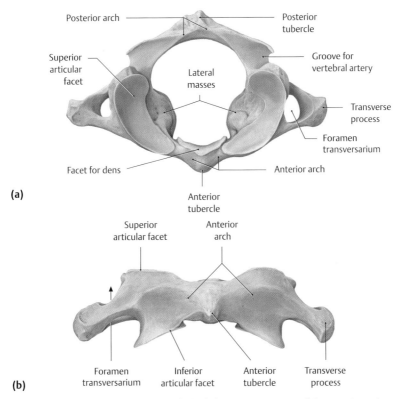

Fig. 1.14 First cervical vertebra (atlas): **(a)** Superior view. **(b)** Anterior view. (From: Schuenke M, Schulte E, Schumacher U. THIEME Atlas of Anatomy. Head, Neck, and Neuroanatomy. Illustrations by Voll M and Wesker K. © Thieme 2020.)

Second Cervical Vertebra (Axis)

It can be easily identified from the rest of the vertebrae because of the presence of *dens* or *odontoid* process. The dens is a blunt, conical, toothlike process which projects superiorly from the body of the vertebra (**Fig. 1.15a**). The spinous process is long, strong, and bifid, and projects posteriorly. The superior articular facets are situated lateral to the odontoid process (**Fig. 1.15b, c**). The transverse processes are small and lie lateral to the superior articular facets. The pedicle, lamina, and bifid spine are massive and very strong.

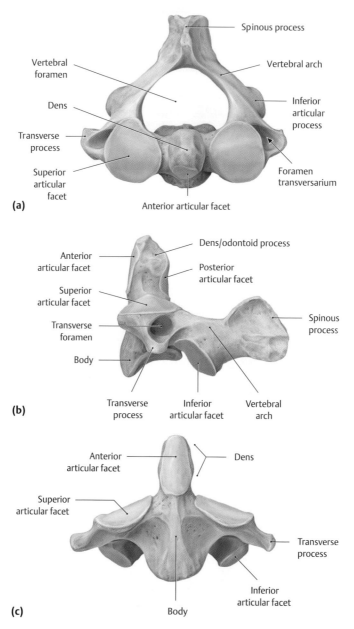

Fig. 1.15 Second cervical vertebra (axis): **(a)** Superior view. **(b)** Left lateral view. **(c)** Anterior view. (From: Schuenke M, Schulte E, Schumacher U. THIEME Atlas of Anatomy. Head, Neck, and Neuroanatomy. Illustrations by Voll M and Wesker K. © Thieme 2020.)

Seventh Cervical Vertebra

This vertebra is easily identified from the other cervical vertebra due to the presence of a very long, horizontal spinous process, which is not bifid (ends in a single tubercle). The transverse processes are large and the foramen transversarium is small because it does not provide passage to the vertebral artery (**Fig. 1.16**).

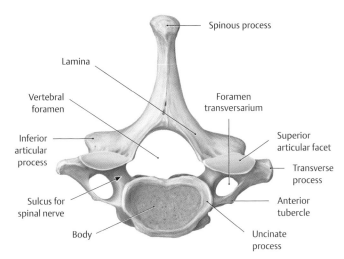

Fig. 1.16 Seventh cervical vertebra (vertebra prominens): Superior view. (From: Schuenke M, Schulte E, Schumacher U. THIEME Atlas of Anatomy. Head, Neck, and Neuroanatomy. Illustrations by Voll M and Wesker K. © Thieme 2020.)

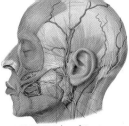

Learning Objectives

At the end of the dissection of the scalp and superficial temporal region, you should be able to identify, understand, and correlate the following clinical aspects:

- Layers of the scalp: Skin, superficial fascia, galea aponeurotica, loose connective tissue layer, and pericranium.
- Nerves: Supratrochlear, supraorbital, auriculotemporal, lesser occipital, and great auricular.
- Vessels: Supratrochlear, supraorbital, superficial temporal, posterior auricular, and occipital.
- Muscle: Occipitofrontalis muscle and epicranial aponeurosis.
- Extension of galea aponeurotica (epicranial aponeurosis), or superficial temporal fascia.
- Temporal fascia, or deep temporal fascia.

Scalp

Introduction

The scalp is defined as the soft tissue covering the vault of the skull. Anteroposteriorly, it extends from the eyebrows to the external occipital protuberance and superior nuchal lines. On the lateral sides, it extends up to the right and left superior temporal lines.

Surface Landmarks

Before starting the dissection, you should quickly identify the following surface landmarks on the cadaver:

1. *Supraorbital margin and glabella*: Palpate the supraorbital margin deep to the eyebrow and glabella between the two eyebrows in midline (just above the root of the nose).

2. *Superciliary arches*: The superciliary arch can be palpated just above the supraorbital margin.

3. *Frontal eminence*: Feel this superolateral prominence on the right and left sides of the forehead.

4. *External occipital protuberance, highest nuchal lines, and superior nuchal lines*: Feel this protuberance on the posterior aspect of the head (in midline, at the junction of the head and neck). Try to palpate the superior nuchal lines on either side of the occipital protuberance.

5. *Superior temporal line*: It will be difficult to feel the superior temporal line on the cadaver. You may clench your teeth repeatedly and feel the contraction at the upper border of the temporalis muscle. The upper border of this muscle will give an idea of the temporal line.

6. *Zygomatic arch:* Palpate this bone between auricle and cheek bone (zygomatic bone).

Dissection and Identification

A. Skin incision and reflection.

1. Shift the head end of the supine cadaver on the edge of the dissection table and place a wooden block under the cervicothoracic junction. This will give you a clear space to work on the occipital region as well.

2. Give a median incision "A" from the root of the nose to the external occipital protuberance. Give a coronal incision "B" starting at the middle of incision "A" up to the auricle on both sides. From the auricle, extend this incision behind up to the mastoid process and in front up to the root of zygoma (**Fig. 2.1a, b**).

3. Before reflecting the skin, you should know the location of blood vessels and nerves in the superficial fascia of the scalp so that you are careful to protect these structures while reflecting the skin.

4. Reflect the skin in four flaps, beginning at the midline (at the junction of the coronal and midline incisions). Proceed toward the periphery up to the zygomatic arch on either side, eyebrows anteriorly and occipital protuberance posteriorly. You may give additional coronal incisions to reflect the skin in smaller flaps.

5. Reflect the skin carefully as superficial fascia (second layer of the scalp) is very dense at the vertex (because dense strands of fibrous tissue traverse the superficial fascia connecting the undersurface of the skin to the epicranial aponeurosis). It will be really difficult to separate the first three layers and find the nerves and vessels in the second layer (superficial fascia). Therefore, the upper three layers of the scalp may often come together.

B. Exposure of muscles, blood vessels, and nerves beneath the skin of forehead.

1. Now this is the time to expose the upper part of the orbicularis oculi muscle and frontal belly of the occipitofrontalis muscle beneath the skin of forehead.

2. Identify the nerves and vessels of the scalp as they are running in the second layer of the scalp. It will be really difficult to trace these nerves as they run in dense connective tissue.

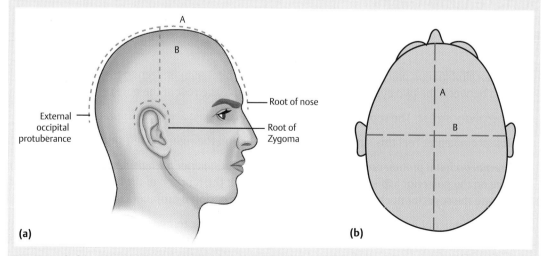

(a)   (b)

Fig. 2.1   (a,b)   Skin incisions for scalp dissection.

3. The location of the nerves and vessels can be assessed as follows:

    a. Supratrochlear nerve and vessels are located at a fingerbreadth away from the glabella.

    b. Feel the supraorbital notch/foramen and then trace the supraorbital nerve and vessels from here, as they pass upward into the scalp.

    c. Feel the zygomatic arch near the auricle and then trace the auriculotemporal nerve and superficial temporal artery from here, as they pass upward into the scalp.

C. Exposure of occipital bellies of occipitofrontalis muscle, nerves, and vessels behind the ear.

1. Turn the cadaver to prone position (face facing downward) so that the posterior part of scalp can be dissected easily.

2. Separate the skin from superficial fascia toward the nuchal lines and external occipital protuberance.

3. Identify the nerves and vessels present in superficial fascia behind the ear. Similarly, see the origin of occipital bellies of occipitofrontalis muscle from highest nuchal lines. Observe the attachment of epicranial aponeurosis to external occipital protuberance. Similarly, trace the attachment of the frontal and occipital bellies with the epicranial aponeurosis.

Layers of the Scalp (Video 2.1)

The scalp consists of five layers (**Fig. 2.2**):

1. *Skin*: Note that the skin is thick and adherent to the third layer (epicranial aponeurosis). As the skin of the scalp is hairy, it contains lots of sebaceous glands.

2. *Superficial fascia*: This layer is dense and fibrous. The fibrous strands bind the skin to the epicranial aponeurosis and contain a number of spaces filled with fat. This layer contains the blood vessels and nerves of the scalp.

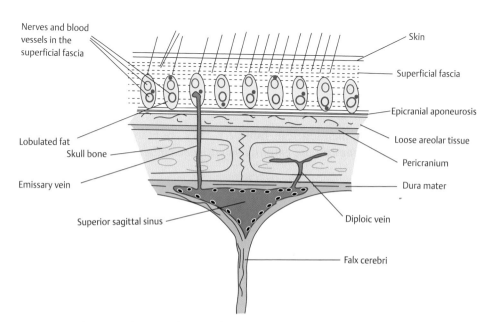

Fig. 2.2 Schematic drawing showing layers of the scalp as seen in the coronal section passing through the scalp and skull (also refer to **Fig. 12.5**).

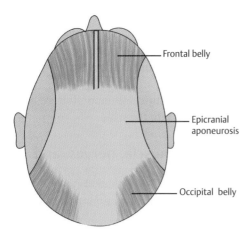

Fig. 2.3 Occipitofrontalis muscle.

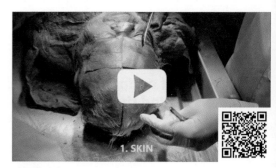

Video 2.1 Layers of scalp.

3. *Occipitofrontalis muscle and epicranial aponeurosis* (**Fig. 2.3**): The flat epicranial aponeurosis is the tendon uniting the frontal and occipital bellies of the occipitofrontalis muscle. The frontal bellies take origin from the skin of the forehead mingling with the upper part of the orbicularis oculi and corrugator supercilii. They are partly united at the midline. The origin has no attachment to the bone. Frontal belly is attached posteriorly to the epicranial aponeurosis. The aponeurosis is attached posteriorly to the external occipital protuberance and the medial part of the highest nuchal lines. The occipital bellies originate from the lateral part of the highest nuchal lines on either side and are inserted on the aponeurosis. On each of the lateral sides, the aponeurosis is attached partly to the temporal line. From here it extends downward as superficial temporal fascia to get attachment on zygomatic arch. The aponeurosis can slide freely on the pericranium (fifth layer of the scalp). The frontal and occipital parts of muscle can move the scalp forward and backward over the vault of the skull.

Note: The above three layers (which are firmly attached to each other) are sometimes called as *scalp proper*.

4. *Layer of loose areolar tissue*: This layer of loose connective tissue is placed between the third and fifth layer of the scalp and extends throughout the scalp. This layer gives a passage to the emissary veins.

5. *Pericranium*: This layer is formed by the periosteum of the cranial bones of the vault.

Blood Vessels of the Scalp

Blood vessels of the scalp are mentioned in **Table 2.1**. They are branches from the external and internal carotid arteries and anastomose extensively with each other in the scalp (**Fig. 2.4**).

Table 2.1 Blood vessels of the scalp

Name	Source
1. Supratrochlear artery	Branch from the ophthalmic artery (branch of internal carotid artery)
2. Supraorbital artery	Branch from the ophthalmic artery (branch of internal carotid artery)
3. Superficial temporal artery	Branch from the external carotid artery
4. Posterior auricular artery	Branch from the external carotid artery
5. Occipital artery	Branch from the external carotid artery

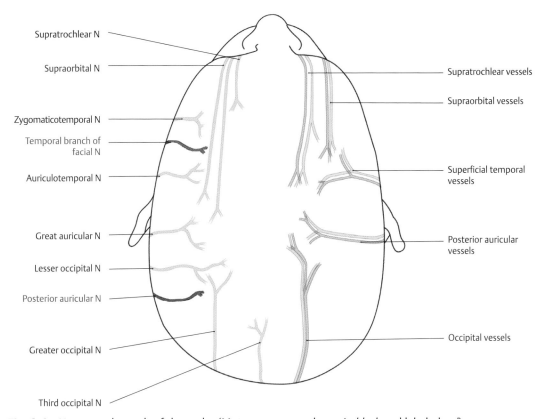

Fig. 2.4   Nerves and vessels of the scalp. (Motor nerves are drawn in *black* and labeled *red*).

The names of the veins of the scalp correspond to that of the arteries. They run along with the corresponding arteries. Students should note that these blood vessels run from the periphery toward the vertex and form an extensive anastomotic network in the scalp. Thus, the scalp is richly supplied with blood and sensory nerves.

Nerves of the Scalp

Motor Nerves

The facial nerve (cranial nerve [CN] VII) supplies the motor fibers to the occipitofrontalis muscle. Its temporal branch is present in front of the auricle and innervates the frontal belly, whereas its posterior auricular branch is present behind the auricle and supplies the occipital belly (refer to **Fig. 2.4**).

Sensory Nerves

The sensory nerves which supply the skin of the scalp in front of the auricle are branches of the trigeminal nerve. While the nerves which supply the skin of scalp behind the ear are branches from the spinal nerves (C2 and C3) (**Table 2.2**; also refer to **Fig. 2.4**).

Table 2.2   Sensory nerves of the scalp

Name	Source	Area supplied
Sensory nerves present in front of the auricle		
1. Supratrochlear	Branch from the ophthalmic division of the trigeminal nerve (CN V)	Skin of the forehead near midline
2. Supraorbital	Branch from the ophthalmic division of the trigeminal nerve (CN V)	Skin of the forehead and the scalp up to the vertex
3. Zygomaticotemporal	Branch from the maxillary division of the trigeminal nerve (CN V)	Skin of the anterior part of the temporal region
4. Auriculotemporal	Branch from the mandibular division of the trigeminal nerve (CN V)	Upper part of the auricle, part of the external acoustic meatus, and side of the head
Sensory nerves present behind the auricle		
1. Great auricular nerve	Branch from the cervical plexus (ventral ramus of C2 and C3)	Its posterior branch supplies a small area of the scalp just behind the auricle adjacent to the mastoid process
2. Lesser occipital	Branch from the cervical plexus (ventral ramus of C2)	It supplies the posterior aspect of the scalp region posterior to the mastoid process
3. Greater occipital	It is the medial branch of the dorsal ramus of the C2 spinal nerve	It supplies the back of the scalp up to the vertex
4. Third occipital	It is the dorsal ramus of the C3 spinal nerve	It supplies the skin covering the external occipital protuberance and the neighboring area

Abbreviation: CN, cranial nerve.

Deeper Dissection

Once you have dissected and seen the structures related to the three layers of the scalp, it is time to study the fourth and fifth layers.

1. Make a small cruciate incision in the epicranial aponeurosis near the vertex. Introduce a metallic probe through this incision deep to the aponeurosis. Your probe is now in the fourth layer of the scalp (layer of the loose areolar tissue) and above the pericranium. The probe will be obstructed posteriorly near the nuchal lines as the aponeurosis is attached to the highest nuchal line. Similarly, the probe will be obstructed laterally as the aponeurosis is adherent to the temporal lines on the lateral side. There is no obstruction to the extent of the fourth layer anteriorly.

2. Make the median and coronal incisions in the occipitofrontalis and epicranial aponeurosis similar to skin incisions (refer to **Fig. 2.1**). Reflect the muscle and aponeurosis to expose the loose areolar tissue layer completely.

3. Note the pericranium covering the various bones of the vault. Also, see various sutures on the vault.

▌Clinical Notes

The clinical anatomy of scalp is described layer by layer (refer to Figs. 2.2 and 2.5):

1. *Skin:* Because of the presence of a lot of sebaceous glands, which are associated with hair follicles, *multiple sebaceous cysts* and *infected sebaceous glands* are commonly found in the skin of the scalp. Various types *of tumors* (benign and malignant) may also arise from the skin.

2. *Superficial fascia (dense connective tissue layer):* As this layer is made up of dense connective tissue-, *there is limited space and, therefore, infection of this layer is limited to a small area.* Due to the same reason, increased pressure on the nerve leads to *severe pain.*

   Wounds of the scalp bleed profusely because of two reasons. First, it is richly supplied with blood vessels and, second, when a blood vessel is cut the fibrous strands of the second layer hold the lumen of the vessel open leading to excessive bleeding. Bleeding can be arrested by applying pressure on the vessels.

3. *Epicranial aponeurosis:* As the skin is firmly attached to the aponeurosis by fibrous strands of the second layer, the upper three layers of the scalp are fused and act as a single layer. A wound of the scalp extending through these three layers will gape when the aponeurosis is cut in the transverse direction. However, the wound will not gape when the aponeurosis is cut in the anteroposterior direction. This is because the pull of the occipitofrontalis muscle is in the anteroposterior direction (**Fig. 2.3**).

   If a portion of the scalp is torn off due to an injury and if it is stitched back, it will heal well due to the profuse blood supply and extensive arterial anastomosis.

4. *Layer of the loose areolar tissue:* The presence of the loose connective tissue layer allows the first three layers of the scalp to slide freely on the pericranium. As the emissary veins pass through this layer, they may bleed, and the infection may pass on to the cranial cavity through these emissary veins.

   The loose connective tissue layer is also known as the *dangerous area of the scalp* because bleeding and infection can spread widely (due to its extensiveness) within this layer. Anteriorly, the bleeding may reach to the orbital margin, eyelid (leading to the formation of *black eye* due to clotting of blood deep to the eyelid).

5. *Pericranium:* It is the periosteum lining the outer aspect of the cranial vault. The bleeding deep to the pericranium (*cephalohematoma*) does not extend beyond the margin of the bone as the pericranium at the margins of the bone is attached to the sutural ligaments. The shape of the bleeding resembles the shape of the bone.

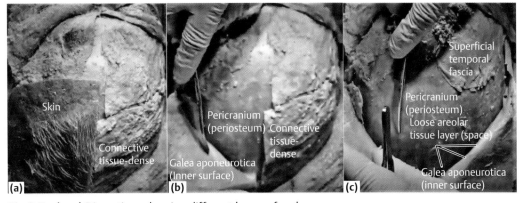

Fig 2.5   (a–c) Dissections showing different layers of scalp.

Superficial Temporal Region (or Temple)

The temporal region extends between the temporal line (above) and the zygomatic arch (below). It contains the temporalis muscle covered by the temporal fascia.

Dissection and Identification

1. We have already reflected the skin from the temple region while dissecting the scalp.

2. In the superficial fascia, look for the nerves and vessels (superficial temporal artery and vein, auriculotemporal nerve, temporal branch of facial nerve, and zygomaticotemporal nerve) (refer to **Fig. 2.4**).

3. Clean the temporal fascia (deep temporal fascia) covering the temporalis muscle and note its attachments above the temporal line and below the zygomatic arch.

You should note that we shall dissect the temporal fossa (structures deep to temporal fascia) with the dissection of the temporal and infratemporal region. (Refer to Chapter 9.)

Layers of the Superficial Temporal Region (Video 2.2)

The superficial temporal region presents six layers of the soft tissues:

1. *Skin:* The skin of the temple region is soft and thin as compared to the scalp.

2. *Superficial fascia:* Superficial fascia contains fat and loose connective tissues. The dense connective tissue of the scalp is absent in this region. This region contains the super-ficial temporal artery (terminal branch of the external carotid artery), the superficial temporal vein, and the auriculotemporal nerve (sensory branch of the mandibular nerve). The anterior part of this region also contains superficial branches of the facial nerve (motor nerve) and the zygomaticotemporal nerve (sensory branch from the maxillary nerve). Referring to **Fig. 2.4**, identify these structures in the cadaver.

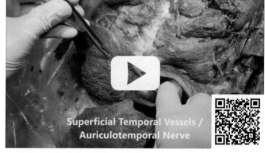

Video 2.2 Dissection of superficial temporal region.

3. *Extension of epicranial aponeurosis and auricular muscles:* A thin extension of the aponeurosis occurs from the superior temporal line toward the ear and zygomatic arch. This thin extension of fascia is sometimes called as *"Superficial temporal fascia."* This lies superficial to deep tempo-ral fascia. There are three extrinsic auricular muscles, that is, anterior, superior, and posterior auricularis.

4. *Temporal fascia (deep temporal fascia):* It is very tough and extends from the superior temporal line to the zygomatic arch covering the temporalis muscle located just deep to it. Temporalis muscle takes origin from its deep surface.

5. *Temporal muscle:* It is a fan-shaped muscle lying deep to the temporal fascia, occupying the temporal fossa. Its thick tendon passes downward behind the zygomatic arch to be inserted into the coronoid process of the mandible.

6. *Pericranium:* It is the periosteum lining the bones of the temporal fossa.

▌Clinical Note

The superficial temporal artery is often used for palpation by an anesthetist when a surgery is performed below the neck region.

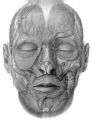
Learning Objectives

At the end of the dissection of the face, you should be able to identify the following:

- Surface landmarks of the face.
- Subcutaneous muscles of the face and the masseter muscle.
- Motor and sensory nerves of the face, that is, branches of the facial (motor) nerve and cutaneous branches of the ophthalmic, maxillary, and mandibular nerves (sensory) on the face.
- Facial artery and its branches; facial vein and its tributaries.
- Parotid gland and parotid duct.

Introduction

Face is the front aspect of the head. It is usually oval in shape. Vertically, it extends from hairline of the forehead above to the chin below. The forehead is common to the face and scalp. On the sides, the face extends from one ear (tragus of external ear) to the other. Face bears the openings of nose, mouth, and eyes. The orbital openings for eyes are present just below the forehead, one on each side of the upper end of the nose. The opening of mouth (oral fissure) is bounded by upper and lower lips and cheeks. Face has no deep fascia because muscles of the face originating from bones of the face are attached to the undersurface of the skin of the face. Therefore, the contraction of these muscles produces various kinds of facial expressions. The skin of the face is richly supplied by arteries and sensory nerves, mainly cranial nerve (CN) V.

Surface Landmarks

On the cadaver, palpate the following surface landmarks by applying deep pressure with your fingers:

Supraorbital margin just deep to the eyebrow, *zygomatic bone* (malar prominence) just below the lateral end of the eye, *zygomatic arch* in front of the external ear, *nasal bones* in the median area, *alveolar process of maxilla* deep to upper lip, *mental protuberance* of mandible in midline, **and palpate the** angle of mandible **located anteroinferior to auricle.**

Dissection and Identification (Video 3.1)

A. Skin incision and reflection.

1. For dissection of the face, the cadaver should be in the supine position. Raise the head by placing a wooden block under the head.

2. Give a circular incision in the skin close to the eyelids (A in **Fig. 3.1**) and another similar incision close to the red margins of upper and lower lips (B in **Fig. 3.1**).

3. Give a midline incision from the root of the nose to the point of the chin (C in **Fig. 3.1**).

4. Give a horizontal incision from the lateral end of the circular incision around the margin of the eyelids and extend it to the front of the auricle (D in **Fig. 3.1**).

5. Give another horizontal incision from the angle of the mouth and extend it up to the posterior border of mandible (E in **Fig. 3.1**).

6. Start reflecting the upper flap from midline and go backward, together with the flap of the scalp, till you reach just anterior to the auricle. Similarly, reflect the lower flap downward till you reach the lower margin of mandible below the auricle. Now carefully reflect the skin from the eyelids.

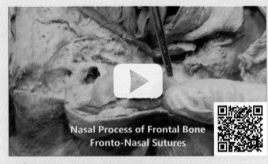

**Nasal Process of Frontal Bone
Fronto-Nasal Sutures**

Video 3.1 External nose.

B. Muscles of the facial expression.

1. Note that the skin of the face (unlike that of the scalp) is thin and mobile except at the nose where it is firmly attached to the deeper cartilage. However, as the muscles of the facial expression are attached to the undersurface of the skin, they are easily damaged during the reflection of the skin. Hence, many of these muscles will be difficult to identify. Therefore, utmost care should be taken to prevent damage to the muscles of the facial expression. If you are unable to find and identify some of these muscles, you are suggested to look at **Fig. 3.2a, b** to learn about the location of these muscles.

2. After reflection of the skin, you are in the superficial fascia which contains loose connective tissues, and fat in which subcutaneous muscles of face, parotid gland, vessels, and nerves are present.

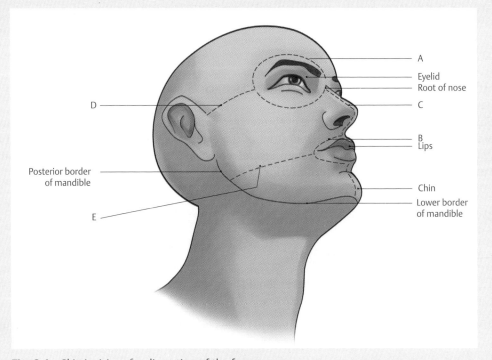

Fig. 3.1 Skin incisions for dissection of the face.

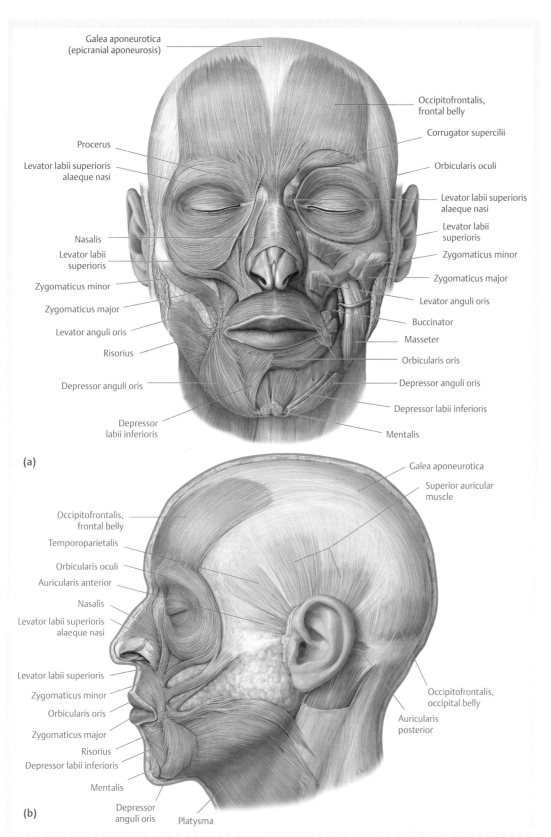

Fig. 3.2   Muscles of facial expression: **(a)** Anterior view. **(b)** Left lateral view. (From: Schuenke M, Schulte E, Schumacher U. THIEME Atlas of Anatomy. Head, Neck, and Neuroanatomy. Illustrations by Voll M and Wesker K. © Thieme 2020.)

3. In the lower part of the face, examine the platysma muscle which is attached to the mandible, skin of cheek, angle of mouth, and orbicularis oris muscle. Reflect this muscle from the angle of the mouth toward the mandible to expose deeper structures such as facial artery and vein.

C. Parotid gland, parotid duct, branches of facial nerve.

1. With the help of forceps, carefully remove the loose connective tissue and fat of superficial fascia to expose parotid duct, masseter muscle, parotid gland, branches of facial nerve (**Fig. 3.3**), various muscles of the face (**Fig. 3.3**), facial artery and vein, and infraorbital and mental nerves.

2. Identify the parotid duct lying on the masseter muscle about 2 cm inferior to the zygomatic arch. Trace the duct backward to reach the anterior margin of the parotid gland. Similarly, trace the parotid duct anteriorly till it pierces the buccinator muscle to drain into oral cavity. You will have to remove the buccal pad of fat to expose the buccinator muscle of the cheek.

3. At the anterior margin of the parotid gland, find the branches of the facial nerve (refer to **Fig. 3.3**). These branches are very thin, and you will have to remain very careful while tracing them superiorly, anteriorly, and inferiorly as they come out from the margin of parotid gland.

D. Facial artery and vein, orbicularis oris and orbicularis oculi muscles, and cutaneous branches of trigeminal nerve.

1. After seeing the zygomaticus major and minor and levator labii superioris (**Fig. 3.2**), cut them at the middle and reflect them upward and downward to expose the facial artery and vein. These vessels are running in the face from the lower border of mandible (close to the anterior margin of masseter muscle) toward the lateral side of root of the nose. Clean the tortuous facial artery as it lies close to the angle of mouth. Identify superior and inferior labial arteries. Find the facial vein which lies away from the artery, close to the anterior margin of masseter muscle (**Fig. 3.3**).

2. This is the time to study the orbicularis oris, orbicularis oculi, and buccinator muscles. The orbicularis oris has no well-defined margins as many muscles approaching upper and lower lips fuse with it. Identify two parts of orbicularis oculi (palpebral and orbital) and medial palpebral ligament (refer to **Fig.3.2a**).

3. At the end, with the help of a forceps, dissect the *infraorbital nerves* and *vessels* as they come out of infraorbital foramen located just below the inferior border of orbital opening and *mental nerve* coming out through the mental foramen of mandible (**Fig. 3.3b**). We have already dissected the *supratrochlear* and *supraorbital nerves* and vessels, in the region of forehead, while dissecting the scalp.

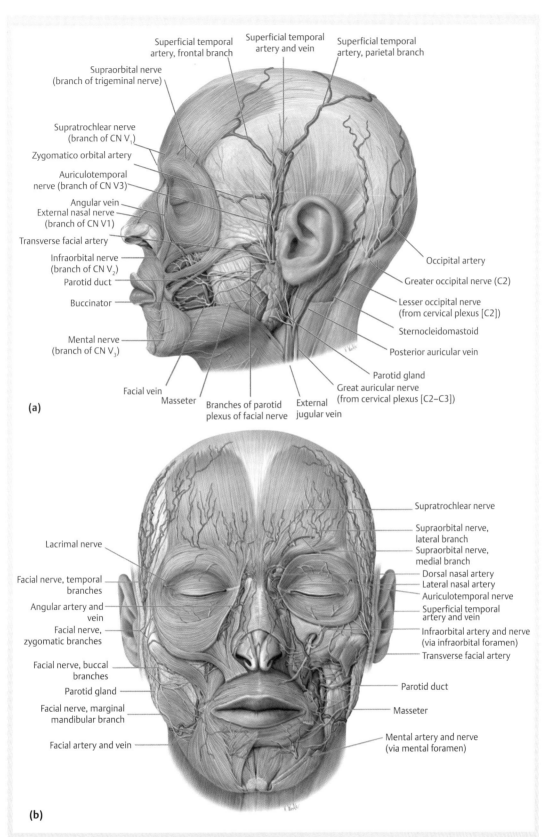

Fig. 3.3 Superficial nerves and vessels **(a)** on the lateral side of head and face. **(b)** Anterior aspect of the head and face. (From: Schuenke M, Schulte E, Schumacher U. THIEME Atlas of Anatomy. Head, Neck, and Neuroanatomy. Illustrations by Voll M and Wesker K. © Thieme 2020.)

Nerve Supply of the Skin of the Face (Sensory Innervation)

The face is supplied by three divisions of *trigeminal* (CN V) nerve (*ophthalmic*, *maxillary*, and *mandibular*) and *great auricular* nerve which originates from spinal nerves with root value C2 and C3. This is depicted in **Fig. 3.4a, b** and **Table 3.1**.

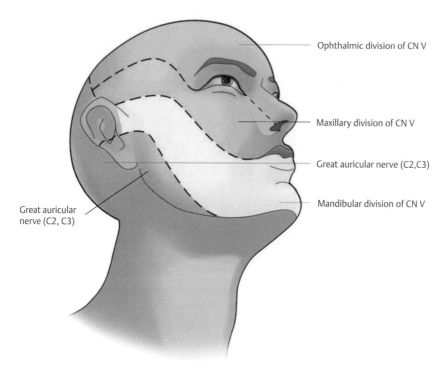

(a)

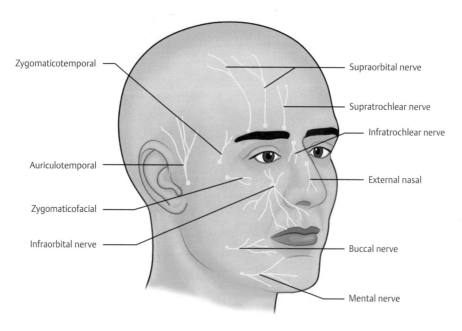

(b)

Fig. 3.4 **(a)** Cutaneous innervation of the face. Three dermatomes supplied by the trigeminal nerve are indicated by different shadings. Skin over the angle of mandible and lower part of auricle is supplied by great auricular nerve (C2 and C3). **(b)** Cutaneous (sensory) innervations of face. Note the branches of ophthalmic, maxillary, and mandibular nerves innervating the area of the skin of face. Correlate the branches with area shown in **a**.

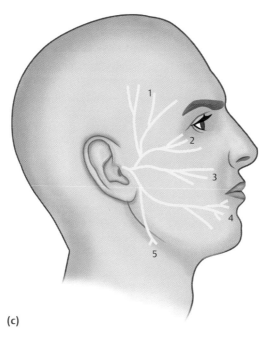

(c)

Fig. 3.4 **(c)** Branches of facial nerve (motor innervation of face). 1, Temporal; 2, zygomatic; 3, buccal; 4, mandibular; 5, cervical.

Table 3.1   Sensory innervations of the face

Nerves	Branches
1. Ophthalmic division of CN V	Supratrochlear, supraorbital, infratrochlear, external nasal and palpebral branch of lacrimal
2. Maxillary division of CN V	Infraorbital, zygomaticofacial, and zygomaticotemporal
3. Mandibular division of CN V	Auriculotemporal, buccal, and mental
4. Great auricular nerves (C2 and C3 spinal nerves)	It ramifies into many unnamed branches, one of which supplies the skin over the angle of mandible

Abbreviation: CN, cranial nerve.

Muscles

Students should note that as there is an absence of deep fascia in the face, muscles originating from the bone are inserted into the undersurface of the skin of the face. Because of this, they are mostly damaged during the reflection of skin and, hence, many are not identified properly. Students should identify these muscles (refer to **Fig. 3.2a, b**). All the muscles of facial expression are supplied by the facial nerve (CN VII). **Table 3.2** summarizes three important muscles of the face, that is, orbicularis oculi, orbicularis oris, and buccinator.

Table 3.2   Important muscles of facial expression

Muscle	Origin	Insertion	Action
1. Orbicularis oculi (orbital, palpebral, and lacrimal parts)	1. The *orbital part* arises from the medial palpebral ligament, the frontal process of maxilla, and adjoining frontal bone 2. The *palpebral part* arises from the medial palpebral ligament and neighboring bone 3. The *lacrimal part* lies behind the lacrimal sac and originates from the crest of lacrimal bone	1. These fibers form a loop around orbit and are inserted on the same point of origin 2. Fibers run in upper and lower eyelids and are attached to the lateral palpebral raphe 3. It divides into upper and lower slips to insert on tarsal plates and lateral palpebral raphe	The orbital and palpebral parts contract together to close the eyelids tightly. Palpebral part closes the lids lightly, whereas lacrimal part contracts to dilate the lacrimal sac
2. Orbicularis oris (sphincter muscle of upper and lower lip)[a]	This intrinsic muscle arises from mucous membrane of the lip and bone of upper and lower jaws opposite to incisor teeth	Muscle fibers pass laterally in upper and lower jaws to insert on the skin of lips	Orbicularis oris acts as sphincter of the mouth
3. Buccinator	It takes origin from mandible and maxilla opposite the molar teeth. It also arises from the pterygomandibular raphe	The upper and lower fibers pass in the corresponding lip, whereas the intermediate fibers decussate at the lateral angle of mouth to go to upper and lower lips	The muscle helps in clearing the food from vestibule. It also helps in sucking, blowing, and whistling

[a] The orbicularis oris has an extrinsic and intrinsic portion. The intrinsic portion is described in the table. The extrinsic portion is contributed by muscles of upper and lower lips and buccinator (students should learn about the extrinsic muscles of lips from a textbook of gross anatomy). Both the extrinsic and intrinsic parts form the main substance of lips and cheek. Extrinsic muscles (**Fig. 3.2a, b**) are responsible for a variety of movements which are seen in the lips.

Branches of the Facial Nerve (Motor Innervations of the Face)

With the help of **Figs. 3.3 and 3.4c**, identify the following branches of facial nerve which innervates all the muscles of facial expression: *temporal, zygomatic, buccal, mandibular,* and *cervical.* The *posterior auricular* and *digastric branches* of the facial nerve will not be seen in the area of the dissection of the face.

Arterial Supply of the Face

The face is richly supplied by the arteries. The facial artery is the main artery to supply blood to the face. There are many other minor branches of arteries contributing to the blood supply (see **Fig. 3.5** and **Table 3.3**).

Table 3.3   Blood supply of the face

Artery	Branch
1. Facial artery • Inferior labial • Superior labial • Lateral nasal • Angular	Branch of the external carotid artery
2. Supraorbital, supratrochlear, and dorsal nasal arteries	Branches of the ophthalmic artery
3. Transverse facial artery	Branch of the superficial temporal artery
4. Infraorbital artery	Branch of the maxillary artery
5. Mental artery	Branch of the inferior alveolar artery

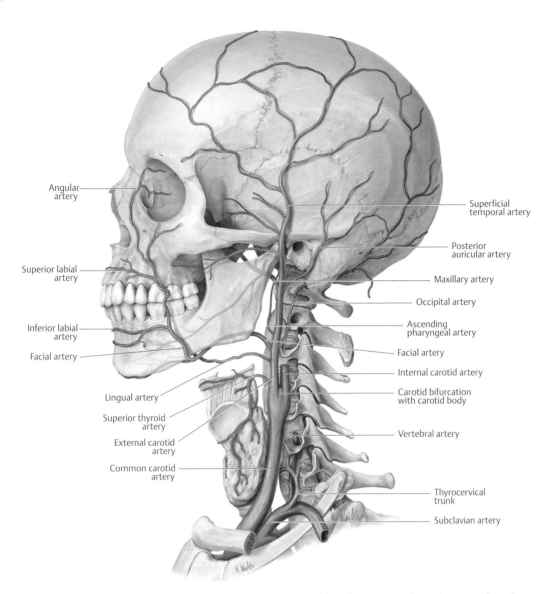

Angular artery

Superior labial artery

Inferior labial artery

Facial artery

Lingual artery

Superior thyroid artery

External carotid artery

Common carotid artery

Superficial temporal artery

Posterior auricular artery

Maxillary artery

Occipital artery

Ascending pharyngeal artery

Facial artery

Internal carotid artery

Carotid bifurcation with carotid body

Vertebral artery

Thyrocervical trunk

Subclavian artery

Fig. 3.5 Arterial supply of the face. Note the branches of facial artery on face. (From: Schuenke M, Schulte E, Schumacher U. THIEME Atlas of Anatomy. Head, Neck, and Neuroanatomy. Illustrations by Voll M and Wesker K. © Thieme 2020.)

Venous Drainage of the Face

The venous blood is drained mainly by the facial vein. The facial vein is formed by the union of supraorbital and supratrochlear veins at the medial angle of the eye. At the medial angle of the eye, it is connected to the superior ophthalmic vein. Other veins of the face are shown in **Fig. 3.6**.

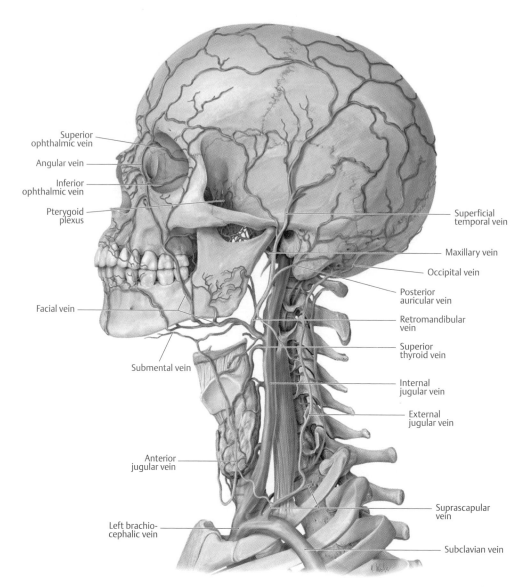

Fig. 3.6 Venous drainage of the face. (From: Schuenke M, Schulte E, Schumacher U. THIEME Atlas of Anatomy. Head, Neck, and Neuroanatomy. Illustrations by Voll M and Wesker K. © Thieme 2020.)

▌Clinical Notes

1. *Trigeminal neuralgia:* In this condition, the patient suffers from bouts of severe pain in the course of distribution of any of the three divisions of the trigeminal nerve (usually the mandibular division).

2. *Bell's palsy:* It is a lower motor neuron type of facial palsy. In this condition, there occurs the unilateral paralysis of muscles of facial expression that are supplied by the facial nerve. Bell's palsy most commonly results due to inflammation of the facial nerve in the facial canal just above the stylomastoid foramen. As the patient is unable to close eyes, tears dribble on the face. There is loss of wrinkles on the affected side of forehead, as well as dribbling of saliva from the affected side. Food tends to accumulate in the vestibule of the mouth because of paralysis of the cheek muscle—the buccinator. There is facial asymmetry, the mouth is displaced toward the normal side due to unopposed action of healthy muscles on the opposite side (**Fig. 3.7**).

3. *Dangerous area of the face:* As veins of the face are without valves, blood can flow in any direction. The facial veins communicate with the cavernous sinus through the superior ophthalmic and deep facial vein. Thus, the infection of face may reach the cavernous sinus, leading to infection and thrombosis of the cavernous sinus or meningitis. The infection and thrombosis of the cavernous sinus usually occur after pressing the pimples located on the upper lip and by the side of the nose. Thus, these areas are often known as *dangerous areas of the face* (**Fig. 3.8a, b**, also refer to **Fig. 14.8**).

4. *Bleeding from the face:* Face has a rich supply of blood. Similar to the arteries of the scalp, arteries of the face anastomose freely. Therefore, the wounds of the face bleed profusely but heal quickly.

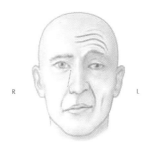

Fig. 3.7   Bell's palsy (right side). (From: Schuenke M, Schulte E, Schumacher U. THIEME Atlas of Anatomy. Head, Neck, and Neuroanatomy. Illustrations by Voll M and Wesker K. © Thieme 2020.)

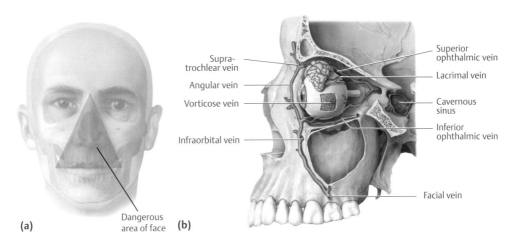

Fig. 3.8   (a,b) Dangerous areas of the face. (From: Schuenke M, Schulte E, Schumacher U. THIEME Atlas of Anatomy. Head, Neck, and Neuroanatomy. Illustrations by Voll M and Wesker K. © Thieme 2020.)

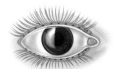

Eyelids and Lacrimal Apparatus

Introduction

Eyelids are soft tissue flaps placed in front of the eyeball. They serve two important functions: (1) protecting the eye from injury and excessive light and (2) spreading the lacrimal fluid on the surface of the cornea and conjunctiva with each blink. Blinking not only helps in spreading the tears on the cornea but also in pushing the lacrimal fluid toward the medial angle of the eye from where it is drained. The lacrimal fluid is drained by the lacrimal canaliculi to the lacrimal sac, which transmits it to the nose via the nasolacrimal duct. The upper eyelid is larger and more mobile than the lower eyelid. The two eyelids meet at the medial and lateral angles. The elliptical opening between the eyelids is called the palpebral fissure. It provides entrance to the conjunctival sac (i.e., the space between the eyelids and eyeball). When the eye is open, the upper eyelid covers the upper margin of the cornea while the lower eyelid lies just below the cornea.
Students are suggested to read the details of the eyelid and lacrimal apparatus from the textbook of gross anatomy before they dissect these structures.

Surface Landmarks

Students are suggested to look at a dry skull at the medial and lateral wall of the orbit to identify the site of attachment of the medial and lateral *palpebral ligaments*, *lacrimal groove (lacrimal fossa)*, and anterior and posterior *lacrimal crests* (refer to **Fig. 1.8a–c**). Similarly, see the opening of the *nasolacrimal duct* in the inferior meatus, at the lateral wall of the nose, by passing a flexible wire downward in the fossa for the lacrimal sac (refer to **Fig. 1.8b**). In the eye of a living person, see the attachment of the *eyelashes (cilia)* at the outer margin of the eyelid and identify the *palpebral fissure*, which is the opening between the upper and lower eyelids. At the medial angle of the eye, identify a small pink bump, the *lacrimal caruncle* (**Fig. 4.1**). This caruncle is surrounded by a small triangular space, known as the *lacus lacrimalis*, in which tears collect at the medial angle of the eye. Note a small elevation/bump on the medial end of the margin of each eyelid which is known as the *lacrimal papilla*. On the top of each lacrimal papilla, there is a small opening called *lacrimal punctum* which drains the tears to the *lacrimal canaliculi*. If possible, evert the upper or lower eyelid in a living person and note many vertical yellowish parallel streaks. These are the *tarsal glands* whose ducts open on the posterior (inner) edge of the lid margin posterior to the attachment of the eyelashes (**Fig. 4.1**).

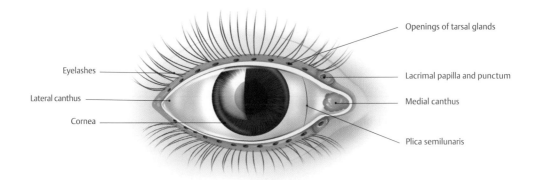

Fig. 4.1   Margin of eyelid everted to show its features.

Dissection and Identification

1. At the medial end of the eyelid margin, insert the needle of a syringe in the lacrimal puncta and inject few milliliters of water. If there is no blockage in the nasolacrimal duct, the water will come out through the nose. This will give an idea about the drainage of tears from the conjunctival sac to the nasal cavity.

A. Orbicularis oculi muscle, orbital septum, and nerves.

1. A circular incision on the lids close to their edges has already been given (refer to **Fig. 3.1**). Now reflect the skin from the eyelids and expose both the palpebral and orbital parts of the orbicularis oculi muscle (**Fig. 4.2**).

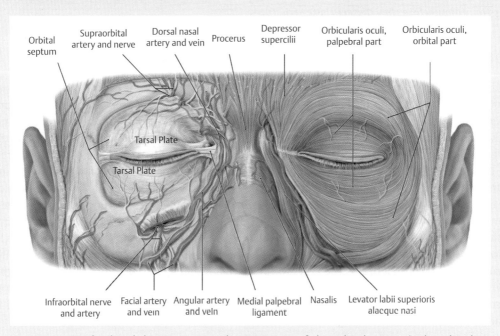

Fig. 4.2   Superficial and deep neurovascular structures of the orbital region (right orbicularis oculi removed). (From: Schuenke M, Schulte E, Schumacher U. THIEME Atlas of Anatomy. Head, Neck, and Neuroanatomy. Illustrations by Voll M and Wesker K. © Thieme 2020.)

2. Separate the palpebral part from the orbital part by giving a circular incision at the junction of the palpebral and orbital parts. Reflect the palpebral part first toward the margin of the eyelid and then toward the medial angle of the eye. This will expose *the tarsal plate* and *orbital septum* (orbital fascia) in the upper and lower eyelids (**Fig. 4.2**).

3. See the attachment of the orbital septum to the periosteum at the margin of the orbit opening. The other end of the septum is attached to the upper and lower tarsal plates (**Fig. 4.2**). Trace these tarsal plates medially and laterally where they fuse to form the medial and lateral palpebral ligaments. Note the attachment of the medial palpebral ligament on the anterior lacrimal crest in front of the lacrimal sac (**Fig. 4.2**).

4. This is the time to see the supraorbital, supratrochlear, infratrochlear, and palpebral branches of the lacrimal nerves. Look for the palpebral branch of the infraorbital nerve going toward the lower eyelid (**Fig. 4.2**).

B. Lacrimal gland and lacrimal sac.

1. With the help of a knife give a horizontal incision in the superolateral part of the orbital fascia to dissect the lacrimal gland (**Fig. 4.3**). With the help of fine forceps pull the gland downward; if possible, see the fine ducts of the gland going toward the superior fornix of the conjunctiva.

2. Identify the lacrimal sac. To expose the sac completely give a cut in the medial palpebral ligament at the site of its attachment on the anterior lacrimal crest. Pull the ligament laterally to see the lacrimal sac (**Fig. 4.3**). Now make a vertical incision in the lacrimal sac. Through this incision, pass a probe downward in the nasolacrimal duct.

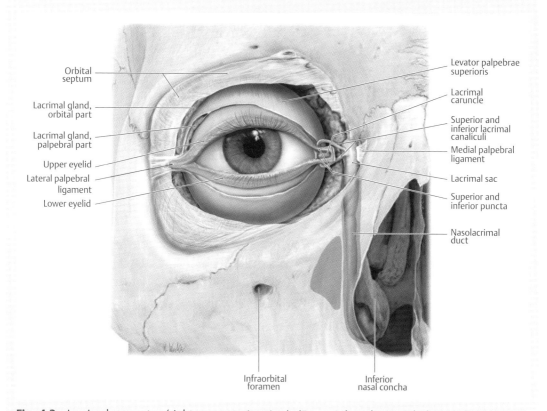

Fig. 4.3 Lacrimal apparatus (right eye, anterior view). (From: Schuenke M, Schulte E, Schumacher U. THIEME Atlas of Anatomy. Head, Neck, and Neuroanatomy. Illustrations by Voll M and Wesker K. © Thieme 2020.)

Eyelids

From superficial to deep, the eyelid consists of the following five layers (**Fig. 4.4**):

1. *Skin*: It is very thin.

2. *Superficial fascia*: It is made up of loose connective tissue. There is no fat in the superficial fascia of the lid.

3. *Muscle layer*: It consists of the palpebral part of the orbicularis oculi (**Fig. 4.2**). The connective tissue deep to this layer of muscle is continuous with the fourth layer of the scalp (layer of loose areolar tissue). Hence, blood from the fourth layer of the scalp may track the eyelid.

4. *Layer of tarsus and orbital septum*: These two structures together form the fourth layer of the eyelid (**Fig. 4.2**). The tarsal plate is present in the upper and lower eyelids. It is made up of condensed fibrous tissue and provides support to the eyelid. The tarsal plate of the upper eyelid is larger and almond shaped, whereas that of the lower eyelid is smaller and rod shaped. The medial and lateral ends of the tarsal plates are connected to the orbital margin by fibrous band known as medial and lateral *palpebral ligaments*. The tarsi are connected to the orbital margin by the palpebral fascia called the orbital septum. The tarsal glands (*meibomian glands*) are embedded in the deep surface of the tarsal plate. Sebaceous glands of the eyelashes are known as the glands of Zeis. The orbital septum (palpebral fascia) is the layer of connective tissue bridging the

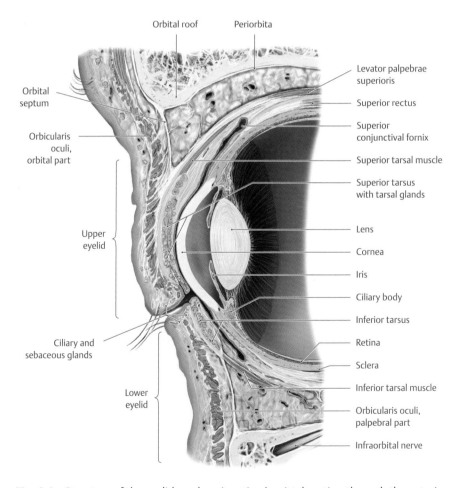

Fig. 4.4 Structure of the eyelids and conjunctiva (sagittal section through the anterior orbital cavity). (From: Schuenke M, Schulte E, Schumacher U. THIEME Atlas of Anatomy. Head, Neck, and Neuroanatomy. Illustrations by Voll M and Wesker K. © Thieme 2020.)

gap between the orbital margin and the tarsal plates of the upper and lower eyelids (**Fig. 4.2**). In the upper eyelid, there is a presence of tendon of levator palpebral superiors in this layer (refer to **Fig. 4.4**). A slip of smooth muscle (*Müller muscle*) arises from the undersurface of the tendon of levator palpebral superioris and is inserted on the tarsal plate. It is supplied by the sympathetic nerve.

5. *Layer of palpebral conjunctiva*: This is made up of transparent mucous membrane lined by the stratified squamous epithelium.

Nerve supply: The upper eyelid is supplied by the supraorbital, supratrochlear, infratrochlear, and palpebral branches of the lacrimal nerves, while the lower eyelid is supplied by the palpebral branch of the infraorbital nerve (sensory) (refer to **Fig. 4.2**). The orbicularis oculi muscle is supplied by the facial nerve (motor).

Blood supply: Superior lid gets its blood supply from the lateral palpebral branches of the lacrimal artery and medial palpebral branches of the ophthalmic artery. The inferior lid is also supplied by the palpebral branch of the infraorbital artery (branch of the maxillary artery) (refer to **Fig. 4.2**).

Lacrimal Apparatus (Video 4.1)

The lacrimal apparatus is concerned with the secretion of tears (lacrimal fluid) by the lacrimal gland and lacrimal passages (lacrimal canaliculi, lacrimal sac, and nasolacrimal duct) which drain the excessive fluid into the nasal cavity. Thus, the lacrimal apparatus consists of the following parts:

1. Lacrimal gland.

2. Conjunctival sac.

3. Lacrimal punctum.

4. Lacrimal canaliculus.

5. Lacrimal sac.

6. Nasolacrimal duct.

The lacrimal gland is about the size and shape of an almond and consists of orbital and palpebral parts. The large orbital part is located in a shallow orbital fossa in the anterolateral part of the orbit near the roof (refer to **Fig. 4.3**). The small palpebral part is located in the lateral part of the upper eyelid. The secretomotor fibers to the gland are supplied by the parasympathetic nerve derived from the greater petrosal branch of the facial nerve.

The conjunctiva is a transparent mucous membrane which covers the sclera (bulbar part) and also lines the inner surface of the eyelids (palpebral part). The fornices are produced when the conjunctiva from sclera is reflected on the inner surface of the eyelid (refer to **Fig. 4.4**). *Conjunctival sac* is the space between the bulbar and palpebral parts of the conjunctiva, which is closed when the eye is shut. Tears pass from the lateral side of the conjunctival sac to its medial side due to capillary action and blinking of the eyelids.

Each *lacrimal canaliculus* begins with the punctum. Each canaliculus measures about 8 mm and opens in the lacrimal sac behind the medial palpebral ligament.

The *lacrimal sac* lies in the lacrimal fossa located in the anterior part of the medial wall of the orbit. It lies behind the medial palpebral ligament. It measures about 15 mm in length and 6 mm in width. Inferiorly, it opens into the nasolacrimal duct (refer to **Fig. 4.3**).

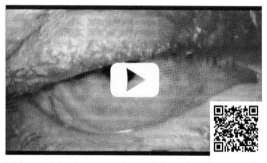

Video 4.1 Layers of eyelid, orbicularis oculi muscle, and lacrimal gland.

The nasolacrimal duct is about 18 mm long, narrow membranous passage. It starts at the lower end of the lacrimal sac and terminates at the inferior meatus of the nose. At its lower end, it is guarded by the membranous valve known as the *valve of Hasner*, which prevents the backward flow of the fluid from the nose.

▌Clinical Notes

Partial ptosis (drooping) of upper eyelid: This occurs due to the paralysis of the Müller muscle (a smooth muscle part of the levator palpebrae superioris) supplied by the sympathetic fibers from the upper cervical sympathetic ganglion as in the case of *Horner syndrome*.

Stye: It is the inflammation followed by the collection of pus in the gland of Zeis (sebaceous gland associated with the eyelashes).

Chalazion: It is the infection and formation of a cyst in the Meibomian gland (tarsal gland) due to obstruction in the duct of the gland.

Epiphora: In this condition, there occurs the overflow of tears from the conjunctival sac. The epiphora may result either due to the excessive secretion of tears as in the case of weeping or due to obstruction in the canaliculi, lacrimal sac, or nasolacrimal duct. Overflow of tears may also occur in old age because of the eversion of the lower punctum due to laxity of the lid (known as *ectropion*).

Dacryocystitis: This condition is due to the inflammation of the lacrimal sac. The patient complains of pain, redness, and swelling at the medial angle of the eye.

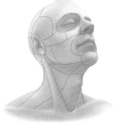

Learning Objectives

At the end of the dissection of the posterior triangle, you should be able to identify the following:

- Borders of the posterior triangle.
- General investing layer of the deep cervical fascia forming the roof of the triangle.
- Cutaneous branches of the cervical plexus.
- Subdivisions of the posterior triangle.
- Spinal accessory nerve.
- Trunks of the brachial plexus.
- Muscles forming the floor.

Introduction

The side of the neck is divided into an anterior and a posterior triangle by the sternocleidomastoid muscle. The posterior triangle is subdivided into *occipital* and *subclavian* (*omoclavicular*) triangles with the help of the inferior belly of the *omohyoid* muscle (**Fig. 5.1**). The roof of the posterior triangle is formed by the investing layer of the deep cervical fascia stretching between the posterior border of the sternocleidomastoid muscle and the anterior border of the trapezius muscle. The roof is pierced by four cutaneous nerves (the supraclavicular, lesser occipital, great auricular, and transverse cervical) (**Fig. 5.2**). These cutaneous nerves arise from the cervical plexus. The triangle also contains the spinal accessory nerve. The floor of the triangle is formed by many muscles. The subclavian part of the triangle contains many important neurovascular structures.

Students should note that though the deep fascia was absent in the face, the muscles and other structures of the neck are tightly covered by deep fascia (cervical fascia). The deep fascia of the neck is present in three layers, that is, general investing layer, a prevertebral layer, and a pretracheal layer. Students are suggested to learn about the cervical fascia from a textbook of anatomy before they start the dissection of the neck.

Surface Landmarks

Identify the medial and lateral ends and superior surface of the *clavicle* bone. Similarly, in a skull, look for the *mastoid process* and *superior nuchal line* (refer to **Fig. 1.2**). On a living person, identify the posterior border of the *sternocleidomastoid* muscle and the anterior border of the *trapezius*. Palpate the mastoid process and, if possible, the superior nuchal line. Also, palpate the sternal and lateral ends of the clavicle. Look for the *sternal* and *clavicular* heads of origin of the sternocleidomastoid muscle (**Fig. 5.1**). If the person is thin, you may also see the inferior belly of the *omohyoid*. Try to find the *external jugular vein* as it crosses the sternocleidomastoid muscle obliquely from above in a downward direction (refer to **Fig. 5.4**).

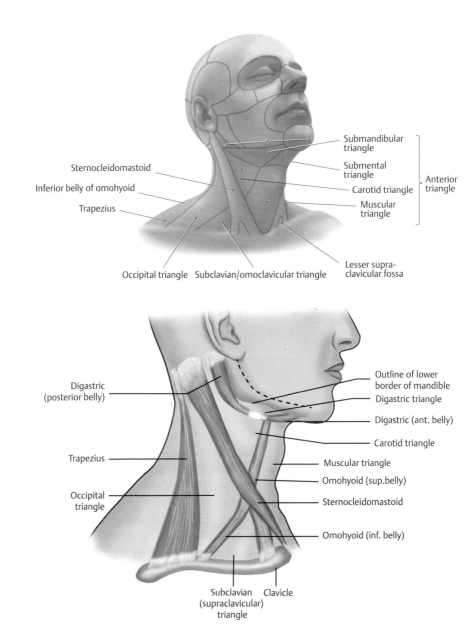

Fig. 5.1 **(a)** Triangles of the neck. The posterior triangle (*light blue shade*) and anterior triangle (*light green shade*). **(b)** Muscles forming the boundaries of various triangles of the neck. Posterior triangle consists of two subdivisions, i.e., occipital and supraclavicular/subclavian. (Figure a: From: Schuenke M, Schulte E, Schumacher U. THIEME Atlas of Anatomy. Head, Neck, and Neuroanatomy. Illustrations by Voll M and Wesker K. © Thieme 2020.)

Dissection and Identification

A. Incision and reflection of skin.

1. The body should remain in a supine position. Give a very careful shallow longitudinal skin incision 'A' superficial to the middle of the sternocleidomastoid muscle extending from the mastoid process to the sternum (**Fig. 5.2**). Your incision should not go deep in the superficial fascia as many structures cross the sternocleidomastoid muscle. The *second incision* 'B' should be made just posterior to the anterior border of the trapezius muscle extending between the

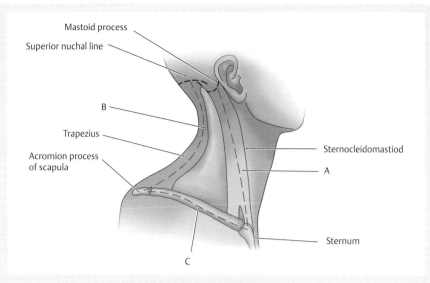

Fig. 5.2   Incision lines to dissect the posterior triangle.

superior nuchal line and the acromion process of the scapula. The *third incision* 'C' should be given between the lower ends of both the above incisions. This incision will pass in front of the clavicle and again should be shallow as the cutaneous supraclavicular nerves lie over the clavicle here.

2. Carefully reflect the skin from the superficial fascia. Identify the thin subcutaneous platysma muscle extending from the clavicle to the mandible after crossing the lower part of the sternocleidomastoid muscle (**Fig. 5.3**). Remove the muscle from the field of dissection as delicate nerves and vein lie deep into it. With the help of forceps, remove the fat and connective tissue from the area to expose various cutaneous nerves and the external jugular vein. These cutaneous nerves will be piercing the deep cervical fascia (roof of the posterior triangle) at various points. The external jugular vein will disappear after piercing the deep fascia just above the clavicle to drain into the subclavian vein (**Fig. 5.4**).

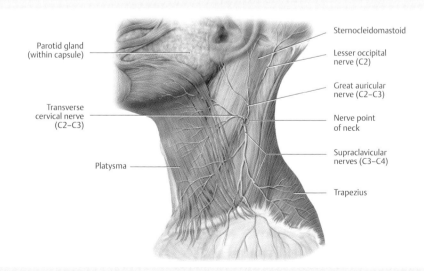

Fig. 5.3   Platysma. (From Schuenke M, Schulte E, Schumacher U. THIEME Atlas of Anatomy Third Edition, Vol 3. © Thieme 2020. Illustrations by Markus Voll and Karl Wesker.)

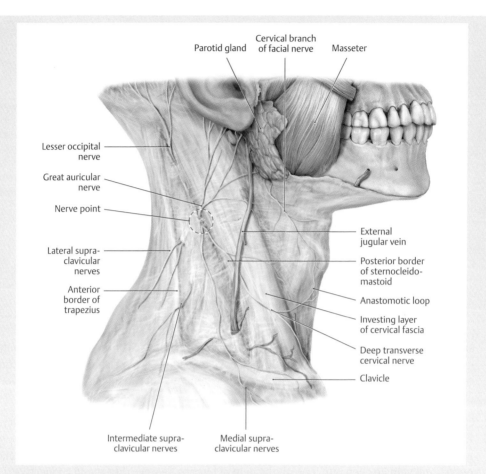

Fig. 5.4 Boundaries and structures piercing the roof of the posterior triangle. (From: Schuenke M, Schulte E, Schumacher U. THIEME Atlas of Anatomy. Head, Neck, and Neuroanatomy. Illustrations by Voll M and Wesker K. © Thieme 2020.)

B. Boundaries of posterior triangle and cutaneous nerves.

1. Identify the boundaries of the posterior triangle, that is, posterior border of the sternocleidomastoid anteriorly, anterior border of the trapezius posteriorly, and the clavicle below (**Fig. 5.4**). Clean the investing layer of the deep cervical fascia (roof) which splits to enclose both these muscles.

2. Using the combination of blunt dissection and scissors remove the investing layer of the deep cervical fascia which forms the roof of the triangle. Also, remove this fascia from both the muscles (i.e., the sternocleidomastoid and trapezius) forming the boundaries of the posterior triangle (**Fig. 5.5**).

3. With the help of blunt dissection, carefully clean the area near the midpoint of the posterior border of the sternocleidomastoid muscle. From this point, various cutaneous nerves of the cervical plexus emerge *(this is also known as the nerve point of the neck)*. Follow the course of each nerve in the triangle (**Fig. 5.6a**).

C. Occipital and subclavian triangles.

1. Clean the lower area of the triangle to identify the inferior belly of the omohyoid which divides the posterior triangle into two subtriangles, that is, *occipital* and *subclavian* (**Fig. 5.1**).

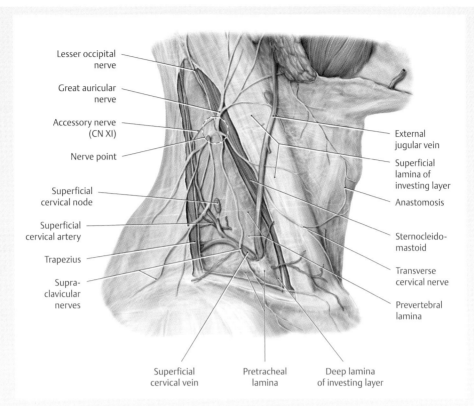

Fig. 5.5 Structures piercing the roof of the posterior triangle exposed. Note the prevertebral lamina (fascia/fascial carpet) covering the muscles of the floor. (From: Schuenke M, Schulte E, Schumacher U. THIEME Atlas of Anatomy. Head, Neck, and Neuroanatomy. Illustrations by Voll M and Wesker K. © Thieme 2020.)

2. Now identify the superficial branches of the transverse cervical artery and vein. Also, look for the accessory nerve as it passes from the posterior border of the sternocleidomastoid to the deep surface of the trapezius (refer to **Fig. 5.6a**). The accessory nerve is accompanied by the C2 and C3 nerves.

D. Floor of posterior triangle, phrenic nerve, brachial plexus, and subclavian vessels.

1. This is the time to identify the prevertebral layer of the deep cervical fascia, which covers the muscles of the floor of the posterior triangle. Remove this layer of the cervical fascia by using the blunt dissection and scissors to expose the muscles of the floor of the posterior triangle. Identify these muscles from above in downward direction as the splenius capitis, levator scapulae, scalenus medius, and part of scalenus anterior (refer to **Fig. 5.6b**).

   a. Cut through the clavicular origin of the sternomastoid and expose the deeper structures by removing the fat and connective tissues. Expose the scalenus anterior muscle completely.

   b. Identify the phrenic nerve as it lies on the scalenus anterior muscle. Also, search for the roots and trunks of the brachial plexus between the scalenus anterior and the scalenus medius.

   c. You shall see the subclavian artery between the scalenus anterior and the scalenus medius in the subclavian triangle. Also, look for the subclavian vein which lies anterior to the scalenus anterior and posterior to the clavicle.

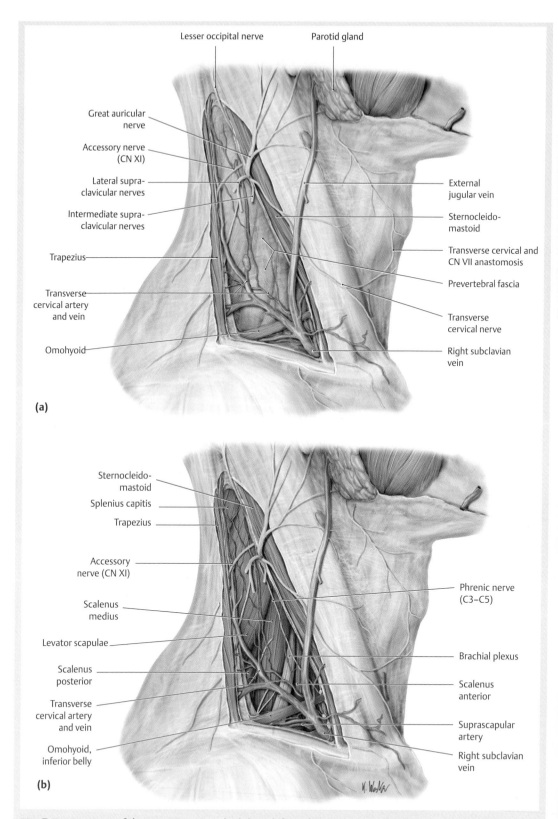

Fig. 5.6 Contents of the posterior triangle. **(a)** With fascial carpet intact. **(b)** With fascial carpet removed. (From: Schuenke M, Schulte E, Schumacher U. THIEME Atlas of Anatomy. Head, Neck, and Neuroanatomy. Illustrations by Voll M and Wesker K. © Thieme 2020.)

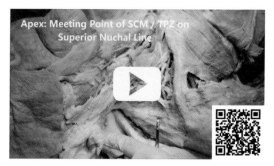

Video 5.1   Posterior triangle of neck.

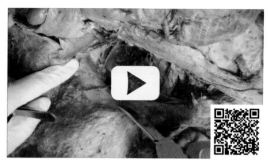

Video 5.2   Lateral aspect of neck, external jugular vein variant, cervical plexus, CN XI, and scalene triangle.

Description of Posterior Triangle (Videos 5.1 and 5.2)

The posterior triangle is described under the following heads, i.e., boundaries, roof, floor, and contents:

Boundaries: The posterior triangle is bounded.
- Anteriorly—by the *posterior border of the sternomastoid.*
- Posteriorly—by the *anterior border of the trapezius.*
- Inferiorly (base)—by the *middle third of the clavicle.*
- Superiorly (apex)—by the *meeting point of the sternomastoid and trapezius.*

The triangle is subdivided by the inferior belly of the *omohyoid* into an upper-*occipital* and a lower-*subclavian triangle* (refer to **Fig. 5.1b**).

Roof: From superficial to deep, it is formed by the skin, superficial fascia (which contains the platysma muscle in the anteroinferior part of the triangle), and investing layer of the deep cervical fascia (refer to **Fig. 5.5**).

Floor: From above downward, it is formed by the *semispinalis capitis, splenius capitis, levator scapulae,* and *scalenus medius* (refer to **Fig. 5.6b**).

(Note: Please note that the scalenus posterior is seen occasionally between the levator scapulae and the scalenus medius. Semispinalis capitis may be or may not be seen near the apex of the triangle. Similarly, scalenus anterior will become visible only after detaching the clavicular head of the sternocleidomastoid at its origin. In the true sense, the scalenus anterior muscle and subclavian vein are not a part of the posterior triangle.)

Contents: The following structures are present in the posterior triangle (**Fig. 5.6a, b**):
- *Nerves*: Branches of the cervical plexus are lesser occipital, great auricular, transverse cervical, and supraclavicular (**Figs. 5.3** to **5.5**). It also contains trunks of the brachial plexus and few branches arising from this plexus (dorsal scapular [C5], nerve to subclavius [C5 and C6], suprascapular [C5 and C6], and long thoracic nerve [C5, C6, and C7]). Spinal accessory and C2 and C3 cross the posterior triangle from the posterior surface of the sternomastoid to the deep surface of the trapezius. The details of these nerves are given in **Table 5.1** (refer **Fig. 5.6a, b**).
- *Arteries* (occipital artery, transverse cervical, suprascapular, and third part of the subclavian artery): The occipital artery is present near the apex of the triangle and is a branch from the external carotid. Transverse cervical and suprascapular arteries are present in the subclavian triangle and are branches of the thyrocervical trunk which itself arises from the first part of the subclavian artery (refer to **Fig. 5.6a, b**). The third part of the subclavian artery lies lateral to the scalenus anterior along with the trunks of the brachial plexus in the subclavian triangle.
- *Veins* (external jugular [terminal part], transverse cervical, and suprascapular veins): External jugular vein is formed behind the angle of the mandible and the parotid gland by the union of

Table 5.1 Nerves of the posterior triangle

Source	Motor/sensory	Innervation
A. Branches from the cervical plexus 1. Lesser occipital (C2) 2. Great auricular (C2, C3) 3. Transverse cervical (C2, C3) 4. Supraclavicular (C3, C4)	*Sensory to skin (exteroceptive sensation, i.e., pain, touch and temperature)*	1. Skin of auricle, mastoid process, and neck 2. Skin of auricle, over mastoid, over angle of mandible, and parotid gland 3. Skin on side and front of neck 4. Skin over upper part of front of the chest and upper half over the deltoid muscle
B. Spinal accessory (CN XI)	*Motor to muscles*	Motor to the sternomastoid and trapezius muscles
C. Branches from the spinal nerves C2 and C3	*Sensory (proprioceptive sensation from the muscles)*	C2 is proprioceptive to the sternomastoid and C2, C3 for the trapezius
D. Branches from the brachial plexus 1. Dorsal scapular (C5) 2. Nerve to subclavius (C5, C6) 3. Suprascapular nerve (C5, C6) 4. Long thoracic (C5, C6, and C7)	*Motor to muscles*	1. Motor to the levator scapulae, rhomboids major and minor 2. Motor to the subclavius 3. Motor to the supraspinatus and infraspinatus 4. Motor to the serratus anterior

Abbreviation: CN, cranial nerve.

the posterior division of the retromandibular vein and posterior auricular vein on the surface of the sternomastoid. It runs vertically downward in the superficial fascia deep to the platysma. It pierces the deep fascia about 2 to 3 cm above the clavicle. It crosses the brachial plexus and third part of the subclavian artery to open in the subclavian vein behind the clavicle. Tributaries to the external jugular veins are the suprascapular, transverse cervical, and anterior jugular veins (**Fig. 5.6a, b**).

Transverse cervical and suprascapular veins are present in the subclavian triangle.

- *Muscle* (the inferior belly of the omohyoid): It arises from the superior border of the scapula and the transverse scapular ligament. It runs anterosuperiorly to form the intermediate tendon (deep to the sternomastoid), which links it with the superior belly. The intermediate tendon is attached below to the clavicle by the fibrous pulley derived from the investing layer of the deep cervical fascia. The muscle is supplied by the inferior root (C2 and C3) of the ansa cervicalis. It acts to depress the hyoid bone during speaking and swallowing.

- *Lymph nodes*: Many lymph nodes are present in small groups, that is, at the apex of the triangle, along the posterior border of the sternomastoid, along the spinal accessory nerve, and above the clavicle (supraclavicular group).

▌Clinical Notes

1. Venous pressure increases in heart failure. This leads to increased distension of the external jugular vein in the neck.

2. The supraclavicular nerves (that supply the skin of the shoulder region) and phrenic nerve (that supply the diaphragm) both are derived from the same spinal segments (C3 and C4). Irritation of the diaphragm is carried by the phrenic nerve and is referred as pain to the area of the shoulder supplied by the supraclavicular nerve.

3. Incision to drain the subcutaneous abscess, at the posterior border of the sternomastoid and in the posterior triangle, should be made carefully as it may damage the spinal accessory and other nerves.

Back of the Neck and Suboccipital Triangle

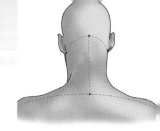

Introduction

The back of the neck is limited above by the external occipital protuberance and superior nuchal lines, one on either side of this protuberance. Below, the neck extends till the level of the spine of the seventh cervical vertebra and the tip of the shoulder, on either side. At the back of the neck, the following layers of soft tissues are seen from superficial to deep, that is, *skin, superficial fascia, deep fascia* (investing layer of the deep cervical fascia), first layer of the muscles (*trapezius* and *sternomastoid*), enclosing an area near the apex of the posterior triangle, second layer of the muscles (*splenius capitis* and *levator scapulae*), and third layer of the muscles (*semispinalis capitis* and *longissimus capitis*). Reflection of the third layer of the muscle exposes the *suboccipital triangle* which is bounded by many small muscles and contains the third part of the *vertebral artery*, *suboccipital nerve* (dorsal ramus of the first cervical spinal nerve), and *suboccipital plexus of vein*. The semispinalis cervicis and multifidus lie deep to the semispinalis capitis muscle. Fibers of the multifidus slope downward and medially from the transverse processes to the spines.

Suggestions to Students

1. Review the bones of the occipital region at the back of the neck.
2. On a dry skull, look for the external occipital protuberance, superior and inferior nuchal lines, external occipital crest, and mastoid process.
3. On the posterior aspect of the cervical vertebrae, look for the transverse processes and spines of all cervical vertebrae (**Fig. 6.1**).
4. See the various bony features of C1 and C2 cervical vertebrae with the help of **Figs. 1.14** and **1.15**. Identify the posterior tubercle, posterior arch, and transverse process of the atlas. Look for the foramen transversarium and groove for the vertebral artery on the superior surface of the posterior arch of the atlas. See the massive lamina and spine of C2 vertebra.

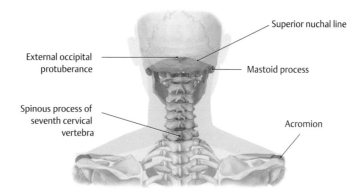

External occipital protuberance

Superior nuchal line

Mastoid process

Spinous process of seventh cervical vertebra

Acromion

Fig. 6.1 Surface landmarks on the back of the neck.

Surface Landmarks

Before starting the dissection, students should identify the following surface landmarks on the cadaver or on a living person:

1. External occipital protuberance: It is felt as a bony knob in the median line where the back of the head joins the back of the neck.

2. Inion: It is the apex of the external occipital protuberance.

3. Acromion process: It is subcutaneous and can be palpated on the top of the shoulder.

4. Mastoid process: It is palpated as a smooth rounded bone behind the lower part of the auricle.

5. Nuchal furrow: It is the median furrow at the back of the neck, deep to which lay the ligamentum nuchae.

6. On either side of this median furrow, a rounded ridge is seen that is produced due to the vertical course of the semispinalis capitis muscle fibers which run parallel to the vertebral column.

7. Spine of the seventh cervical vertebra (vertebra prominence): It is felt as a bony tubercle in the lower part of the nuchal furrow. The bony landmarks are shown in **Fig. 6.1**.

Dissection and Identification

A. Incision and reflection of skin.

1. Make a vertical skin incision (A) extending from the external occipital protuberance to the tip of the spine of the seventh cervical vertebra. Make a horizontal incision (B) from the seventh cervical spine to the acromion process on either side (**Fig. 6.2**). We have already given a skin incision just posterior to the anterior border of the trapezius muscle while dissecting the posterior triangle. Reflect the skin downward on either side. The skin at the back of the neck is relatively thick.

2. Remove the tough fibrofatty tissues of the superficial fascia and search for the greater occipital nerve, third occipital nerve, and occipital artery close to the superior nuchal line (**Fig. 6.3**).

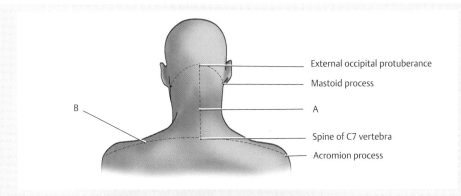

Fig. 6.2   Skin incisions for dissection of the back of the neck.

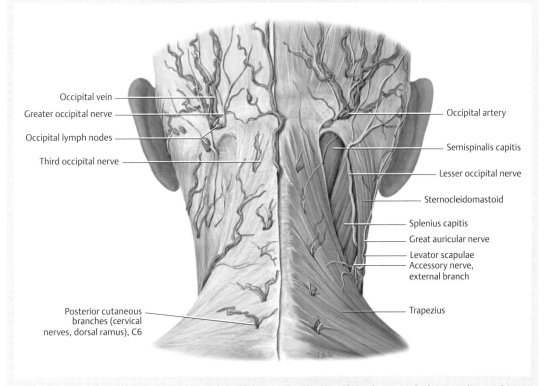

Fig. 6.3   Superficial dissection of the back of the neck. (From: Schuenke M, Schulte E, Schumacher U. THIEME Atlas of Anatomy. Head, Neck, and Neuroanatomy. Illustrations by Voll M and Wesker K. © Thieme 2020.)

B. Exposure and reflection of trapezius.

1. Reflect the deep fascia from the anterior border of the trapezius muscle toward the midline. See the attachment of the deep fascia to the ligamentum nuchae. Once again, identify the semispinalis capitis, splenius capitis, and levator scapulae in the floor of the posterior triangle. We have already exposed these muscles during the dissection of the posterior triangle (refer to **Fig. 6.4**).

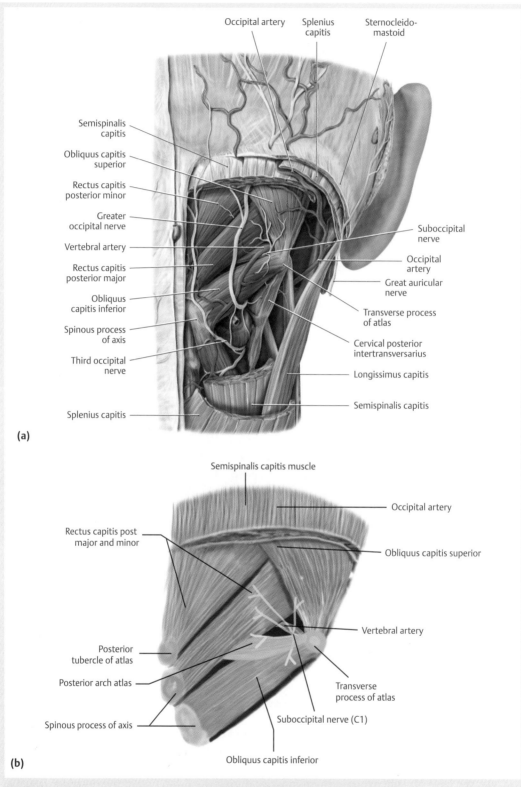

Fig. 6.4 **(a)** Deep dissection on the back of the neck showing suboccipital triangle. Within the triangle, note the presence of the third part of vertebral artery and suboccipital nerve. **(b)** Note the presence of suboccipital nerve (C1 dorsal ramus) and vertebral artery (third part) above the posterior arch of atlas. The posterior atlanto-occipital membrane is not seen as it lies deep to rectus capitis posterior major and minor muscles. (Figure a: From: Schuenke M, Schulte E, Schumacher U. THIEME Atlas of Anatomy. Head, Neck, and Neuroanatomy. Illustrations by Voll M and Wesker K. © Thieme 2020.)

2. Reflect the trapezius muscle downward by giving a horizontal incision near the superior nuchal line and a vertical incision near the midline. On its deep surface look for the spinal accessory, C2 and C3 nerves, and transverse cervical artery. Reflection of the trapezius will expose the splenius capitis and part of the semispinalis capitis.

C. Semispinalis capitis and greater occipital nerve.

1. Detach the splenius capitis muscle from its vertebral attachment and reflect it upward toward the mastoid process. This will expose the semispinalis capitis and longissimus capitis muscles. Semispinalis capitis is pierced by the greater occipital nerve. You will have to make a careful blunt dissection to save the greater occipital nerve as it is passing through the substance of the muscle. Once the nerve is safely dissected, then detach the semispinalis capitis muscle from the occipital bone and reflect it downward. Similarly, reflect the longissimus capitis from the skull downward and trace the occipital artery as it lies deep to the mastoid process (**Fig. 6.4**).

D. Muscles forming the boundaries of suboccipital triangle, C1 spinal nerve, and vertebral artery.

1. Reflection of the semispinalis capitis and longissimus capitis will expose the suboccipital triangle of muscles. However, this triangle is difficult to dissect because it is filled with dense connective tissue that overlaps the boundaries and contents of the triangle.

2. Refer to **Fig. 6.4** to clean the muscles forming the boundaries of the suboccipital triangle. To expose the triangle, you will have to separate (pull) these muscles away from each other (as shown in Fig. 6.4b).

3. The fine branches of the dorsal ramus of C1 spinal nerve (suboccipital nerve) and venous plexus are embedded in the dense connective tissue. Very carefully remove this dense connective tissue in piecemeal and preserve the branches of the nerve.

4. In the floor of the triangle, search for the third part of the vertebral artery (refer **Fig. 6.4**) and posterior atlanto-occipital membrane.

5. The reflection of the semispinalis capitis downward will expose the muscle semispinalis cervices below C4 level and its reflection will expose the deepest muscle of the multifidus.

Description of the Suboccipital Triangle

It is present at the lower part of the back of the neck between the occipital bone and axis and atlas vertebrae.

Boundaries of the triangle are as follows:

1. *Superomedially*: Rectus capitis posterior major and rectus capitis posterior minor.

2. *Superolaterally*: Superior oblique muscle (obliquus capitis superior).

3. *Below and laterally*: Inferior oblique muscle (obliquus capitis inferior).

Roof: Semispinalis capitis muscle.
Floor: Posterior atlanto-occipital membrane and posterior arch of the atlas.

Contents: The triangle contains fibrofatty tissue, third part of the vertebral artery, suboccipital nerve, and suboccipital venous plexus.

Some of the contents of the suboccipital triangle can be described as follows:

The third part of the vertebral artery courses from the foramen transversarium of the atlas to the lateral edge of the posterior atlanto-occipital membrane. The artery runs behind the superior articular process of the atlas (facet) and lies in the sulcus of the vertebral artery. In the sulcus, it lies above the suboccipital nerve (C1 spinal nerve).

The suboccipital nerve (dorsal ramus of C1 spinal nerve) enters the suboccipital triangle between the posterior arch of the atlas and the vertebral artery. It breaks into many branches to supply the four muscles forming the boundaries and part of one muscle forming the roof of the triangle. It has no cutaneous branches.

Muscles at the Back of the Neck

The important muscles are described in **Table 6.1**.

Table 6.1   Important muscles at the back of the neck

Name of the muscle	Origin	Insertion	Nerve supply	Action
Trapezius (cervical part only)	Superior nuchal line, external occipital protuberance, ligamentum nuchae spine of the seventh cervical vertebra	Posterior surface of the lateral half of the clavicle and medial border of the acromion	Spinal accessory (motor), branch from C3 and C4 (proprioceptive)	Extension of the neck, elevation of the acromion
Splenius capitis	Ligamentum nuchae (lower part), spine of the seventh cervical vertebra and spines of the upper thoracic vertebrae	Mastoid process and below the lateral part of the superior nuchal line	Dorsal ramus of C3–C6 spinal nerves, part of it is also supplied by suboccipital nerve (dorsal ramus of C1)	Rotation of the head to turn the face to the same side
Levator scapulae	From transverse processes of the upper four cervical vertebrae	At the medial border of the scapula between superior angle and spine	Ventral rami of C3 and C4 nerves	Elevation and rotation of the scapula
Semispinalis capitis	From articular processes of the lower four cervical and transverse process of the upper six thoracic vertebrae	On the occipital bone, in the medial area between superior and inferior nuchal lines	Dorsal rami of the cervical and thoracic nerves	Extension of the head and rotation of the face to the opposite side
Longissimus capitis	Upper five thoracic transverse process and lower four cervical articular processes	On the mastoid process below the attachment of the splenius capitis	Dorsal ramus of the lower cervical and upper thoracic spinal nerves	Extension of the head and turning of the head to the same side
Rectus capitis posterior major	Spine of the second cervical vertebra	In the lateral part below the inferior nuchal line	Dorsal ramus of C1 (suboccipital nerve)	Extends the head and rotates the head to the same side
Rectus capitis posterior minor	From the posterior tubercle of the atlas near the midline	In the medial part below the inferior nuchal line	Dorsal ramus of C1	It extends the head

Name of the muscle	Origin	Insertion	Nerve supply	Action
Superior oblique	Upper surface of the transverse process of C1 vertebra	Lateral area between superior and inferior nuchal line	Dorsal ramus of C1 spinal nerve	Posterolateral flexion of the head
Inferior oblique	Lateral surface of the spine of C2 vertebra	On the posterior and inferior side of C1 transverse process	Dorsal ramus of C1 spinal nerve	It rotates the head to the same side

∎ Clinical Notes

1. *The dizziness following the rotation of the head*: The prolonged rotation of the head to look backward during driving may lead to stretching and kinking of the third part of the vertebral artery, especially in old people suffering from arteriosclerosis and spondylosis. This leads to a reduction in blood flow to the brainstem causing dizziness.

2. *Cisternal puncture*: It is done in the suboccipital region by introducing a needle just above the spine of axis, in forward and upward direction, to withdraw cerebrospinal fluid from the cerebromedullary cistern.

3. *Spasm of muscles of the back of the neck*: The extensor muscles of the neck may go in spasm secondary to irritation of the nerve roots due to meningitis causing retrocolitis (drawing of head backward).

7 Anterior Triangle of the Neck

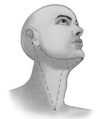

Learning Objectives

At the end of the dissection of anterior triangle, you should be able to identify the followings:

- Muscles forming the boundaries of anterior triangle and its subdivisions.
- Submandibular gland, submandibular lymph nodes, facial artery and facial vein.
- Carotid sheath and its contents (internal jugular vein, common and internal carotid arteries, vagus nerve); branches arising from external carotid artery; hypoglossal nerve; ansa cervicalis and branches of vagus nerve in the carotid triangle.
- Infrahyoid muscles covering the thyroid gland.
- Mylohyoid and constrictor muscles of the pharynx forming the floor.

Introduction

Anterior triangle of the neck is present on the anterior aspect of the neck. It is bounded *medially* by midline extending from chin to suprasternal notch, *above* by the base of mandible and line extending from base of the mandible to the mastoid process and *laterally* by the anterior border of sternocleidomastoid muscle. Anterior triangle is subdivided into *submental (only half), muscular, digastric,* and *carotid* triangles (**Fig. 7.1**). The anterior region of the neck between two sterno-cleidomastoid muscles is divided into suprahyoid and infrahyoid regions. The suprahyoid region includes digastric and submental triangles, while infrahyoid region includes carotid and muscular triangles.

Submental triangle: It lies between two anterior bellies of digastric muscles and hyoid bone: *Apex* at symphysis menti, *base* at hyoid bone, *sides* at anterior bellies of digastric muscles.

Digastric triangle: It is located between the base of mandible and anterior and posterior bellies of digastric muscles: *Superior boundary*—base of mandible, *anteroinferior*—anterior belly of digastric, *posteroinferior*—posterior belly of digastric. The digastric triangle contains facial artery, facial vein, submandibular gland, and submandibular lymph nodes.

Carotid triangle: It is bounded by three muscles, that is, *superior*—posterior belly of digastric; *anteroinferior*—superior belly of omohyoid; and *posterior*—sternocleidomastoid (**Fig. 7.1**). The carotid triangle contains carotid sheath which encloses internal jugular vein, common and internal carotid arteries, and vagus nerve. It also contains external carotid artery, carotid sinus, and carotid body. External carotid artery gives many branches in this triangle.

Muscular triangle: It lies below the hyoid bone and contains an infrahyoid group of muscles which overlie the thyroid gland and trachea. *Boundaries: Posterosuperior*—superior belly of omohyoid; *posteroinferior* —anterior border of sternocleidomastoid; *anterior*—midline extending from hyoid to sternum.

The *floor* of most of these triangles is formed by mylohyoid and constrictors of pharynx on which the contents of triangle lie.

The *roof* of all these triangles is formed by skin, superficial fascia, and investing layer of deep (cervical) fascia of the neck.

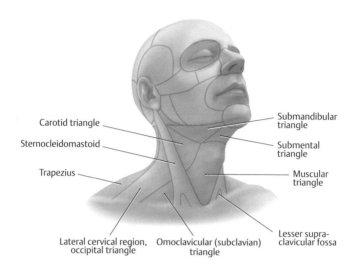

Carotid triangle

Sternocleidomastoid

Trapezius

Submandibular triangle

Submental triangle

Muscular triangle

Lesser supra-clavicular fossa

Lateral cervical region, occipital triangle   Omoclavicular (subclavian) triangle

Fig. 7.1 Anterior triangle and its subdivisions. (From: Schuenke M, Schulte E, Schumacher U. THIEME Atlas of Anatomy. Head, Neck, and Neuroanatomy. Illustrations by Voll M and Wesker K. © Thieme 2020.)

Surface Landmarks

Advice: Before marking the surface landmarks, students are advised to review the lower border of body and ramus of the mandible and look for digastric fossa near symphysis menti (refer to **Fig. 1.10**). Similarly, with the help of **Fig. 1.11,** review the features of hyoid bone.

1. *Symphysis menti:* In a living person, or on your own body, palpate the symphysis menti in the midline of mandible.

2. *Hyoid bone:* Trace your finger downward about 5 cm below the chin to locate the hyoid bone. The U-shaped hyoid bone can be gripped between thumb and index finger just above the laryngeal prominence. Palpate the body and greater horns of hyoid bone.

3. *Thyroid cartilage:* The prominence of thyroid cartilage (Adam's apple) can be palpated in midline below the hyoid bone.

4. *Cricoid cartilage and tracheal rings:* Move your finger down below the Adam's apple and trace to palpate the rounded arch of cricoid cartilage and rings of trachea that are located above the sternal notch.

Dissection and Identification

A. Incision and reflection of the skin.

1. Note that we have already given the skin incision (A) along the lower border of mandible extending posteriorly up to the mastoid process and incision on the skin along the anterior border of sternocleidomastoid.

2. Now give a midline incision (B) from chin to sternal notch and reflect skin flaps downward both on right and left side (**Fig. 7.2**).

3. You are now in superficial fascia which contains a variable amount of fat. It is quite loosely connected to the skin and deep fascia. Find the *platysma* muscle and reflect it upward toward the lower border of the mandible.

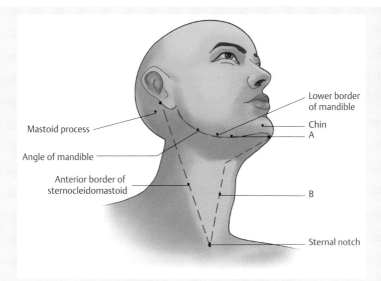

Fig. 7.2 Skin incisions for dissection of anterior triangle of the neck.

B. Nerves and veins in superficial fascia of anterior triangle.

Identify the cervical branch of *facial nerve* below the angle of mandible and the *transverse cervical* nerve as it crosses the sterno-mastoid and comes in anterior triangle (refer to **Fig. 5.6a**). Also, find the *anterior jugular vein* (**Fig. 7.3**) close to midline and trace it downward till it pierces the deep fascia. Give a small horizontal cut in deep fascia just above sternum to expose the *suprasternal space* in which terminal ends of right and left anterior jugular veins lie. Look for *jugular arch.*

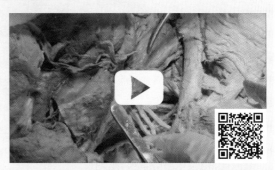

Video 7.1 Anterior triangle of neck.

C. Exposure of submental and digastric triangles (Video 7.1).

1. This is the time to remove the deep fascia (investing layer of cervical fascia) from the anterior triangle. Carefully remove the deep fascia from both the anterior bellies of digastrics and from the area between the two. This will expose the *mylohyoid* muscle in submental triangle.

2. Now cut the deep fascia from the lower border of mandible but preserve the facial artery and vein as they lie on lower border of mandible. Reflect the deep fascia toward posterior belly of digastrics. This will expose a part of *submandibular gland*. Now pull the submandibular gland laterally to expose the intermediate tendon of digastrics and *stylohyoid muscle*. In the posterior part of the digastric triangle, try to find posterior border of *mylohyoid* and part of *hyoglossus muscle*. With the help of blunt dissection, find the *hypoglossal nerve* in this area.

D. Dissection of muscular triangle (Video 7.2).

Now remove the deep fascia from the area between hyoid bone and sternum on either side of midline (area of *muscular triangle*). Clean *infrahyoid muscles* and identify them. Once you have identified these muscles, cut the *sternohyoid* muscle from middle and reflect the cut ends

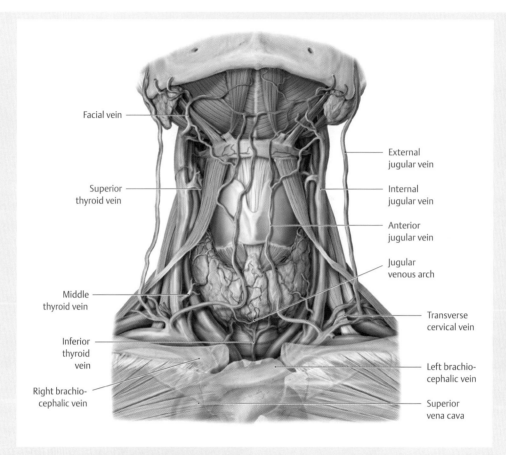

Fig. 7.3 Superficial veins on the anterior aspect of the neck. (From: Schuenke M, Schulte E, Schumacher U. THIEME Atlas of Anatomy. Head, Neck, and Neuroanatomy. Illustrations by Voll M and Wesker K. © Thieme 2020.)

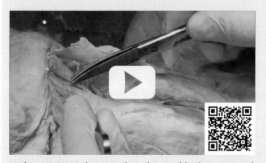

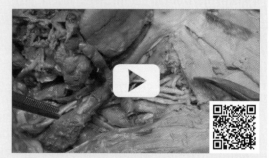

Video 7.2 Submental, submandibular, carotid and muscular triangles.

Video 7.3 Carotid triangle.

upward and downward (**Fig. 7.4a, b**). This will expose *sternothyroid* and *thyrohyoid* muscles. Look for *median thyrohyoid ligament, laryngeal prominence, cricothyroid ligament,* and *cricothyroid muscle.* Identify the isthmus of thyroid gland and pretracheal fascia covering the trachea.

E. Dissection of carotid triangle (Video 7.3).

1. You should now remove the deep fascia from the area of carotid triangle, that is, begin from the posterior belly of digastric and superior belly of omohyoid and go backward toward anterior border of sternomastoid muscle. Reflection of deep fascia will expose the *carotid sheath.* Carefully dissect the carotid sheath (as you will have to preserve *hypoglossal nerve* and

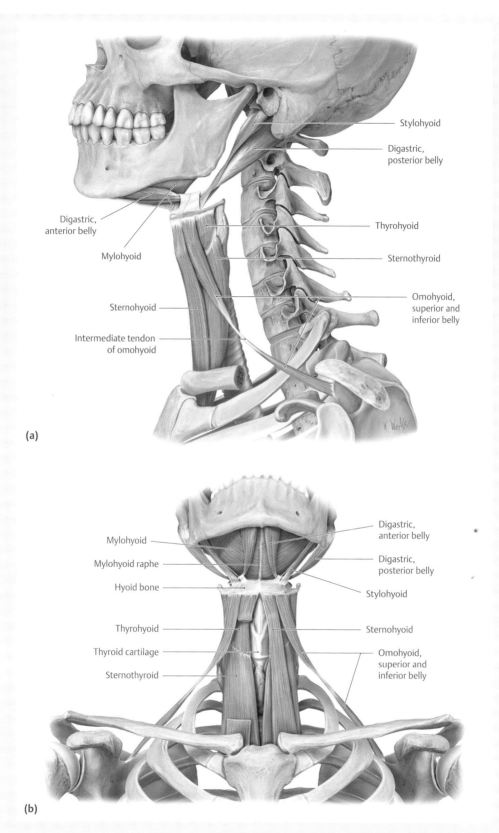

(a)

(b)

Fig. 7.4 Supra- and infrahyoid muscles. **(a)** Left lateral view. *(Continued)* **(b)** Anterior view. (From: Schuenke M, Schulte E, Schumacher U. THIEME Atlas of Anatomy. Head, Neck, and Neuroanatomy. Illustrations by Voll M and Wesker K. © Thieme 2020.)

superior root of ansa cervicalis). This dissection will expose *internal jugular vein* laterally, common and internal carotid arteries medial to vein. The external carotid artery lies anteromedial to internal carotid artery. Look for *vagus nerve* between artery and vein.

2. External carotid artery gives many branches (*ascending pharyngeal, superior thyroid, lingual, facial,* and *occipital*) in the carotid triangle. Dissect and identify each (**Fig. 7.5**).

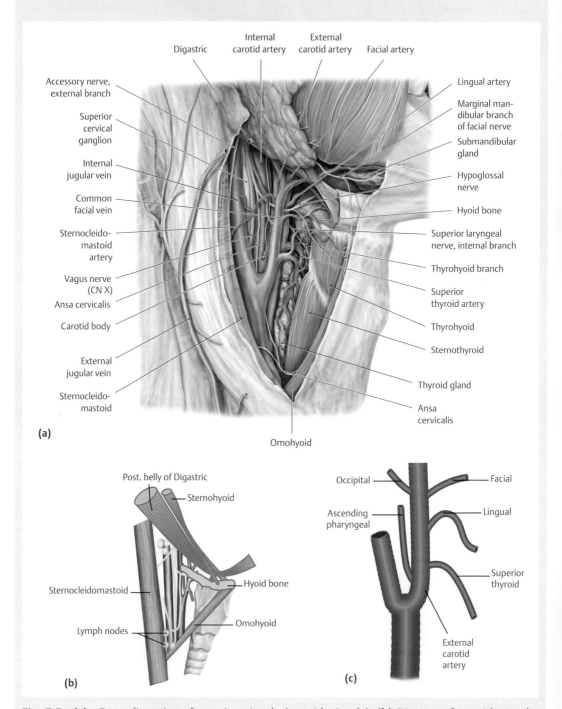

Fig. 7.5 **(a)** Deep dissection of anterior triangle (carotid triangle). **(b)** Diagram of carotid triangle. **(c)** Branches of external carotid artery in carotid triangle. (Figure a: From: Schuenke M, Schulte E, Schumacher U. THIEME Atlas of Anatomy. Head, Neck, and Neuroanatomy. Illustrations by Voll M and Wesker K. © Thieme 2020.)

Muscles Related to the Anterior Triangle

A brief description of the muscles related to anterior triangle is given in **Table 7.1** (also refer to **Fig. 7.4a, b**). Students are suggested to study the details of these muscles from the textbook of gross anatomy.

Table 7.1   Muscles related to anterior triangle

Muscle	Origin	Insertion	Nerve supply	Action
Platysma	From *fascia* over deltoid and pectoralis major muscle at the level of the second rib	Anterior fibers to mandible and posterior fibers to the skin near the angle of mouth	Cervical branch of facial nerve	Produces tension in the skin of the neck and pulls the angle of mouth downward
Sterno-cleidomastoid	From upper and anterior surface of manubrium sterni and from the superior surface of medial one-third of clavicle	On mastoid process and superior nuchal line	Spinal root of accessory nerve (motor) and C2–C4 spinal nerve (sensory)	Protraction of head (or lifting of head from pillow) when both muscles are acting/tilting of head on the same side and turning of face to the opposite side
Digastric	Anterior belly from digastric fossa of mandible and posterior belly from mastoid notch of mastoid process	Intermediate tendon of two bellies is attached to hyoid bone by a fascial sling	Anterior belly by mylohyoid branch of inferior alveolar (mandibular nerve) and posterior belly of facial nerve	Depression of mandible and elevation of hyoid bone
Mylohyoid	From mylohyoid line of mandible	On median fibrous raphe (stretching from symphysis menti to hyoid bone) and on anterior aspect of hyoid bone	Mylohyoid branch of inferior alveolar	Elevation of hyoid in swallowing and speech and depression of mandible
Stylohyoid	From posterior aspect of styloid process	Body of hyoid bone at its junction with greater cornua	Facial nerve	Elevation and retraction of hyoid bone
Sternohyoid	From the posterior surface of manubrium and posterior surface of sternal end of clavicle	Body of hyoid bone	From ansa cervicalis (C1–C3)	Depresses the hyoid bone as in swallowing
Superior belly of omohyoid	From the lower border of body of hyoid bone	At intermediate tendon	From the superior root of ansa cervicalis	Depression and retraction of hyoid bone
Sternothyroid	Posterior surface of manubrium sterni and edge of the first costal cartilage	On the oblique line of thyroid cartilage	Ansa cervicalis	Muscle depresses the larynx
Thyrohyoid	From the oblique line of thyroid cartilage	Inferior border of body and greater cornu of hyoid bone	Fibers from C1 through hypoglossal nerve	Elevation of larynx and depression of hyoid

Arteries of the Anterior Triangle

Arteries of the anterior triangle have been depicted in **Table 7.2** and **Fig. 7.5a–c**.

Table 7.2   Arteries of the anterior triangle

Name of the artery	Origin	Termination	Branches
Common carotid	The cervical part begins behind the sternoclavicular joint	At the upper border of thyroid cartilage where it bifurcates in external and internal carotid	It does not give any branch in the neck
Internal carotid	From bifurcation of common carotid at the superior border of thyroid cartilage	It enters in carotid canal in petrous temporal bone	It does not give any branch in the neck
External carotid	From bifurcation of common carotid at the superior border of thyroid in carotid triangle	Behind the neck of mandible by terminating in maxillary and superficial temporal	It gives many branches in carotid triangle: ascending pharyngeal, superior thyroid, lingual, facial, occipital, and posterior auricular (occasional)
1. Ascending pharyngeal	Arises as the first branch from the medial aspect of ext. carotid in carotid triangle	Ends near the base of skull by giving many branches by the side of pharynx	Pharyngeal, inferior tympanic, and meningeal arteries
2. Superior thyroid	Arises from anterior aspect of ext. carotid in carotid triangle	Terminates in muscular triangle by dividing into many branches	Branch to thyroid, infrahyoid branch, superior laryngeal, sternomastoid branch, and cricothyroid artery
3. Lingual	Arises from the anterior aspect of ext. carotid in carotid triangle at the tip of greater cornu, above superior thyroid	Terminates in tongue	Suprahyoid, dorsal lingual, sublingual arteries
4. Facial	Arises from the anterior aspect of ext. carotid in carotid triangle above lingual	Terminates in face medial to eye	Ascending palatine, tonsillar, submental, glandular, inferior labial, superior labial, and angular arteries
5. Occipital	Arises from the posterior aspect of ext. carotid in carotid triangle	Ends in the posterior part of scalp	Lower and upper sternomastoid branches, auricular branch, and mastoid branch

Veins of the Anterior Triangle

The internal jugular vein is the largest vein of the neck that runs in the carotid sheath. It begins at the jugular foramen and terminates behind the medial end of clavicle by joining subclavian vein to form innominate vein. Its main tributaries in the anterior triangle are lingual vein, facial vein, and superior thyroid vein (**Fig. 7.3**).

Important Nerves of Anterior Triangle

1. *Vagus nerve*: After coming out from jugular foramen, it runs in carotid sheath, posterolateral to internal and common carotid arteries. It has the following main branches in anterior triangle:

   a. *Pharyngeal branch*: It joins the pharyngeal plexus on the middle constrictor of pharynx to supply muscles of pharynx.

   b. *Superior laryngeal branch*: This divides into external and internal laryngeal branches. The internal laryngeal is sensory after piercing thyrohyoid membrane and it supplies the mucosa above vocal cord. The external laryngeal is motor and supplies the cricothyroid and inferior constrictor muscle.

2. *Accessory nerve*: It is present in the upper part of the carotid triangle (**Fig. 7.5**).

3. *Hypoglossal nerve*: It lies in the carotid triangle between the internal jugular vein and the internal carotid artery. It then crosses both the carotid arteries and loop of the lingual artery. In the carotid triangle, it gives the superior root of ansa cervicalis (C1 root value) and nerve to thyrohyoid (C1) (**Fig. 7.5**).

Lymph Nodes

The upper deep cervical group of lymph nodes lies on the internal jugular vein in carotid triangle (**Fig. 7.6**).

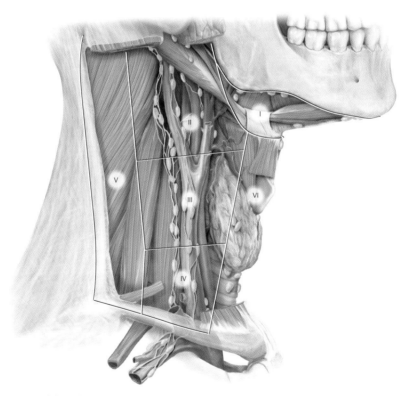

Fig. 7.6   Deep cervical lymph nodes. **I**, Submental and submandibular lymph nodes; **II, III,** and **IV,** jugular or deep cervical group of lymph nodes (jugulodigastric and jugulo-omohyoid); **V,** posterior cervical group of lymph nodes; **VI,** anterior cervical group of lymph nodes. (From: Schuenke M, Schulte E, Schumacher U. THIEME Atlas of Anatomy. Head, Neck, and Neuroanatomy. Illustrations by Voll M and Wesker K. © Thieme 2020.)

▮ Clinical Notes

1. *Ludwig's angina*: The investing layer is attached above to the base of the mandible and below to the hyoid bone. Because of these attachments, infection in the submandibular region produces a triangular swelling, known as Ludwig's angina.

2. *Enlargement of submental lymph node in the submental triangle* is observed after infection or tumor of tip of tongue, floor of mouth, or lower incisor teeth.

3. Deep cervical group of lymph nodes is located close to the internal jugular vein in the carotid triangle. In case of their enlargement, secondary to tumor, nodes are removed carefully preserving the vein or along with the vein.

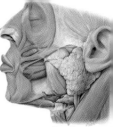

© THIEME Atlas of Anatomy

Introduction

The parotid bed (retromandibular fossa) is an irregular wedge-shaped area bounded *above* by the external auditory meatus, *posteriorly* by the mastoid process, *anteriorly* by the ramus of mandible, and *medially* by the styloid process. The parotid bed is made soft by muscles attached to the mastoid process, styloid process, and ramus of mandible. The parotid gland is enclosed within the parotid sheath which is formed by the investing layer of deep cervical fascia. The gland is in close contact with nerves, vessels, muscles, bones, and ligaments in this region. The parotid duct crosses the lateral surface of masseter muscle about 2 cm inferior to the zygomatic arch. If present, the accessory parotid gland lies above or on the parotid duct on the masseter.

Surface Landmarks

Before marking the surface landmarks, students are advised to review the following bony features of parotid bed (retromandibular fossa) in the skull (with articulated mandible):

- Look for the stylomastoid foramen, between styloid and mastoid processes (refer to **Fig. 1.5**). This foramen gives passage to the facial nerve.
- Look for the mastoid process, external acoustic meatus, tympanic plate, and styloid process (refer to **Fig. 1.4**).
- In the mandible, review the head, neck, angle, and posterior border of ramus (refer to **Fig. 1.10**).
- In a living person or a cadaver, palpate the area between the neck of mandible and ear.

1. The anterior border of the sternomastoid muscle, zygomatic arch, and posterior border of ramus of mandible can be easily palpated.
2. The anterior margin of masseter muscle can be easily palpated by clenching the teeth of upper and lower jaw.
3. *Mastoid process:* It can be felt as a round, bony prominence behind the lower part of the auricle.
4. *Head and neck of mandible:* Place your finger in front of tragus and then open and close the mouth, the head of mandible is felt gliding downward and forward.
5. The styloid process lies deep in the retromandibular fossa.

Dissection and Identification

A. Exposure of parotid gland and parotid duct/Stensen duct (Video 8.1).

1. As the parotid region is present on the lateral aspect of face in front and below the auricle, we have already reflected the skin from this area while dissecting the region of the face. We have also examined the anterior border of parotid gland while following the branches of facial nerve in the face (**Figs. 8.1a, 8.2,** and **8.3**).

2. Identify the parotid duct on the surface of masseter muscle and follow it anteriorly till it turns inward and disappears in buccinator muscle and posteriorly till the anterior border of parotid gland (**Fig. 8.3**).

3. With careful dissection, remove the parotid fascia (parotid sheath) from the lateral surface of the gland.

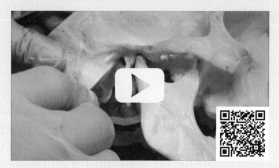

Video 8.1   Parotid gland and Parotid duct/Stensen duct.

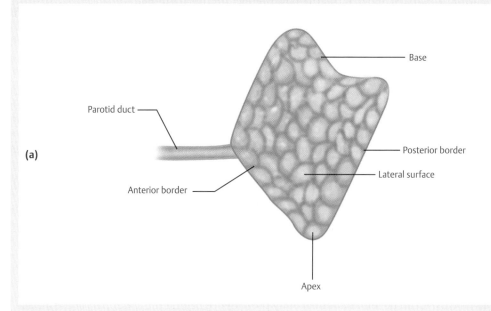

(a)

Fig. 8.1   (a) Line diagram showing parotid gland from its lateral surface. Note base, apex, and anterior and posterior borders.

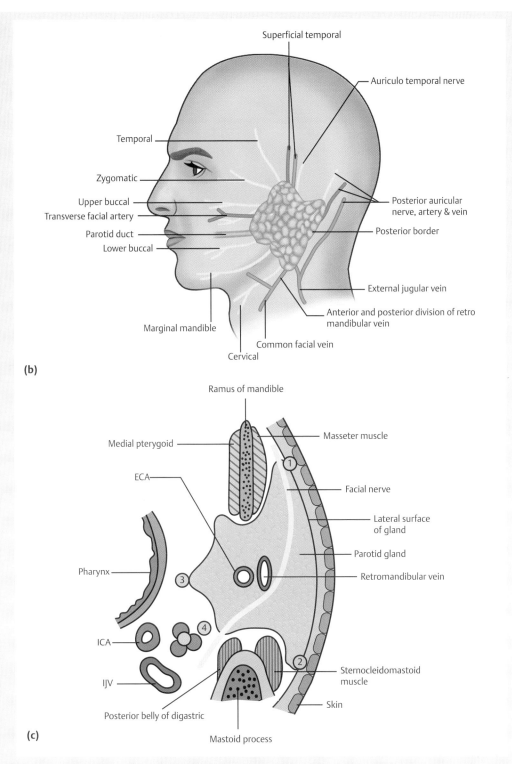

(b)

(c)

Fig. 8.1 **(b)** Diagram showing the lateral surface of parotid gland. Note the various structures emerging from its base, apex, and anterior border. Branches of facial nerve are emerging from the anterior border of the gland. **(c)** The schematic diagram of cross-section of parotid gland showing relations of anterior (1), posterior (2), and medial (3) borders. The anteromedial, posteromedial, and lateral surfaces lie between these borders. (4) The cross-section of styloid process and muscles attached to it (stylopharyngeus, stylohyoid, and styloglossus). ECA, external carotid artery; ICA, internal carotid artery; IJV, internal jugular vein.

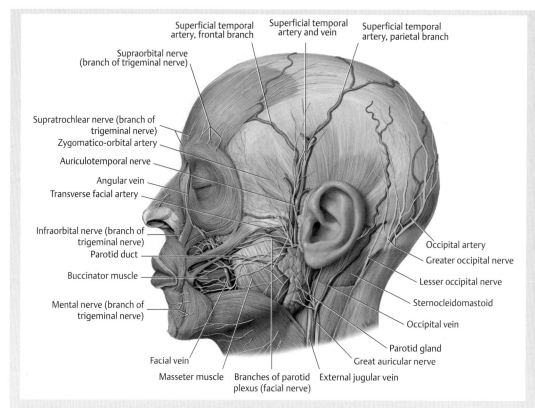

Fig. 8.2 Superficial dissection of the parotid region. Note the branches of facial nerve emerging at the anterior border of the parotid gland. (From: Schuenke M, Schulte E, Schumacher U. THIEME Atlas of Anatomy. Head, Neck, and Neuroanatomy. Illustrations by Voll M and Wesker K. © Thieme 2020.)

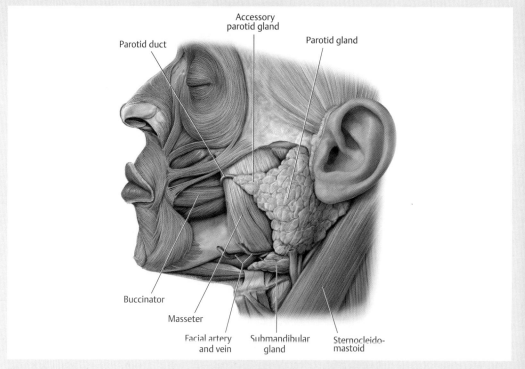

Fig. 8.3 Complete exposure of the parotid gland. Note the presence of accessory parotid gland lying on the parotid duct. (From: Schuenke M, Schulte E, Schumacher U. THIEME Atlas of Anatomy. Head, Neck, and Neuroanatomy. Illustrations by Voll M and Wesker K. © Thieme 2020.)

Parotid Gland and Parotid Duct

The shape of the gland is roughly like an inverted pyramid (apex lies below and base above). It has an apex, base, three surfaces, that is, lateral, anteromedial, and posteromedial. These surfaces are separated by three borders, i.e., anterior, posterior, and medial (**Fig. 8.1a–c**).

Relations of Parotid Gland

Relations of parotid gland are complicated because of irregular parotid region; thus, the shape of the gland is also irregular.

- *Apex*—It lies at the level of posterior belly of digastric and may extend in the upper part of carotid triangle.
- *Base*—It is concave and related to external acoustic meatus and posterior aspect of temporo-mandibular joint.
- *Lateral surface*—It is covered by skin, superficial fascia, platysma, great auricular nerve, investing layer of fascia (parotid fascia), and lymph nodes.
- *Anteromedial surface*—Temporomandibular joint, masseter muscle, posterior border of ramus, medial pterygoid muscle, and stylomandibular ligament. The branches of facial nerve emerge from this surface, close to the anterior border.
- *Posteromedial surface*—It is related to mastoid process, sternomastoid, and the posterior belly of digastrics. Styloid process with stylohyoid, stylopharyngeus, and styloglossus muscle is attached to it. Facial nerve after emerging from stylomastoid foramen enters the gland on this surface. The internal jugular vein and internal carotid artery along with wall of pharynx lies deep to the styloid process (**Fig. 8.1c**).
- *Anterior border*—This border is related to branches of facial nerve, parotid duct, and transverse facial vessels (**Fig. 8.1a**).
- *Posterior border*—It is related to sternomastoid muscle.
- *Medial border*—It is related to lateral wall of pharynx (**Fig. 8.1c**).

Within the substance of the parotid gland lie the branches of facial nerve; tributaries and branches of retromandibular vein; external carotid artery and its terminal branches and auriculotemporal nerve. Facial nerve is most superficial, followed by retromandibular vein, and the external carotid artery is the deepest, within the substance of the gland. The plane of passage of branches of facial nerve artificially divides the gland into superficial and deep lobes joined by the isthmus in the middle.

Dissection and Identification

B. Dissection of facial nerve.

1. Identify the buccal branches of facial nerve which lie close to duct and follow it posteriorly into the substance of gland. Carefully remove the substance of gland in small pieces till this branch joins other branches of facial nerve and its trunk.

2. In the same way, clean the other branches of facial nerve, such as temporal, zygomatic, marginal mandibular and cervical, and find the trunk of the nerve. The branches of facial nerve on the face often join with each other to form parotid plexus of facial nerve. Trace the trunk of facial nerve posteriorly to stylomastoid foramen. At this level, try to find the posterior auricular branch, and branch to stylohyoid and posterior belly of digastric (**Fig. 8.4**).

3. Between the head of mandible and external acoustic meatus, find the auriculotemporal nerve, which lies within the substance of the parotid gland (refer to **Figs. 8.2, 8.4**, and **8.5**).

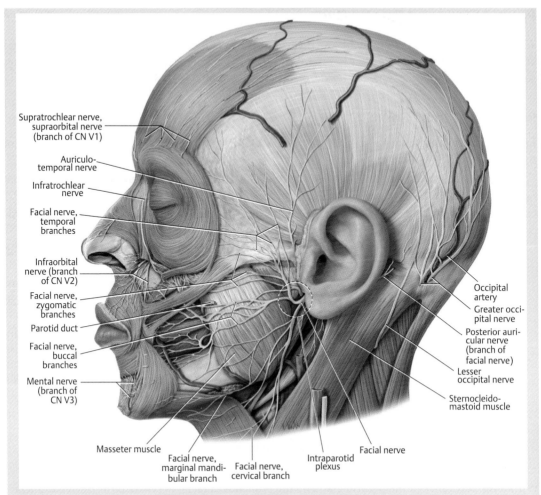

Fig. 8.4 Nerves of the parotid region. (From: Schuenke M, Schulte E, Schumacher U. THIEME Atlas of Anatomy. Head, Neck, and Neuroanatomy. Illustrations by Voll M and Wesker K. © Thieme 2020.)

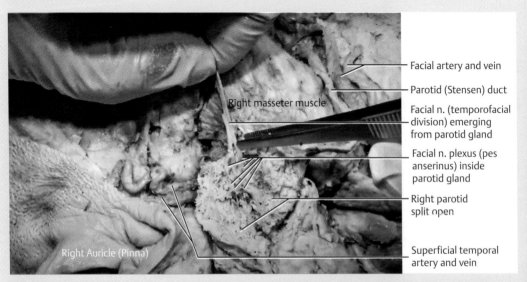

Fig. 8.5 Facial nerve in the parotid region.

Nerves of the Parotid Region

Facial nerve: The facial nerve emerges, at the base of the skull, through stylomastoid foramen. It then binds around the lateral aspect of the styloid process and internal jugular vein to enter the posteromedial surface of parotid gland. However, before entering the gland, facial nerve divides into two nerves, that is, posterior auricular nerve which innervates occipitofrontalis and auricular muscles and a nerve which innervates the posterior belly of digastric and the stylohyoid muscle. Within the parotid gland, it divides into five terminal branches (temporal, zygomatic, buccal, marginal mandibular, and cervical) which innervate the muscles of facial expressions. We have already studied and identified these branches in the superficial dissection of the face.

Auriculotemporal nerve: It is a branch of mandibular division of trigeminal nerve (CN V). It innervates the skin of the ear and temporal region. As it lies in the substance of gland, it delivers postganglionic parasympathetic (secretomotor) fibers to parotid gland, which it receives from the otic ganglion. This nerve also carries the sensation from parotid gland.

Great auricular nerve: It originates in the cervical plexus (C2 and C3) and one of its branches supplies the skin over the parotid region (near the angle of mandible) and the ear.

Dissection and Identification

C. Dissection of external carotid artery and its terminal branches and retromandibular vein.

1. Now from the upper part of the carotid triangle, with the help of the blunt dissection, follow the external carotid artery upward in the substance of parotid gland. The artery will lie close to posterior border of the ramus of mandible. Posterior to the neck of mandible, it will terminate by dividing into two branches, superficial temporal and maxillary. Follow the superficial temporal upward, but do not follow the maxillary artery as it will be dissected later (**Fig. 8.6**).

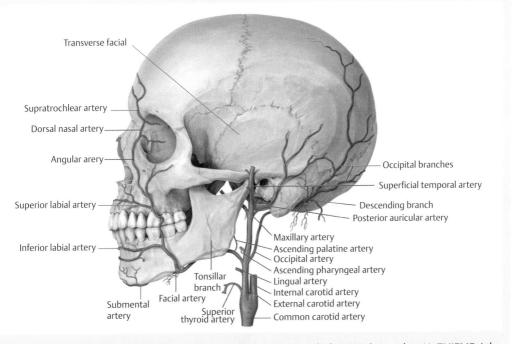

Fig. 8.6   Arteries of the parotid region. (From: Schuenke M, Schulte E, Schumacher U. THIEME Atlas of Anatomy. Head, Neck, and Neuroanatomy. Illustrations by Voll M and Wesker K. © Thieme 2020.)

2. Deep to these branches of facial nerve, remove the parotid gland piece by piece to dissect the retromandibular vein which lies deep into the branches of facial nerve. Follow the retromandibular vein upward where it is formed by joining the maxillary and superficial temporal vein (**Fig. 8.7**).

3. Remove the remaining part of the gland piece by piece and expose the attachment of sternomastoid, posterior belly of digastric on the mastoid process.

4. If possible, dissect deep to find the styloid process and stylomandibular ligament. This ligament separates the parotid and submandibular gland.

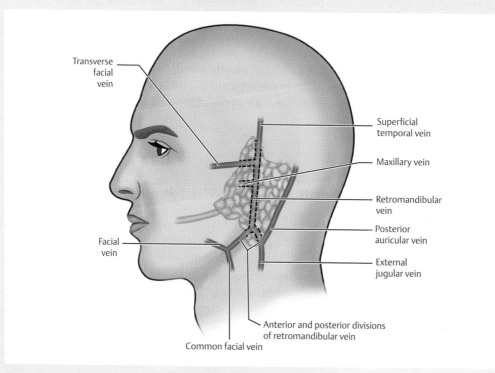

Fig. 8.7   Veins of the parotid region.

Arteries of the Parotid Region

Arteries of the parotid region are external carotid, superficial temporal, maxillary, and transverse facial arteries (**Fig. 8.6**).

Veins of the Parotid Region

Veins of the region are embedded within the substance of the gland and are as follows: superficial temporal, transverse facial, maxillary, retromandibular, and its anterior and posterior divisions (**Fig. 8.7**).

Muscles Related to the Parotid Region

Three muscles, that is, sternomastoid, posterior belly of digastric, and stylohyoid are in immediate relation to the parotid gland. We have already reviewed these muscles during the dissection of anterior triangle (refer to Chapter 7).

Parotid Lymph Nodes

The parotid region contains superficial and deep groups of parotid lymph nodes. These are embedded in the gland, especially near its superficial surface. From these groups, lymph is drained to deep cervical group of lymph nodes (**Fig. 8.8**).

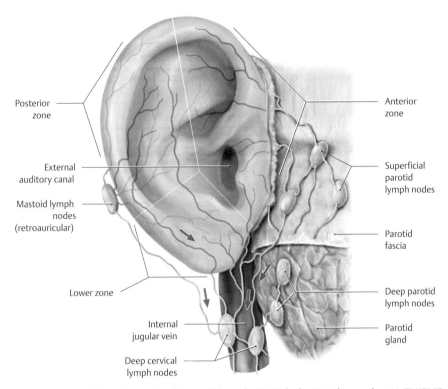

Fig. 8.8 Parotid lymph nodes. (From: Schuenke M, Schulte E, Schumacher U. THIEME Atlas of Anatomy. Head, Neck, and Neuroanatomy. Illustrations by Voll M and Wesker K. © Thieme 2020.)

▌ Clinical Notes

1. *Mumps or other infections of gland*: Mumps is a viral infection (called mumps virus) of parotid gland. As the parotid gland is enclosed by the tough inelastic investing layer of deep cervical fascia, the gland cannot enlarge during this or any other infection, leading to pressure on nerves. Therefore, mumps is a highly painful condition.

2. *Parotid tumors*: These are very common. Nonmalignant tumors usually occur in superficial lobe (part of gland superficial to facial nerve branches), while malignant tumors are common in the deep lobe of the gland. The plane of passage of branches of facial nerve helps the surgeon remove the superficial or deep lobes separately without causing damage to the facial nerve.

3. *Parotid abscess*: It is the collection of pus in parotid gland secondary to infection. To drain this pus, a surgeon will always make a transverse incision in the parotid fascia (parallel to the direction of facial nerve branches) to avoid injury to the branches.

Temporal and Infratemporal Regions

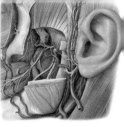

© THIEME Atlas of Anatomy

Introduction

The temporal and infratemporal regions are located on the lateral side of the head. Temporal fossa is an area between the temporal line and zygomatic arch. It contains the temporalis muscle, deep temporal vessels, and nerve. The infratemporal fossa is located below the zygomatic arch and deep to the ramus of the mandible. Within the infratemporal fossa, the medial and lateral pterygoid muscles, maxillary artery, and branches of the mandibular nerve are located. The temporal and infratemporal fossa are in open communication with each other through a gap between the zygomatic arch and lateral surface of the skull.

Infratemporal fossa communicates with the pterygopalatine fossa through the pterygomaxillary fissure. Terminal branches of the maxillary artery are given in this fossa.

Surface Landmarks

Students are suggested to proceed with the dissection of this region only after understanding the bony features of the infratemporal fossa.

1. Examine the lateral aspect of the skull articulated with the mandible (refer to **Fig. 1.4**). Look for the temporal lines, floor of the temporal fossa, and pterion.

2. Put your finger deep into the zygomatic arch; this space communicates between the temporal and infratemporal fossa.

3. Examine the boundaries of the infratemporal fossa. Its *anterior* boundary is formed by the posterior surface of the maxilla, *medial* by the lateral pterygoid plate, *lateral* by the ramus of the mandible, and *roof* by the greater wing of the sphenoid. The floor of the infratemporal fossa is open.

4. Now remove the mandible from the skull and examine the bony structure of the infratemporal fossa: lateral pterygoid plate and posterior surface of the maxilla bone. Look for the pterygomaxillary fissure which lies between the lateral plate of the pterygoid and maxilla. Further deep in this fissure lies a small pterygopalatine fossa.

5. In the anterior part of the infratemporal fossa, look for the inferior orbital fissure. Look at the roof of the fossa and identify two foramina, that is, the foramen ovale and foramen spinosum which are located in the greater wing of the sphenoid bone.

6. This is the time to review the disarticulated mandible. Identify the head, neck, coronoid process, ramus, and angle of the mandible with the help of **Fig. 1.10**. Also, look for the mandibular foramen on the internal surface of the ramus.

7. On your own body, palpate the zygomatic arch, angle, and posterior border of the ramus of the mandible. Palpate the temporalis and masseter muscles by clenching teeth.

Dissection and Identification

A. Dissection to expose the temporalis muscle (Video 9.1).

1. We have already dissected the superficial part of the temporal fossa (refer to **Chapter 2**).

2. Remove the temporal fascia from the superior temporal line to the zygomatic arch to expose the temporalis muscle. It will be difficult to reflect the fascia as the temporalis takes origin from its deep surface. Clean the fibers of the temporalis as they go deep into the zygomatic arch (**Fig. 9.1a**).

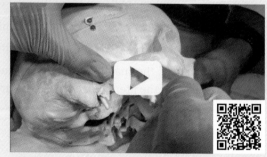

Video 9.1   Infratemporal fossa and pterygomaxillary fissure.

3. Now clean the lateral surface of the masseter muscle and cut the zygomatic arch with the help of a saw, anterior and posterior to the attachment of the masseter. Pull the masseter muscle and cut portion of the zygomatic arch downward toward the angle of the mandible (**Fig. 9.1b**). This will expose the lateral surface of the ramus of the mandible. Look for the masseteric nerve and vessels on the deep surface of the masseter.

4. Note the directions of the muscle fibers of the temporalis as they go toward its tendon. Note the attachment of the tendon of the temporalis on the coronoid process (refer to **Fig. 9.1b**). For seeing the structures of the infratemporal fossa, we shall have to remove the lateral wall (ramus) of the fossa. Pass a forceps or a probe forward and downward through the mandibular notch, deep to the attachment of the temporalis on the coronoid process. Give an oblique cut on the coronoid process, with the help of a saw, along the direction of the probe (**Fig. 9.2a**). Cut the temporalis in the temporal fossa above the zygomatic arch. Find the deep temporal vessels and nerves on the floor of the temporal fossa deep to the temporalis (**Fig. 9.2b**).

B. Dissection to expose the infratemporal fossa.

1. This is the time to remove the upper part of the ramus of the mandible to expose the deeper structures of the infratemporal fossa. Give a horizontal cut at the neck of the mandible (**2 in Fig. 9.2a**) and another cut almost at the middle of the ramus (**3 in Fig. 9.2a**). The level of the lower cut (**3 in Fig. 9.2a**) is determined by the presence of the mandibular foramen through which the inferior alveolar nerve and vessels enter the mandible. To preserve the nerves and vessels, pass a probe or forceps deep to the ramus of the mandible and press it downward till it is arrested by the inferior alveolar nerve and vessels. Give a horizontal cut on the ramus with the help of a saw, just at the level of the probe. Be careful to avoid injury to the underlying nerves and vessels. Remove this piece of bone to expose the infratemporal fossa.

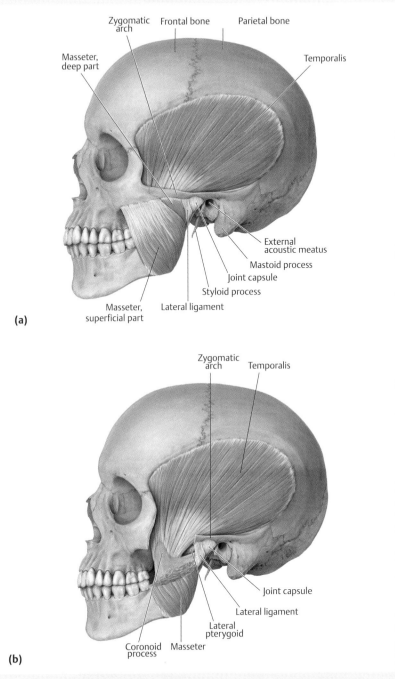

Zygomatic arch   Frontal bone   Parietal bone

Masseter, deep part   Temporalis

External acoustic meatus
Mastoid process
Joint capsule
Styloid process
Masseter, superficial part   Lateral ligament

(a)

Zygomatic arch   Temporalis

Joint capsule
Lateral ligament
Lateral pterygoid
Coronoid process   Masseter

(b)

Fig. 9.1 **(a)** Superficial dissection of the temporal fossa. **(b)** Zygomatic arch removed to show the insertion of the temporalis muscle. (From: Schuenke M, Schulte E, Schumacher U. THIEME Atlas of Anatomy. Head, Neck, and Neuroanatomy. Illustrations by Voll M and Wesker K. © Thieme 2020.)

2. Clean the fat and connective tissues to clear the underlying muscle, nerves, and vessels. You will have to remove the pterygoid plexus of veins along with the fibrofatty tissue to clean the structures of the fossa.

3. Identify the inferior alveolar nerve and vessels as they enter the mandibular foramen. Also, identify the lingual nerve lying anterior to the inferior alveolar nerve.

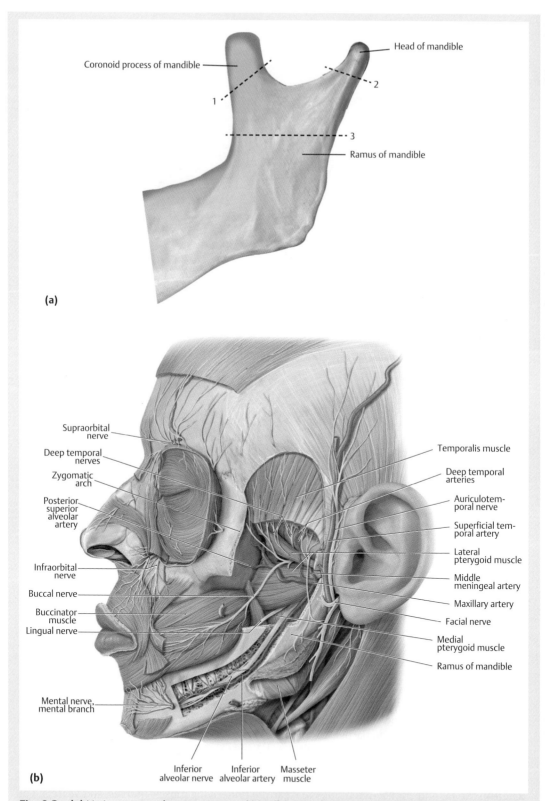

Fig. 9.2 **(a)** Various cuts to be given in mandible. **(b)** Superficial dissection of the infratemporal fossa to expose the lateral pterygoid muscle and related nerve and vessels. (Figure b: From: Schuenke M, Schulte E, Schumacher U. THIEME Atlas of Anatomy. Head, Neck, and Neuroanatomy. Illustrations by Voll M and Wesker K. © Thieme 2020.)

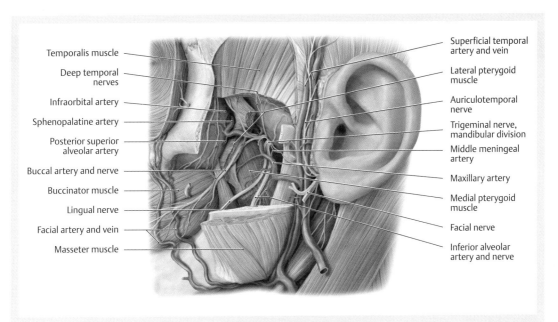

Temporalis muscle

Deep temporal nerves

Infraorbital artery

Sphenopalatine artery

Posterior superior alveolar artery

Buccal artery and nerve

Buccinator muscle

Lingual nerve

Facial artery and vein

Masseter muscle

Superficial temporal artery and vein

Lateral pterygoid muscle

Auriculotemporal nerve

Trigeminal nerve, mandibular division

Middle meningeal artery

Maxillary artery

Medial pterygoid muscle

Facial nerve

Inferior alveolar artery and nerve

Fig. 9.3 Deep dissection of the infratemporal fossa (lateral pterygoid removed) to show the maxillary artery, its branches, and related nerves. (From: Schuenke M, Schulte E, Schumacher U. THIEME Atlas of Anatomy. Head, Neck, and Neuroanatomy. Illustrations by Voll M and Wesker K. © Thieme 2020.)

4. Clean and identify the lateral and medial pterygoid muscles, maxillary artery, and its branches (**Fig. 9.2b**).

5. Follow the maxillary artery toward the pterygopalatine fossa. Here, the artery gives postero-superior alveolar and infraorbital branches before entering the pterygopalatine fossa (refer to **Fig. 9.3**). After entering the pterygopalatine fossa, it divides into terminal branches, that is, the greater palatine and sphenopalatine artery (**Figs. 9.2** and **9.3**).

Muscles Related to the Temporal and Infratemporal Regions

Muscles present in the temporal and infratemporal regions are responsible for movements of the lower jaw at the temporomandibular joint. Therefore, these muscles are also known as *muscles of mastication*. These are the *temporalis*, *masseter* (refer to **Fig. 9.1a, b**), *lateral pterygoid*, and *medial pterygoid* (refer to **Figs. 9.2–9.4**; **Table 9.1**; **Videos 9.2 and 9.3**).

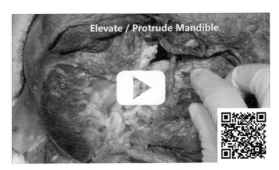

Video 9.2 Infratemporal fossa: Part I

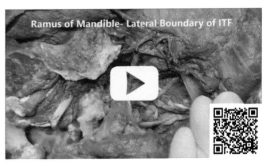

Video 9.3 Infratemporal fossa: Part II

Table 9.1   Muscles of mastication

Muscle	Origin	Insertion	Nerve supply	Action
Temporalis	From the whole of the temporal fossa and undersurface of the temporal fascia	Medial surface and anterior border of the coronoid process	Deep temporal nerves	Anterior fibers elevate the jaw (closure of the mouth); posterior fibers retract the jaw
Masseter	Anterior two-thirds of the zygomatic arch and medial surface of the arch	Outer surface of the ramus and angle of the mandible	Masseteric nerve	Elevation (closure of the mouth) and protraction of the mandible
Lateral pterygoid	Upper head from the infratemporal crest and undersurface of the greater wing of the sphenoid. Lower head from lateral pterygoid plate (lateral surface)	Pterygoid fovea and articular capsule and disc of the temporomandibular joint	A branch from the anterior division of the mandibular nerve	Draw the head of the mandible and disc forward on the articular tubercle (protrudes the mandible and depresses the chin, i.e., opening of the mouth) When a single muscle is acting, the head of the mandible on that side is drawn forward and the chin is tilted to the opposite side
Medial pterygoid	Superficial head is small and arises from the maxillary tuberosity Deep head arises from the medial surface of the lateral pterygoid plate	Medial aspect of the ramus of the mandible below the mandibular foramen	From the trunk of the mandibular nerve	It elevates the mandible and helps in protraction (closure of the mouth)

Dissection and Identification

C. Deep dissection of infratemporal fossa.

1. To see the deeper part of the infratemporal fossa, we shall remove the lateral pterygoid muscle in small pieces. After giving a cut at its insertion in the neck of the mandible and articular disc, rest of the muscle should be removed in piecemeal (**Figs. 9.3** and **9.4**).

2. Follow the inferior alveolar and lingual nerve upward toward the foramen ovale (**Fig. 9.3**). Look for the union of the chorda tympani and lingual nerve below the roof of the infratemporal fossa. Look for various branches arising from the anterior and posterior divisions of the mandibular nerve (**Fig. 9.5**).

3. See the middle meningeal artery entering the foramen spinosum. Deep into the artery lies the tensor palati muscle.

4. Now lift the trunk of the mandibular nerve laterally to search for the otic ganglion just below the foramen ovale (**Fig. 9.6**).

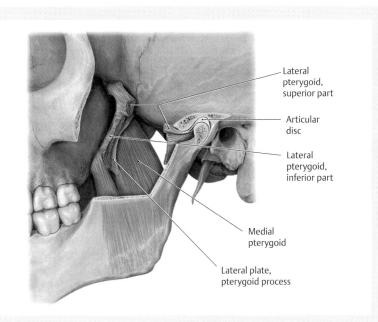

Fig. 9.4 Exposure of the medial pterygoid muscle and temporomandibular joint. (From: Schuenke M, Schulte E, Schumacher U. THIEME Atlas of Anatomy. Head, Neck, and Neuroanatomy. Illustrations by Voll M and Wesker K. © Thieme 2020.)

Labels in Fig. 9.4:
- Lateral pterygoid, superior part
- Articular disc
- Lateral pterygoid, inferior part
- Medial pterygoid
- Lateral plate, pterygoid process

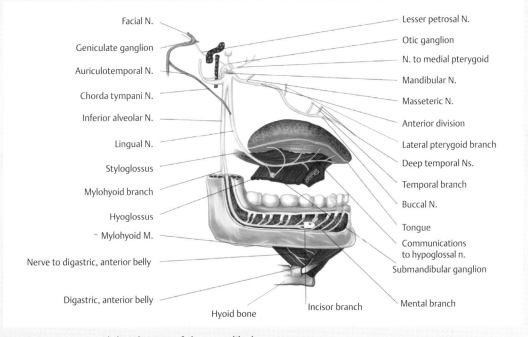

Labels in Fig. 9.5:
- Facial N.
- Geniculate ganglion
- Auriculotemporal N.
- Chorda tympani N.
- Inferior alveolar N.
- Lingual N.
- Styloglossus
- Mylohyoid branch
- Hyoglossus
- Mylohyoid M.
- Nerve to digastric, anterior belly
- Digastric, anterior belly
- Hyoid bone
- Incisor branch
- Lesser petrosal N.
- Otic ganglion
- N. to medial pterygoid
- Mandibular N.
- Masseteric N.
- Anterior division
- Lateral pterygoid branch
- Deep temporal Ns.
- Temporal branch
- Buccal N.
- Tongue
- Communications to hypoglossal n.
- Submandibular ganglion
- Mental branch

Fig. 9.5 Course and distribution of the mandibular nerve.

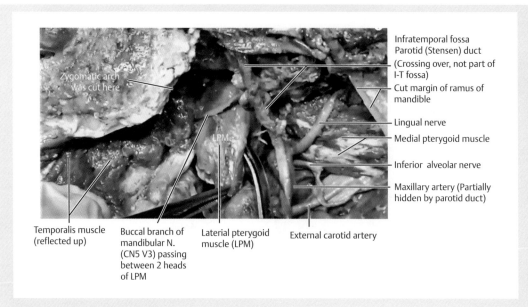

Fig. 9.6   Lateral pterygoid muscle and its relations.

Important Nerves of the Region

The temporal and infratemporal fossa contains the mandibular nerve, chorda tympani nerve, and otic ganglion.

1. The *mandibular nerve* is a division of the trigeminal (fifth cranial) nerve. It is a mixed (motor and sensory) nerve. It has a short trunk which after coming out of the foramen ovale divides into anterior and posterior divisions (**Fig. 9.5** and **Table 9.2**). The mandibular nerve and its branches are given in **Table 9.2**.

Table 9.2   Mandibular nerve and its branches

Trunk/Division	Branches	Motor supply to	Sensory supply to
Trunk	Meningeal branch	——	Dura mater of the middle cranial fossa
	Branch to the medial pterygoid muscle	Medial pterygoid, tensor palatine, and tensor tympani	——
Anterior division	Buccal nerve	——	Skin and mucous membrane of the cheek
	Nerve to the lateral pterygoid	Lateral pterygoid muscle	——
	Deep temporal nerves	Temporalis muscle	——
	Nerve to the masseter	Masseter muscle	——
Posterior division	Auriculotemporal nerve	Carries the secretomotor fibers from the otic ganglion to the parotid gland	Skin of the temple, ear, and temporomandibular joint
	Inferior alveolar	Nerve to the mylohyoid and anterior belly of the digastric	To the teeth of the lower jaw and skin and mucous membrane over the mandible
	Lingual nerve	Carries the secretomotor fibers for the chorda tympani	General sensation from the anterior two-thirds of the tongue Sense of taste for the chorda tympani

2. The *chorda tympani nerve* is a branch of the facial nerve which joins the lingual nerve about 2 cm below the base of the skull (**Fig. 9.5**). It contains the secretomotor fibers to the submandibular and sublingual salivary glands. It also carries the taste fibers from the anterior two-thirds of the tongue.

3. *Otic ganglion* is a small parasympathetic ganglion for relay of the secretomotor fibers to the parotid gland (**Fig. 9.5**). It is located below the foramen ovale deep into the trunk of the mandibular nerve but superficial to the tensor palati muscle.

Arteries of the Region

The artery of the infratemporal fossa is the maxillary artery, which is one of the terminal branches of the external carotid artery. It begins posteromedial to the neck of the mandible. The artery is divided into three parts for descriptive purposes (refer to **Figs. 9.2 and 9.3**; **Table 9.3**):

1. The *first part* of the artery lies below the lower border of the lateral pterygoid muscle.

2. The *second part* lies on the superficial surface of the lateral pterygoid muscle.

Table 9.3   Branches of the maxillary artery

Parts of the maxillary artery	Branches	Passes through	Distribution
First part	Anterior tympanic	Petrotympanic fissure	Middle ear and inner aspect of the tympanic membrane
	Deep auricular	Cartilage of the auricle	Temporomandibular joint, external auditory meatus, and external surface of the tympanic membrane
	Middle meningeal	Foramen spinosum	Dura mater
	Accessory meningeal	Foramen ovale	Dura mater, trigeminal ganglion, and mandibular nerve
	Inferior alveolar	Mandibular canal	Mandible, teeth of the lower jaw, skin of the chin, and mucous membrane
	Deep temporal	Ascends deep to the temporalis muscle	To the temporalis muscle
Second part	Artery to the masseter	Passes above the mandibular notch	To the masseter muscle
	Pterygoid arteries		To the pterygoid muscles
	Buccal artery		Skin and mucosa of the cheek
Third part	Posterosuperior alveolar (**Fig. 9.3**)	Enters the posterior surface of the maxilla	Supply the upper molar and premolar teeth
	Infraorbital	Infraorbital fissure and then the infraorbital foramen	Orbit and skin of the face
	Greater palatine	Greater palatine canal	Hard palate, floor of the nasal cavity, tonsil, and soft palate
	Artery of the pterygoid canal	Pterygoid canal	Pharynx, pharyngotympanic tube, and tympanic cavity
	Sphenopalatine	Sphenopalatine foramen	Mucosa of the nasal cavity
	Pharyngeal branch	Palatinovaginal canal	Roof of the nasopharynx, auditory tube, and sphenoidal air sinus

3. The *third part* enters the pterygomaxillary fissure to give terminal branches in the pterygopalatine fossa.

Veins of the Region

Veins of the infratemporal fossa form a venous plexus around the lateral pterygoid muscle. Veins of the pterygoid plexus are derived from the corresponding branches of the maxillary artery. The venous plexus forms one or two short maxillary veins which pass to the parotid gland and drain into the retromandibular vein (**Fig. 9.7**).

Communications of the pterygoid venous plexus are:

1. Cavernous sinus via emissary veins passing through the foramen lacerum and ovale.

2. Ophthalmic veins passing through the inferior orbital fissure.

3. Facial vein passing through the deep facial vein.

4. Plexus drains to the maxillary vein.

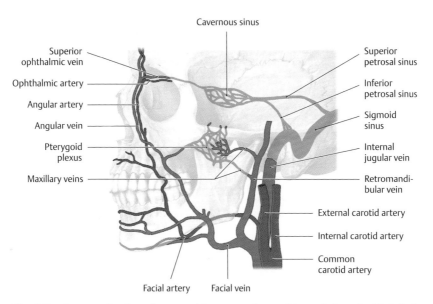

Fig. 9.7   Communication of pterygoid venous plexus. (From: Schuenke M, Schulte E, Schumacher U. THIEME Atlas of Anatomy. Head, Neck, and Neuroanatomy. Illustrations by Voll M and Wesker K. © Thieme 2020.)

▌Clinical Notes

1. *Anesthetic block of the inferior alveolar nerve*: It is performed by inserting a needle lateral to the pterygomandibular raphe. The needle is carried further backward till the middle of the medial aspect of the ramus. The anesthetic is injected into the area of the mandibular foramen. This will anesthetize all the teeth of the lower jaw, lower lip, and skin of the chin.

2. *Referred pain in the ear*: The skin of a portion of the ear is supplied by a branch of the mandibular nerve, which also supplies the teeth of the lower jaw. Hence, the pain of the infection of the lower tooth may be referred to the ear.

10 Temporomandibular Joint

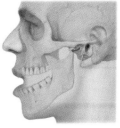

© THIEME Atlas of Anatomy

At the end of the dissection of the temporomandibular (TM) joint, you should be able to identify the following:

- *Ligaments*: Capsular ligament, lateral ligament of the TM joint, and sphenomandibular and stylomandibular ligaments.
- *Articular surfaces*: Articular surface of the head of the mandible and mandibular fossa covered by the fibrocartilage.
- *Articular disc*: Articular disc of the TM joint. Attachment of the tendon of the lateral pterygoid muscle to the articular disc and capsule of the TM joint.

Introduction

The TM joint is present in the infratemporal fossa. It is a synovial type of joint between the head of the mandible below and mandibular fossa and articular tubercle of the temporal bone above. The joint cavity is divided by an articular fibrocartilaginous disc into two compartments, upper and lower. The joint is supported by only one true ligament, that is, the TM ligament or lateral ligament of the TM joint. It has two accessory ligaments (the sphenomandibular and stylomandibular) which are away from the joint. The fibrous capsule of the joint is attached close to the articular margins on both the articulating bones. The articular disc is concavoconvex on its superior surface but concave on its lower surface. The disc around its periphery is attached to the inside of the fibrous capsule. Various kinds of masticatory movements of the lower jaw are possible at the TM joint.

Surface Landmarks

Before marking the surface landmarks, students are advised to look for the following bony features on the skull:

1. On the external surface of the base of the skull, look for the root of the zygoma, articular tubercle, and mandibular fossa in the squamous temporal bone (**Fig. 10.1**).

2. Note the tympanic plate forming the posterior nonarticular part of the mandibular fossa.

3. Also, look for the spine of the sphenoid and styloid process.

4. In a disarticulate mandible, see the shape of the head of the mandible (**Fig. 10.2**).

5. *Head of the mandible:* On your own body, palpate the head of the mandible and its movements during slight opening and closing of the mouth or during the chewing movements.

6. *Mandibular fossa:* Put the tip of your finger behind the head of the mandible and now open your mouth widely, your finger will go in a depression in front of the tragus of the ear. Your finger is now in the mandibular fossa as the mandible has vacated the mandibular fossa and moved forward under the articular tubercle.

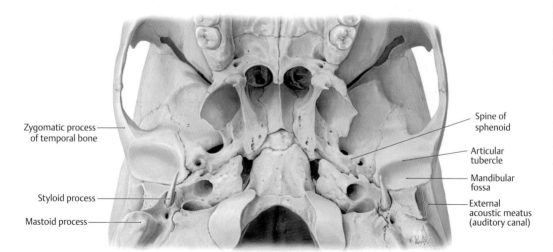

Fig. 10.1 Mandibular fossa and articular tubercle provide the articular area of the temporomandibular (TM) joint. (From: Schuenke M, Schulte E, Schumacher U. THIEME Atlas of Anatomy. Head, Neck, and Neuroanatomy. Illustrations by Voll M and Wesker K. © Thieme 2020.)

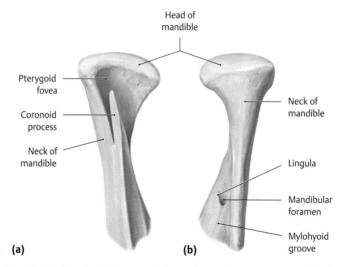

Fig. 10.2 Head of the mandible in the right temporomandibular (TM) joint. **(a)** Anterior aspect and **(b)** posterior aspect. (From: Schuenke M, Schulte E, Schumacher U. THIEME Atlas of Anatomy. Head, Neck, and Neuroanatomy. Illustrations by Voll M and Wesker K. © Thieme 2020.)

Dissection and Identification

A. Dissection of joint cavity and exposure of articular disc

1. During the dissection of the infratemporal fossa, we had given a cut at the level of the neck of the mandible. Thus, at present, we only have the head of the mandible and stump of the neck.

2. Clean and identify the lateral ligament of the TM joint. Identify and observe the joint capsule posterior and deep to the lateral ligament.

3. With the help of a scalpel, remove the lateral ligament. Give a vertical cut passing through the joint from above downward (**Fig. 10.3**). This cut will pass through the articular disc and will expose the upper and lower compartments of the joint above and below the disc, respectively.

4. See the concavoconvex upper surface and concave lower surface of the disc (**Fig. 10.3**).

5. Observe the head of the mandible in the lower compartment, below the disc.

6. Also, see the fibers of the tendon of the lateral pterygoid, gaining attachment on the anterior margin of the disc (**Figs. 10.3 and 10.4b, c**).

7. Now trace the middle meningeal artery up to the foramen spinosum and auriculotemporal nerve which is in relation to the medial and posterior surface of the joint capsule.

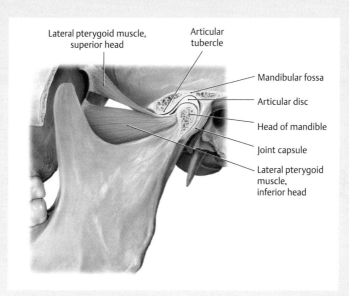

Fig. 10.3 Interior of the temporomandibular (TM) joint. (From: Schuenke M, Schulte E, Schumacher U. THIEME Atlas of Anatomy. Head, Neck, and Neuroanatomy. Illustrations by Voll M and Wesker K. © Thieme 2020.)

Description of the Joint

The bones taking part in the formation of the TM joint are the head of the mandible below and mandibular fossa and articular tubercle of the temporal bone above. The head of the mandible fits in the mandibular fossa. The articulating surfaces of both these bones are covered by the fibrocartilage.

The *fibrous capsule* of the joint is attached above to the margin of the articular area (mandibular fossa and articular tubercle) and below to the neck of the mandible. The *lateral ligament* is attached above to the zygomatic process at the root of the zygoma and below to the lateral aspect of the neck of the mandible (**Fig. 10.5**).

The intra-articular disc is an oval fibrocartilaginous disc, which is concavoconvex at its upper surface and concave at its lower surface. It divides the cavity of the joint into upper and lower compartments. The anterior margin of the disc and adjoining capsule gives attachment to the fibers of the lateral pterygoid (**Figs. 10.3 and 10.4c**).

The main stability of the joint is provided by the muscles as the joint is protected by only one true ligament. The other two ligaments are accessory (sphenomandibular and stylomandibular) and are placed away from the joint (**Fig. 10.6**).

Small branches from the superficial temporal artery and maxillary artery supply blood to the joint. Auriculotemporal, deep temporal, and masseteric nerves supply the joint capsule.

Movements of the Joint

Following movements of the lower jaw occur at the TM joint (**Fig. 10.4**):

1. Protraction and retraction.

2. Depression and elevation.

3. Movements of chewing (grinding).

Protraction (protrusion or forward movement of the jaw): In this movement, the articular disc and head of the mandible both glide forward in the upper compartment of the joint. Muscles producing this movement are lateral and medial pterygoids (**Fig. 10.4a**).

Retraction (retrusion or backward movement): It is the opposite of protraction. In this movement, the head of the mandible along with the articular disc glides back to the original position. The muscle responsible for retraction is the posterior fibers of the temporalis (**Fig. 10.4a**).

Depression (opening of the mouth): In slight opening of the mouth, the head of the mandible rotates forward in the lower compartment (below articular disc) (**Fig. 10.4b**). In wide opening of the mouth, the above hinge-like movement is followed by the forward gliding of the disc and head of the mandible in the upper compartment of the joint (above the articular disc). At the end of this movement, the head comes to lie under the articular tubercle (**Fig. 10.4c**). The muscle responsible is the lateral pterygoid assisted by gravity. In wide opening (or opening against resistance), the main muscle responsible is the lateral pterygoid assisted by the anterior belly of the digastric, mylohyoid, and geniohyoid.

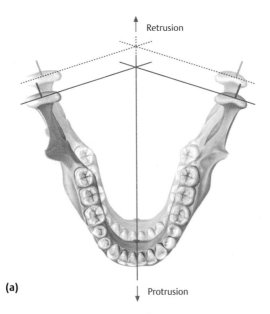

(a)

Fig. 10.4   (a) Protrusion and retrusion movements of the mandible occur at upper compartments of the right and left temporomandibular (TM) joints.

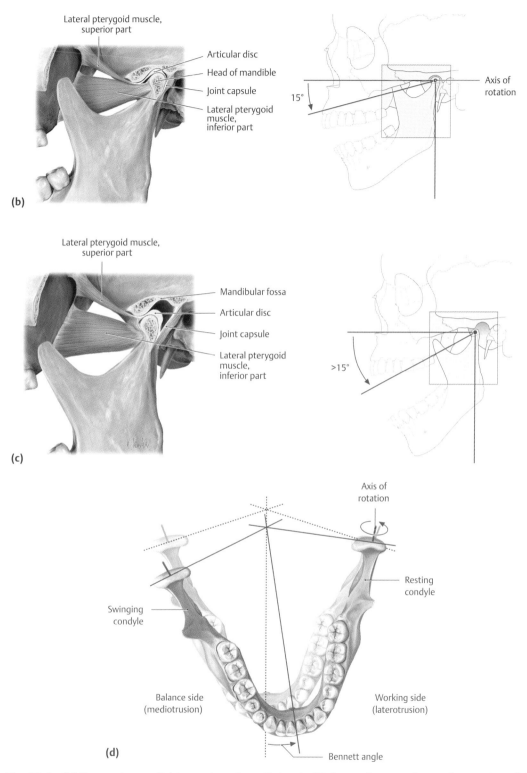

(b)

(c)

(d)

Fig. 10.4 **(b)** Depression or slight opening of mouth (up to 15 degrees) occurs due to the rotation of the head of mandible in the lower compartment of the TM joint. **(c)** In wide opening of the mouth, the above movement is followed by forward gliding of head and disc in the upper compartment. Now the head lies below the articular tubercle. **(d)** In chewing or side-to-side movements of the mandible, forward movement (protrusion) occurs on one side, while rotation of the head of mandible occurs in opposite TM joint. The same movement is now repeated in the TM joint of other side. (From: Schuenke M, Schulte E, Schumacher U. THIEME Atlas of Anatomy. Head, Neck, and Neuroanatomy. Illustrations by Voll M and Wesker K. © Thieme 2020.)

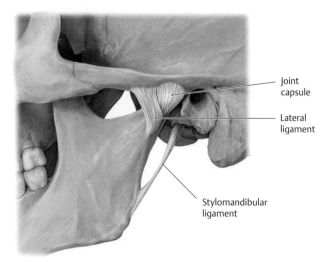

Fig. 10.5 Ligaments of the left temporomandibular (TM) joint. (From: Schuenke M, Schulte E, Schumacher U. THIEME Atlas of Anatomy. Head, Neck, and Neuroanatomy. Illustrations by Voll M and Wesker K. © Thieme 2020.)

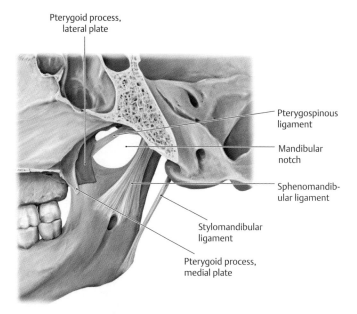

Fig. 10.6 Accessory ligaments of the temporomandibular (TM) joint (as seen on the medial aspect of the ramus of mandible). (From: Schuenke M, Schulte E, Schumacher U. THIEME Atlas of Anatomy. Head, Neck, and Neuroanatomy. Illustrations by Voll M and Wesker K. © Thieme 2020.)

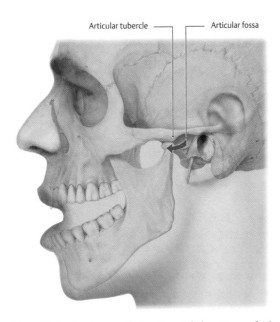

Articular tubercle ——   —— Articular fossa

Fig. 10.7 Locking of the jaw (dislocation of the temporomandibular [TM] joint). (From: Gilroy AM, MacPherson BR, Ross LM. Atlas of Anatomy. Second Edition. Illustrations by Markus Voll and Karl Wesker. © Thieme 2012.)

Elevation (closure of the mouth): This movement is just the reverse of depression. It is produced by backward gliding of the disc and head of the mandible in the upper compartment of the joint. Then it is followed by the backward rotation of the head of the mandible on the undersurface of the disc (in the lower compartment). Elevation is produced by the masseter, superior and anterior fibers of the temporalis, and medial pterygoid.

Chewing movements (side to side movements): The movements of chewing are produced by the medial and lateral pterygoid muscles of each side acting alternatively (**Fig. 10.4d**).

Thus, in summary, we may say that two types of movements occur in the TM joint. The gliding movements occur in the upper compartment between the articular disc and mandibular fossa producing protraction and retraction movements. While in the lower compartment, hinge-like movements occur between the head of the mandible and undersurface of the articular disc, producing elevation and depression.

■ Clinical Notes

Anterior dislocation of mandible (Locking of the jaw): In case of wide opening of the mouth (as in the case of taking a big bite of an apple), the head of the mandible may slip forward, anterior to the articular tubercle, in the infratemporal fossa. This is followed by spasm of muscles, such as the masseter and medial pterygoid. In this position, the jaw remains locked in an open position and the patient cannot close his/her mouth (**Fig. 10.7**). This dislocation can be reduced by applying downward pressure on the mandibular molars and the upward and backward pressure on the chin helps the head of the mandible to come to the original position, that is, the mandibular fossa.

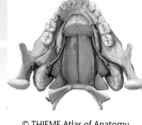

© THIEME Atlas of Anatomy

Introduction

The submandibular region lies between the body of the mandible and hyoid bone and encloses the submental and digastric triangles (**Fig. 11.1**). This region contains the submandibular and sublingual salivary glands, suprahyoid group of muscles, root of the tongue, and floor of the mouth.

This region also contains nerves which innervate the tongue (glossopharyngeal, lingual, and hypoglossal). The submandibular parasympathetic ganglion is related to the lingual nerve in this region. Important vessels of the region are lingual artery and lingual vein. The lymph nodes of this region form a group, that is, the submandibular group of lymph nodes.

Surface Landmarks

Before marking the surface landmarks, students are advised to look for the following bony features:

1. See the medial surface of the body of the mandible and look for the submandibular fossa, mylohyoid line, and mylohyoid groove (refer to **Fig. 1.10**).
2. See the upper and lower genial tubercles near the symphysis menti.
3. Also, review the body and lesser and greater cornu of the hyoid bone (refer to **Fig. 1.11**).
4. On your own body, try to palpate the submandibular salivary gland and submandibular lymph nodes at the lower border of the body of the mandible.
5. Try to grasp the greater cornu of the hyoid bone, between the thumb and finger.

Dissection and Identification

A. Deep dissection of submandibular region

1. We have already dissected two triangles (submental and digastric) in the superficial part of the submandibular region (**Fig. 11.1**). We shall now dissect the deeper part of this region.

2. Detach the anterior belly of the digastric muscle from its attachment on the mandible and turn it downward.

3. Follow and clean the posterior belly of digastric toward its attachment on the mastoid notch. Similarly, clean and follow the stylohyoid muscle to the styloid process (**Fig. 11.2**).

4. Follow the facial artery and facial vein, from the lower border of the mandible, backward toward the posterior end of the submandibular gland.

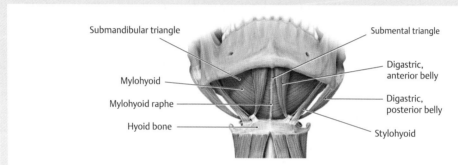

Fig. 11.1   Boundaries of submental and digastric triangles. (From: Schuenke M, Schulte E, Schumacher U. THIEME Atlas of Anatomy. Head, Neck, and Neuroanatomy. Illustrations by Voll M and Wesker K. © Thieme 2020.)

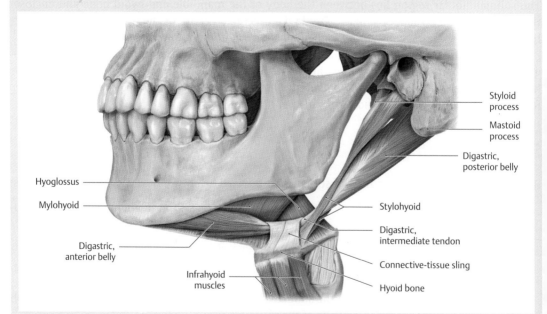

Fig. 11.2   Muscles of the submandibular region (left lateral view). (From: Schuenke M, Schulte E, Schumacher U. THIEME Atlas of Anatomy. Head, Neck, and Neuroanatomy. Illustrations by Voll M and Wesker K. © Thieme 2020.)

5. With the help of a saw, give a median cut in the symphysis menti of the mandible. Be careful not to go deeper than the bone. We had already given a cut in the ramus of the mandible during the dissection of the infratemporal fossa. Now you can easily turn the lower border of the mandible laterally and upward. This will expose the area of the submandibular region for easy dissection.

B. Exposure of submandibular gland

1. Clean the surfaces of the submandibular gland and observe the submandibular group of lymph nodes.

2. Expose the relation of the facial artery with the submandibular gland. Note its submental and glandular branches.

3. Expose and note the deeper part of the gland and continuation of the deeper and superficial parts of the gland around the posterior border of the mylohyoid muscle. Note various surfaces of the superficial part of the gland and their relations.

C. Exposure of mylohyoid muscle

1. Pull the submandibular gland and submental vessels posteriorly to expose the mylohyoid muscle completely. If the mylohyoid muscle is not seen properly, due to the presence of the superficial part of the gland, cut the gland at the junction of the superficial and deep part, near the posterior margin of the mylohyoid. Remove the superficial part of the gland. This will expose the mylohyoid completely. Note the part of the hyoglossus muscle, which lies above the mylohyoid and at its posterior border.

D. Exposure of hyoglossus muscle and its superficial relations

1. Give a cut in the mylohyoid muscle near its origin from the mylohyoid line and also near the midline. Reflect the muscle medially and backward toward the hyoid bone. This will expose the hyoglossus muscle completely.

2. Clean and identify the following structures after removal of the mylohyoid muscle, that is, the hyoglossus, hypoglossal nerve, deep part of the submandibular gland and duct, and lingual nerve and submandibular ganglion. All these structures are superficial to the hyoglossus muscle (**Figs. 11.3** and **11.4**).

3. Clean the structures present anterior to the anterior border of the hyoglossus muscle. These are the sublingual gland (which lies just deep to the mucous membrane of the floor of the mouth), genioglossus, geniohyoid muscles, and lingual artery (which, at the anterior margin of the hyoglossus, is dividing into the sublingual and deep lingual arteries) (refer to **Fig. 11.3**).

E. Dissection of muscles and ligament attached to Styloid process, Genioglossus, Lingual vessels and Glossopharyngeal nerve

1. Trace the hyoglossus muscle toward the tongue where its fibers intermingle with the styloglossus. Follow the styloglossus backward toward the styloid process. Identify the stylohyoid ligament and stylopharyngeus muscle attached to the styloid process. Trace the ligament toward the lesser cornu of the hyoid bone deep to the hyoglossus. Similarly, trace the stylopharyngeus downward and find the glossopharyngeal nerve winding around its lateral

surface before going deep to the hyoglossus. See the upper border of the middle constrictor muscle above the tip of the greater cornu.

2. Now detach the hyoglossus muscle at its origin from the greater cornu and body of the hyoid bone. Reflect it upward and clean the lingual artery and its branches, lingual vein, and posterior part of the genioglossus (**Fig. 11.4**).

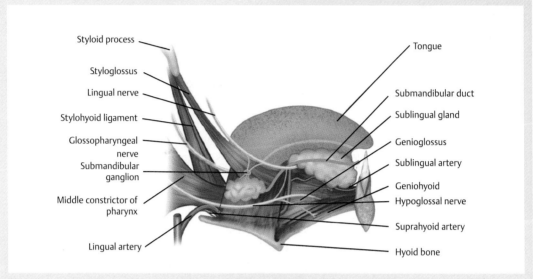

Fig. 11.3   Dissection of submandibular region (structures lying deep to mylohyoid muscle).

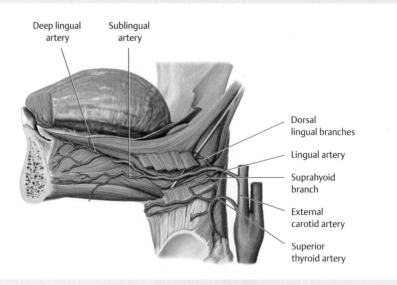

Fig. 11.4   Lingual artery and its branches as seen deep to hyoglossus muscle (left lateral view). (From: Schuenke M, Schulte E, Schumacher U. THIEME Atlas of Anatomy. Head, Neck, and Neuroanatomy. Illustrations by Voll M and Wesker K. © Thieme 2020.)

Muscles of the Submandibular Region (Video 11.1)

We have already learnt about the digastric bellies and mylohyoid and stylohyoid muscles of the submandibular region in Chapter 7 (Anterior Triangle of the Neck). Here, we shall learn about the remaining deep muscles of the submandibular region, that is, the hyoglossus, styloglossus, geniohyoid, and genioglossus muscles (**Fig. 11.5a, b** and **Table 11.1**).

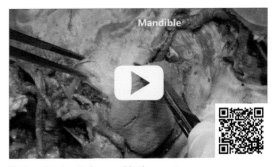

Video 11.1   Submandibular region.

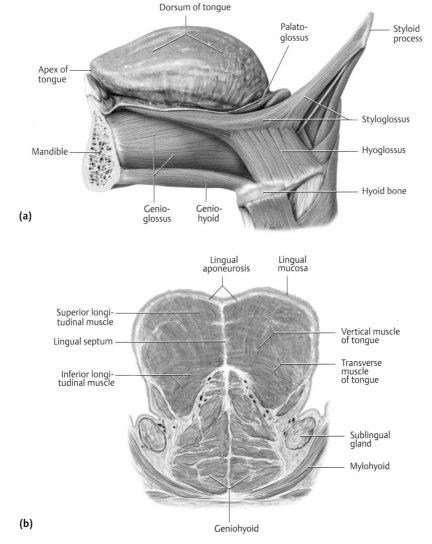

(a)

(b)

Fig. 11.5   (a) Extrinsic muscles of the tongue (left lateral view). **(b)** Intrinsic muscles of the tongue (view in a coronal section). (From: Schuenke M, Schulte E, Schumacher U. THIEME Atlas of Anatomy. Head, Neck, and Neuroanatomy. Illustrations by Voll M and Wesker K. © Thieme 2020.)

Table 11.1   Deep muscles of the submandibular region

Muscle	Origin	Insertion	Nerve supply	Action
Hyoglossus	It arises from the greater cornu and body of the hyoid bone	In the posterior half of side of the tongue	Hypoglossal nerve	It depresses the side of the tongue
Styloglossus	It arises from the tip of the styloid process and adjacent part of the stylohyoid ligament	On the side of the tongue	Hypoglossal nerve	Pulls the tongue posterosuperiorly
Geniohyoid	It arises from the inferior genial tubercle and the posterior aspect of the symphysis menti	On the anterior aspect of the body of the hyoid bone	By C1 fibers traveling through the hypoglossal nerve	Draws the hyoid bone upward and forward and depresses the mandible
Genioglossus	It arises from the upper genial tubercle and the posterior aspect of the symphysis menti	It is inserted on the dorsal aspect of the tongue from the tip to the hyoid bone, close to the median plane	Hypoglossal nerve	Posterior part protrudes the tongue, middle part depresses the central part of the tongue, and anterior fibers retract the tip of the tongue

Important Nerves of the Region

Important nerves of the region (refer to **Fig. 11.3**) include the following:

1. *Glossopharyngeal (ninth cranial) nerve*: It appears in the submandibular region after winding around the stylopharyngeus muscle. It runs forward and lies deep to the stylohyoid ligament and hyoglossus muscle. It terminates by dividing into branches to the tongue. It supplies the posterior one-third of the tongue and carries general sensations and a sense of taste.

2. *Lingual (branch of the mandibular, fifth cranial) nerve*: In the submandibular region, the lingual nerve first lies between the mucous membrane of the mouth and the body of the mandible, posteroinferior to the third molar. Then, it winds around the styloglossus and lies on the upper part of the hyoglossus. Here, it hooks beneath the submandibular duct. The submandibular ganglion is suspended from the lingual nerve by two short branches. From a textbook, read about the details of the submandibular ganglion.

   The lingual nerve supplies the mucous membrane over the anterior two-thirds of the tongue. It carries both general sensations and sensation of taste.

3. *Hypoglossal (twelfth cranial) nerve*: In this region, the nerve lies between the mylohyoid and hyoglossus. On the hyoglossus, it lies between the hyoid bone and submandibular duct. At the anterior margin of the hyoglossus, it pierces the genioglossus muscle and breaks into many branches to supply the extrinsic and intrinsic muscles of the tongue **(Fig. 11.3)**.

Arteries of the Region

Two important arteries, that is, the facial and lingual arteries are present in the submandibular region.

1. *Facial artery*: The facial artery is the branch of the external carotid artery. It arises at the level of the tip of the greater cornu of the hyoid bone. First, it runs upward on the middle and superior

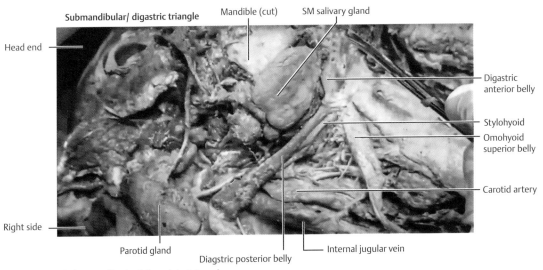

Fig. 11.6   Submandibular/digastric triangle.

constrictors lying deep to the posterior belly of the digastric and stylohyoid muscles. Then, it makes an s-shaped band (**refer to Fig. 8.6**). The first bend (convex upward) lies at the posterior end of the gland. This bend is located between the lateral surface of the gland and medial pterygoid muscle. The second bend is concave upward around the lower margin of the mandible. Here, at the anteroinferior angle of the masseter muscle, it pierces the deep fascia to lie on the face.

In the neck, it gives the following branches (refer to **Fig. 8.6**):

a. Ascending palatine.

b. Tonsillar.

c. Submental: runs in the mylohyoid groove with the nerve to the mylohyoid.

d. Branch to the submandibular gland.

2. *Lingual artery*: It is a branch from the ventral aspect of the external carotid artery. It arises in the carotid triangle at the level of the tip of the greater cornu. With the help of the hyoglossus muscle, for descriptive purposes, it is divided into three parts (refer to **Fig. 11.4**):

a. First part: It extends from the external carotid artery to the posterior border of the hyoglossus muscle. It forms a loop (convex upward) on the tip of the greater cornu.

b. Second part: It lies deep to the hyoglossus and superficial to the middle constrictor muscle. It runs close to the upper border of the greater cornu of the hyoid bone. This part of the artery is separated by the hypoglossal nerve as the nerve lies superficial to the hyoglossus muscle.

c. Third part: It extends from the anterior border of the hyoglossus to the tip of the tongue. This part passes through the substance of the tongue. It lies on the genioglossus muscle and then is seen deep to the mucous membrane on the inferior surface of the tongue.

Branches: These supply the tongue and sublingual salivary gland, that is, the suprahyoid artery, dorsal lingual artery, and sublingual (deep lingual) arteries.

Veins of the Region

The deep vein of the tongue begins at the tip of the tongue and then runs superficial to the hyoglossus muscle below the hypoglossal nerve. The dorsal veins are present near the dorsal surface of the tongue. At the posterior border of the hyoglossus, all veins of the tongue join to form the lingual vein. The lingual vein may join the facial vein or the internal jugular vein.

Glands of the Region

The glands located in the submandibular region are submandibular and sublingual glands.
Submandibular gland: The gland is located in the digastric triangle. It consists of two parts, that is, a large superficial part and a small deep part. The superficial part is wedge shaped and located between the body of the mandible and mylohyoid muscle. The investing layer of the deep cervical fascia splits to enclose the gland.

The superficial part of the gland has three surfaces, that is, the *inferolateral*, *medial*, and *lateral*.

1. The inferolateral surface is covered by the skin, superficial fascia containing the platysma, and cervical branch of the facial nerve and facial vein.

2. The lateral surface is related anteriorly to the body of the mandible and posteriorly to the medial pterygoid muscle and facial artery.

3. The medial surface is related to the mylohyoid and hyoglossus muscles. On the hyoglossus, it is related to the lingual nerve, submandibular ganglion, and hypoglossal nerve. Further posteriorly, the gland is related to the pharynx and hypoglossal nerve and lingual artery (**Fig. 11.3**).

At the posterior margin of the mylohyoid muscle, a small prolongation of the gland, from its medial surface, passes between the mylohyoid and hyoglossus muscles. This is the deep part of the gland (**Figs. 11.7** and **11.8**).

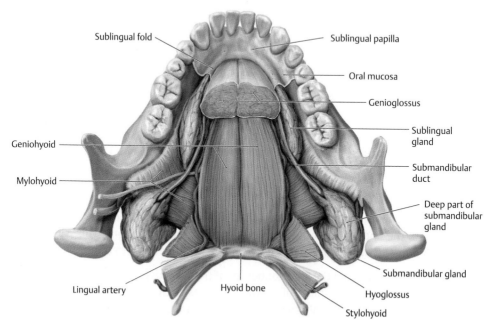

Fig. 11.7 Sublingual and deep part of the submandibular glands and few muscles of submandibular region as seen from above after removal of the tongue. (From: Schuenke M, Schulte E, Schumacher U. THIEME Atlas of Anatomy. Head, Neck, and Neuroanatomy. Illustrations by Voll M and Wesker K. © Thieme 2020.)

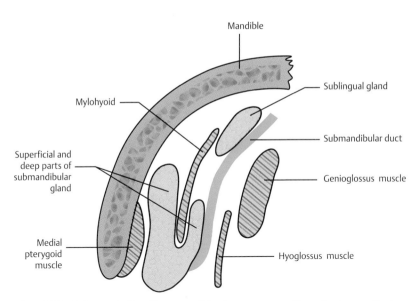

Fig. 11.8 Schematic line diagram of the transverse section of submandibular region to show the relations of submandibular gland.

The submandibular duct (Wharton duct) also emerges from its medial surface and passes antero-superiorly between the mylohyoid and hyoglossus. Later it runs anteriorly between the sublingual gland and genioglossus muscle to open on the sublingual papilla into the oral cavity.

The gland is supplied by the glandular branch of the facial artery. Common facial vein drains the blood. The sensory innervation is from the lingual nerve, and secretomotor fibers come from the submandibular ganglion.

Sublingual gland: It is present in the sublingual fossa of the mandible and lies beneath the mucous membrane of the floor of the mouth (**Figs. 11.7 and 11.8**).

1. It is related *laterally* to the mandible and *medially* to the genioglossus muscle.

2. *Below*: The gland lies on the anterior part of the mylohyoid muscle.

3. *Above*: It is covered by the mucous membrane of the floor of the mouth, on its superior surface.

It pours its secretion on the surface of the lingual fold at the floor of the mouth by 8 to 20 small ducts.

Lymph Nodes

Submandibular and submental groups of lymph nodes are present in this region (**Fig. 11.9**).

Submandibular group of lymph nodes are located in the digastric fossa deep to deep fascia, in relation to the submandibular salivary gland (sometimes they are embedded in the gland). The group consists of four to five lymph nodes. This group drains the lymph from a large area, that is, the middle part of the forehead, medial side of the eye, nose, cheek, and upper lip, lateral part of the lower lip, anterior two-thirds of the tongue, most of the paranasal air sinuses, and gums.

Submental groups of lymph nodes are few and small, which are located in the submental triangle. They drain lymph from the tip of the tongue, median part of the lower lip, and chin.

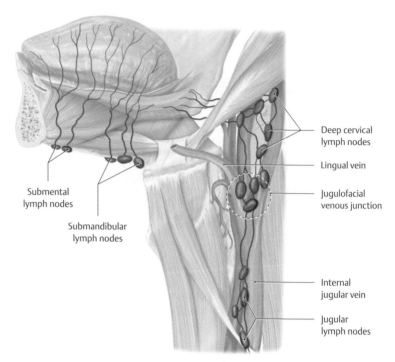

Fig. 11.9 Lymph nodes of the submandibular region. (From: Schuenke M, Schulte E, Schumacher U. THIEME Atlas of Anatomy. Head, Neck, and Neuroanatomy. Illustrations by Voll M and Wesker K. © Thieme 2020.)

▌Clinical Notes

1. *Submandibular lymph nodes and submandibular gland*: As the submandibular group of lymph nodes is embedded in the salivary gland, they need to be removed along with the gland following their enlargement, secondary to the tumor in the area of drainage.

2. *Submandibular duct* (Wharton duct) is a common site of the formation of stones (calculi).

3. *Injury to the lingual nerve*: The lingual nerve lies just posteroinferior to the third molar teeth on the medial surface of the mandible. Sometimes, it may be injured during the extraction of the impacted third molar tooth.

Removal of the Brain from the Cranial Cavity, Cranial Meninges, and Dural Venous Sinuses

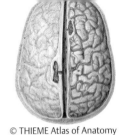

© THIEME Atlas of Anatomy

Introduction

The brain is enclosed in the cranial cavity. It is well protected by the cranial bones, meninges, and cerebrospinal fluid (CSF). In order to study the structures (other than brain) present in the cranial cavity, we need to remove the brain. After removal of the brain, we can study the meningeal vessels, dura mater, dural folds, and dural venous sinuses. Branches of the middle meningeal vessels are present in the extradural space. Dura mater forms many folds such as the falx cerebri, tentorium cerebelli, and falx cerebelli. Two layers of the dura, at places, split to enclose the dural venous sinuses such as the superior and inferior sagittal sinuses and transverse and sigmoid sinuses.

Surface Landmarks

On a dry skull, study the external and internal surface of the calvaria (skull cap) (refer to **Figs. 1.1** and **1.6**). On the external surface of the calvaria, identify the frontal, parietal, and occipital bones. Also, identify the coronal, sagittal, and lambdoid sutures. On the internal surface of the calvaria, note the frontal crest and sagittal sulcus in the midline. Many small depressions (*granular pits*) are observed on each side of the sagittal sulcus. Note the presence of grooves for the meningeal vessels. With the help of **Fig. 1.7,** study the bony features on the internal aspect of the floor of the anterior, middle, and posterior cranial cavities. On the cut edge of the skull cap, look for the outer and inner tables of the compact bone and intervening spongy bone (diploë). On the cadaver, palpate the supraorbital margin and external occipital protuberance.

Dissection and Identification

Note: *Removal of the brain from the cranial cavity is tricky and needs experience. Therefore, you should constantly take the help of your teacher for this dissection and should remove the brain only under his/her supervision; otherwise, the brain may get damaged.*

A. Removal of the skull cap.

1. The cadaver should be in supine position. Place a wooden block under the neck to raise the head.

2. We have already dissected the scalp and reflected it inferiorly from the calvaria (Chapter 2). We have also reflected the temporal muscle from the temporal fossa (Chapter 9).

3. To remove the skull cap, mark a point with the help of a skin-marking pencil, about 1 cm above the supraorbital margin anteriorly and external occipital protuberance posteriorly. Draw a circular line joining these two points (**Fig. 12.1**).

4. Make the cut in the bone by a saw along the marked line. Cut the bone carefully. The cut should reach only up to the diploë and should not cut the inner table of the compact bone; otherwise, the dura mater and brain may get damaged.

5. As you are cutting around the skull, you will have to turn the body from the supine to the prone and again to the supine position.

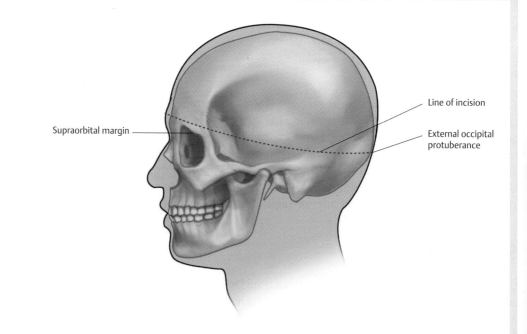

Supraorbital margin

Line of incision

External occipital protuberance

Fig. 12.1 Incision for removal of the skull cap.

6. After giving the complete circumferential cut, you will have to cut the inner table of the cranial bones. This is achieved by gently using the chisel and mallet around the groove produced by the saw cut.

7. Now you are in a position to remove the skull cap from the underlying dura mater. Lift the anterior margin of the skull cap with the help of a chisel blade using the chisel as a lever. Hold the anterior margin of the skull cap with your fingers. Pull the cap from the anterior to posterior, without using much force. Because of the force of pull, the undersurface of the skull cap will get detached from the underlying dura mater. Observe the inner surface of the skull cap (calvaria) for the sagittal sulcus and grooves for the meningeal vessels.

B. Exposure of middle meningeal vessels and dissection of dural venous sinuses and dural folds (Video 12.1).

1. On the outer surface of the dura, examine the branches of the middle meningeal vessels (**Fig. 12.2**). Identify its frontal (anterior) and parietal branches. Note the relation of the anterior branch with the pterion.

2. This is the time to see the dural venous sinus and dural fold. The superior sagittal sinus is present in the midline in the dura. Give a longitudinal incision in the dura mater, in the midline, and expose the superior sagittal sinus (**Figs. 12.2 and 12.3**). The arachnoid granulations may be seen in the lateral side of the sinus lumen.

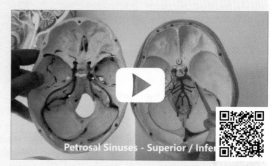

Video 12.1   Intracranial dural venous sinuses.

3. Now use scissors to give two anteroposterior incisions on either side of the superior sagittal sinus. Deep to the sagittal sinus lies a midline dural fold (falx cerebri). Its anterior end is attached to the crista galli. With the help of your teacher, give a cut in this fold at the crista galli. Pull this fold of the dura along with the sagittal sinus upward and backward toward the external occipital protuberance. You will have to cut many veins which are entering the superior sagittal sinus from the brain (see these superior cerebral veins entering the sagittal sinus in **Fig. 12.3**).

C. Exposure of arachnoid mater, subarachnoid space, and brain covered by pia mater.

1. Give a coronal incision, on either side, in the dura to reflect it in the four flaps inferiorly (so that after removal of the brain you can restore the dura covering), or alternately you may give a cut in the dura along the cut edge of the bone (refer to **Fig. 12.3**).

2. This will completely expose the arachnoid mater covering the surface of the brain (see the left half of **Fig. 12.3**).

3. Arachnoid mater is a thin, almost transparent membrane; therefore, the cerebral veins are visible through the arachnoid mater. These veins are present in the subarachnoid space filled with CSF in a living person.

4. Reflect the arachnoid mater which is covering the right half of the brain. You are now in the subarachnoid space. Now observe the vessels on the surface of the brain which itself is

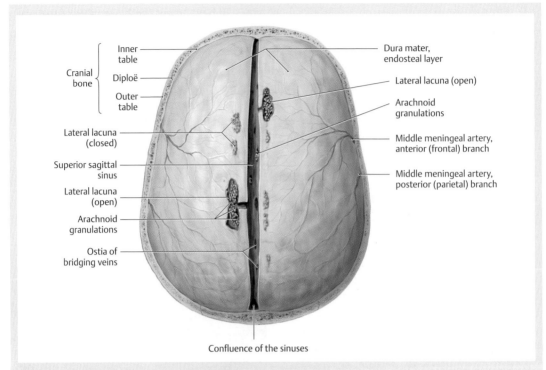

Fig. 12.2 Brain and meninges in situ (superior view). The calvaria has been removed. Note the meningeal vessels. The superior sagittal sinus and its lateral lacunae have been opened. (From: Schuenke M, Schulte E, Schumacher U. THIEME Atlas of Anatomy. Head, Neck, and Neuroanatomy. Illustrations by Voll M and Wesker K. © Thieme 2020.)

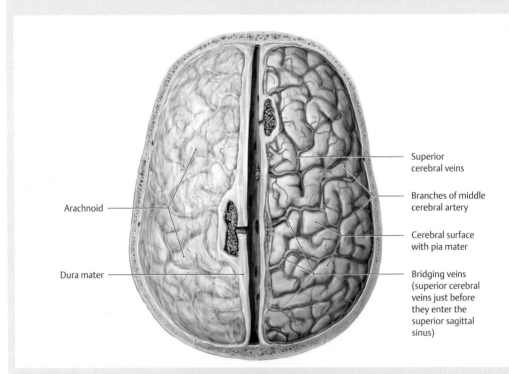

Fig. 12.3 Brain and meninges in situ (superior view). The dura mater has been removed from the surface of the left hemisphere. Dura and arachnoid have been removed from the surface of the right hemisphere. (From: Schuenke M, Schulte E, Schumacher U. THIEME Atlas of Anatomy. Head, Neck, and Neuroanatomy. Illustrations by Voll M and Wesker K. © Thieme 2020.)

covered with the pia mater (refer to the right half of **Fig. 12.3**). The pia mater is firmly adhering to the surface of the brain and cannot be removed from it.

5. Now we can remove the brain from the cranial cavity along with the arachnoid and pia maters. The dura mater remains attached to the cranial cavities as it is firmly attached to the bones.

D. Removal of the brain from cranial cavity with arachnoid and pia maters.

1. Remove the wooden block from the undersurface of the neck; this will allow the head to tilt backward.

2. With your fingers, gently lift the frontal lobes of the brain from the anterior cranial fossa. With the help of a scalpel cut the optic nerves, internal carotid arteries, oculomotor nerves, infundibular stalk, and trochlear nerves, on either side.

3. Now work on the lateral side of the brain and lift the temporal lobe to expose the horizontal fold of the dura, that is, the tentorium cerebelli. Give a cut in this fold of the dura, close to its attachment on the superior border of the petrous temporal bone. The cut should extend from the free margin of the tentorium cerebelli to near the groove for sigmoid sinus. You may give another cut in it, anteroposteriorly, close to the midline (**Fig. 12.4**). This cut will help to deliver the cerebellum which is situated deep to the tentorium cerebelli in the posterior cranial fossa. Now repeat the same procedure (of giving cuts in tentorium cerebelli) on the opposite side also.

4. Now elevate the cerebrum and brainstem gently from the floor of anterior and middle cranial fossae to identify and cut the trigeminal, abducens, facial, vestibulocochlear, glossopharyngeal, vagus, accessory, and hypoglossal nerves on either side. Cut the vertebral arteries as they come in the cranial cavity through the foramen magnum.

5. Pass the scalpel, as far as possible, in the vertebral canal through the foramen magnum, on the ventral aspect of the brainstem and spinal cord. Sever the cervical spinal cord gently.

6. Very carefully, withdraw the brain from the cranial cavity in one piece.

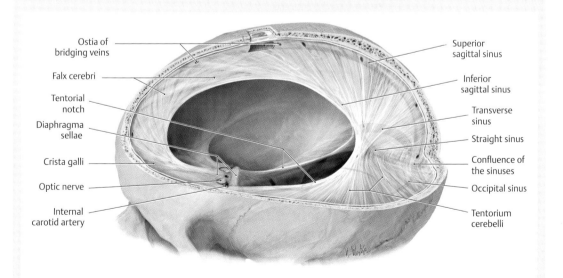

Fig. 12.4 Sagittal section of the calvarium through the skull to the left of the falx cerebri. The brain has been removed to show the dural septa (folds) (left lateral view). (From: Schuenke M, Schulte E, Schumacher U. THIEME Atlas of Anatomy. Head, Neck, and Neuroanatomy. Illustrations by Voll M and Wesker K. © Thieme 2020.)

Middle Meningeal Vessels

After the removal of the skull cap (calvaria), many vessels are seen ascending toward the vertex (refer to **Figs. 12.2 and 13.3**). These vessels are extensively branching on the surface of the cranial (endosteal layer) dura. These are branches of the middle meningeal artery and vein. These vessels are closely applied to the undersurface (inner table) of the skull bones. Therefore, they produce grooves on the internal aspect of the calvaria. Thus, the branches of the middle meningeal vessels are extradural in location.

These vessels supply blood to the diploë, outer and inner tables of the adjacent bones, endocranium and the meningeal layer of the dura.

Cranial Meninges

The meninges surrounding the brain are called the *cranial meninges* and those surrounding the spinal cord are called the *spinal meninges*. Meninges are of three different types: *dura mater, arachnoid mater,* and *pia mater.*

Dura Mater

The dura mater is the outermost thick meningeal layer made up of dense connective tissue. It covers the brain and spinal cord. The dura covering the brain is known as the *cranial/cerebral dura.* The cerebral dura is made up of outer *endosteal (periosteal) layer* and an inner *meningeal layer* (**Fig. 12.5**). The endosteal layer of the dura mater is nothing but the endocranium or the inner periosteum. The endosteal layer is firmly attached to the cranial bones and is continuous with the pericranium or the outer periosteum at the foramina in the skull. The meningeal layer of the dura mater is the membranous layer. It covers the brain and then becomes continuous with the dura mater covering the spinal cord.

The two layers of the dura mater are tightly fused with each other except at a few places where they form the *dural folds* or *dural venous sinuses.* At these places, the meningeal layer separates from

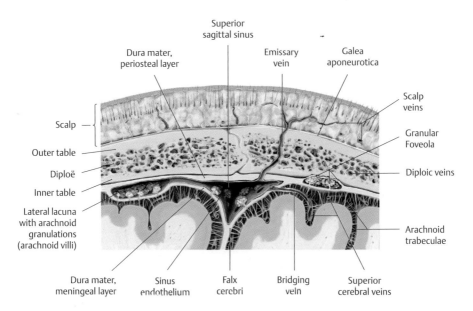

Fig. 12.5 Coronal section through the calvarium, superior sagittal sinus, and brain to show the relationship of the meninges to the brain and calvarium. (From: Schuenke M, Schulte E, Schumacher U. THIEME Atlas of Anatomy. Head, Neck, and Neuroanatomy. Illustrations by Voll M and Wesker K. © Thieme 2020.)

the endosteal layer to form a double-layered fold/partition or *dural venous sinus*. These *folds of the dura mater* extend between the major parts of the brain. For example, in the case of the superior sagittal sinus, the meningeal layer separates from the endosteal layer to form a triangular space, i.e., superior sagittal sinus (refer to **Fig. 12.5**). Here, the internal surface of the dura mater forming the boundary of the sinus is smooth, shining, and lined by the endothelial cells.

Dural Folds

The following folds or septa of the dura mater are formed in the cranial cavity due to duplication of the meningeal layer of the dura (refer to **Fig. 12.4**).

Falx cerebri: It is a sickle-shaped fold placed vertically in the midline between two cerebral hemispheres. Anteriorly, it is attached to the crista galli and posteriorly to the tentorium cerebelli. It encloses the *superior sagittal sinus* at the upper border, *inferior sagittal sinus* at the inferior border, and the *straight sinus* at its junction with the tentorium cerebelli.

Tentorium cerebelli: This tentlike fold of the dura mater forms the roof of the posterior cranial fossa. It is crescent shaped and placed horizontally between the cerebrum and cerebellum. It has a free and an attached margin. Along its attached margin, it encloses the *transverse* and *superior petrosal sinuses* on either side.

Falx cerebelli: It is a sickle-shaped fold present in the posterior cranial fossa between two cerebellar hemispheres. It encloses the occipital sinus.

Diaphragma sellae: It forms the roof of the sella turcica. The pituitary gland is present below it.

Dural Venous Sinuses

The dural venous sinuses drain blood from some cranial bones, meninges, and brain. They ultimately pour the blood into the internal jugular veins (refer to **Figs. 12.4, 12.6,** and **13.5**). The dural venous sinuses are formed due to the separation of the meningeal and endosteal layers. These sinuses can be classified as *paired* or *unpaired*.

1. *Unpaired sinuses* are the superior sagittal, inferior sagittal, straight sinus, occipital sinus, basilar plexus of the veins, and intercavernous sinuses.

2. *Paired sinuses* are the transverse sinuses, sigmoid sinuses, superior petrosal sinuses, inferior petrosal sinuses, sphenoparietal sinuses, and cavernous sinuses.

Unpaired Sinuses

Superior sagittal sinus: It is situated in the midline along the upper border of the falx cerebri. It extends anteroposteriorly from the crista galli to the internal occipital protuberance. It drains the venous blood from the frontal sinus, veins of the nose, and superior cerebral veins. It drains into the right transverse sinus at the internal occipital protuberance.

Inferior sagittal sinus: This fold of the dura is present at the inferior border of the falx cerebri. It drains the falx and medial surface of the cerebral hemisphere. It becomes continuous with the straight sinus, posteriorly.

Straight sinus: The union of the inferior sagittal sinus and great cerebral vein forms the straight sinus at the junction of the falx and tentorium cerebelli. At the internal occipital protuberance, it forms the left transverse sinus.

Occipital sinus: It is present in the posterior edge of the falx cerebelli in the posterior crania fossa. It is connected below to the sigmoid sinuses.

Basilar plexus of the veins: It lies on the clivus of the skull in the posterior cranial fossa.

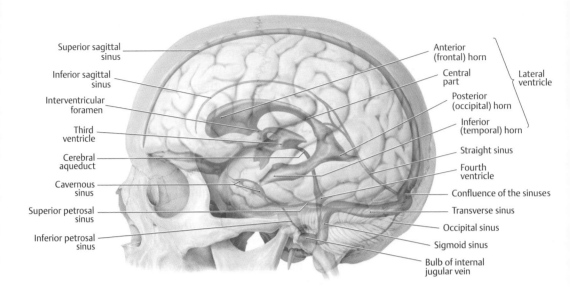

Fig. 12.6 Dural venous sinuses in relation to the brain (left lateral view). (From: Schuenke M, Schulte E, Schumacher U. THIEME Atlas of Anatomy. Head, Neck, and Neuroanatomy. Illustrations by Voll M and Wesker K. © Thieme 2020.)

Paired Sinuses

Transverse sinus: This sinus lies along the posterolateral edge of the tentorium cerebelli and extends from the internal occipital protuberance to the base of the petrous temporal bone. It is formed by the superior sagittal sinus on the right side and on the left by the straight sinus. On each side, it drains in the sigmoid sinus.

Confluence of the sinuses: This is the meeting place of the superior sagittal, straight, right and left transverse sinuses, and occipital sinus at the internal occipital protuberance.

Sigmoid sinus: It is present in the sigmoid sulcus in the posterior cranial fossa. It passes through the jugular foramen to form the internal jugular vein.

Further details of many of the dural sinuses will be given in the next chapter (Cranial Fossae, refer to **Fig. 13.5**).

Arachnoid Mater

Deep to the dura mater, there lies a delicate, thin, and almost transparent membrane known as the *arachnoid mater*. It is separated from the dura mater by a capillary space which is called the *subdural space*. The subarachnoid space lies beneath the arachnoid mater, between the arachnoid and pia mater. It is filled with CSF. The arteries, veins, and cranial nerves lie in the subarachnoid space. Cerebral veins which are present in the subarachnoid space are visible through the arachnoid mater (refer to **Fig. 12.3**). These are present on the cerebral surface, the pia mater. Cerebral veins empty their blood into the superior sagittal sinus.

Sometimes, on the surface of the brain, pia and arachnoid mater are widely separated from each other to form the subarachnoid cisterns. Large cisterns are formed around the brainstem and cerebellum.

Arachnoid Villi and Granulations

The CSF from the subarachnoid space passes into the blood stream of the dural venous sinuses through the arachnoid villi. Arachnoid villi are minute fingerlike elevations of the arachnoid mater that project into the dural venous sinuses (especially the superior sagittal sinus) through apertures in the dura mater. These act as channels of communication between the subarachnoid space and dural venous sinus.

The arachnoid villi become large and globular in shape during old age and they may indent the overlying bone of the skull. These villi are now known as the arachnoid granulation (refer to **Figs. 12.2** and **12.5**). The marks of the indentation are seen as parasagittal depressions on the inner surface of the cranial vault.

Pia Mater

The pia mater is a thin membrane which is firmly attached on the surface of the brain. The pia mater cannot be removed from the surface of the brain.

■ Clinical Notes

1. *Extradural (epidural) hemorrhage*: Epidural hemorrhage occurs due to rupture of the meningeal vessels running between the endosteal and meningeal layers of the dura mater. The most common artery affected is the anterior branch of the middle meningeal artery and vein, which lies in the area of the pterion.

2. *Subdural hemorrhage*: Trauma to the head (forceful movement of the brain within the cranial cavity) may tear the superior cerebral vein(s). This results in the collection of blood in the subdural space.

3. *Thrombosis of the dural venous sinuses*: Though thrombosis is rare, it may occur in the dural venous sinuses. It occurs most commonly in the superior sagittal, cavernous, and sigmoid sinuses.

Cranial Fossae

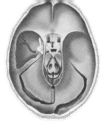

Introduction

The base of the cranial cavity is divided into three large fossae, that is, *anterior, middle,* and *posterior cranial fossae.* The boundary between anterior and middle cranial fossae is formed by the posterior borders of the lesser wing of the sphenoid and anterior clinoid processes. The middle and posterior cranial fossae are separated from each other by superior borders of the petrous temporal bone, posterior clinoid processes, and dorsum sellae. On the floor of the anterior cranial fossa rests the *frontal lobe,* while on the middle fossa rests the *temporal lobe of cerebrum.* The posterior cranial fossa lodges the *cerebellum.* Various *dural venous sinuses* are present in the middle and posterior cranial fossae. They pour their blood in the internal jugular veins. *Cranial nerves I to XII* and few vessels pass through various foramina in the floor of the cranial fossae. *Medulla* of the brainstem passes through the foramen magnum. An important endocrine gland, the *hypophysis cerebri (pituitary),* is present in the middle cranial fossa.

Surface Landmarks

Use the base of the skull to identify the bones forming the base of the anterior cranial fossa (sphenoid, ethmoid, and orbital plate of frontal bone). In the median region of the floor of the anterior cranial fossa, note the frontal crest, crista galli, cribriform plate of ethmoid, and jugum sphenoidale (refer to **Fig. 1.7**).

The floor of the middle cranial fossa is formed by sphenoid, cranial surface of the greater wing of sphenoid, squamous, and petrous parts of the temporal bone. Identify the hypophyseal fossa, superior orbital fissure, the foramen rotundum, foramen ovale, foramen spinosum, and foramen lacerum.

The floor of the posterior cranial fossa is formed by the body of sphenoid, occipital bone, posterior surface of petrous temporal bone, mastoid part of temporal bone, and posteroinferior angle of parietal bone. Identify foramen magnum, internal acoustic meatus, jugular foramen, and transverse sulcus.

Dissection and Identification

*Students are suggested to keep the base of the dry skull and a brain on the dissection table during the dissection of the cranial fossae. With the help of your teacher, study the attachment of cranial nerves on the ventral aspect of the brain. Also, study the bony features at the base of the various cranial fossae (***Fig. 1.7a***). Now keep the brain in the skull to realize that the base of the brain fits well in the cranial fossae.*

A. Anterior cranial fossa (Video 13.1).

1. After keeping the brain in the base of a dry skull, realize that the frontal lobe of the brain rests on the orbital part of the frontal bone.

2. Foramina in the cribriform plate give passage to the *olfactory nerve* (**Fig. 13.1**).

3. Note the attachment of the cut end of *falx cerebri* to the crista galli.

4. Now remove the dura mater from the floor of the anterior cranial fossa, with the help of the toothed forceps and probe *(remove the dura from one side of the cranial cavities, keeping the dura on the other side intact)*.

5. Look for the *sphenoparietal sinus* at the posterior margin of the lesser wing of the sphenoid.

B. Middle cranial fossa (Video 13.2).

1. Middle cranial fossa lodges the *temporal lobe* of the brain.

2. To see the structures of the middle cranial fossa, we shall now remove the dura mater from its floor. Gently start pulling the dura from the posterior border of the lesser wing of the sphenoid. Keep on pulling till you reach the superior border of the petrous temporal bone.

3. Identify the *middle meningeal artery* (**Fig. 13.2**). It will come along with the dura, adhering on its outer surface. Dissect the proximal part of the artery from the dura and leave it near the foramen spinosum.

4. Try to locate the *superior petrosal sinus* at the superior border of the petrous temporal bone.

5. Look for the stump of the internal carotid artery and optic nerve. The optic nerve lies medial to the artery and will be seen passing through the optic canal.

6. Identify the midline region of the hypophyseal fossa. Identify the stump of the *infundibular stalk* as it comes out through the opening in the *diaphragma sellae*. Give radial cuts to the diaphragma sellae and carefully deliver the pituitary gland. Give a sagittal incision in the pituitary gland and observe it under a hand lens.

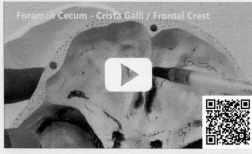

Video 13.1 Cranial venous sinus, superior sagittal sinus (SSS), cavernous sigmoid petrosal dural folds, clinicals.

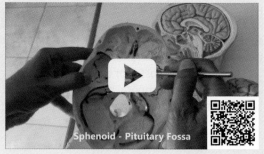

Video 13.2 Cavernous petrosal sinus, origin, tributaries, cavernous sinus (CS) syndrome, carotid-cavernous fistula (CCF), clinicals.

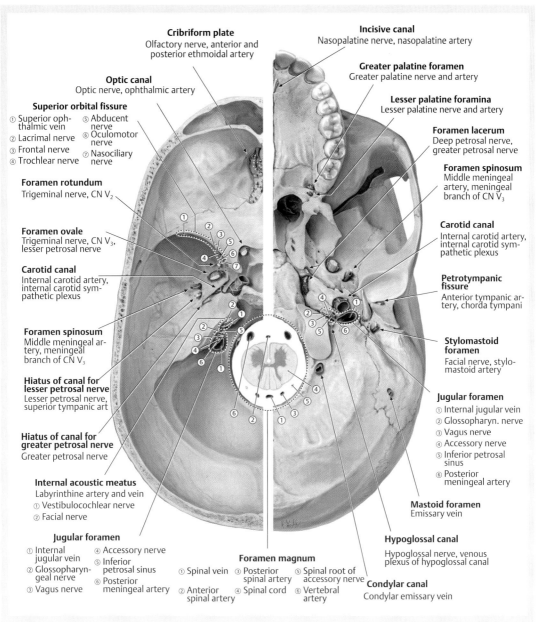

Fig. 13.1 Sites where nerves and vessels pass through the skull base. One half of the figure shows base of the skull from inner aspect (norma basalis interna) while other half of figure shows base from outer aspect (norma basalis externa). (From: Schuenke M, Schulte E, Schumacher U. THIEME Atlas of Anatomy. Head, Neck, and Neuroanatomy. Illustrations by Voll M and Wesker K. © Thieme 2020.)

7. Now clean the structures passing through the *superior orbital fissure*, deep to the posterior border of the lesser wing of the sphenoid (refer to **Figs. 13.1** and **14.9**).

8. Follow the oculomotor, trochlear, ophthalmic, and abducens nerves backward, from the superior orbital fissure to the superior border of the petrous temporal bone. These nerves lie in relation to the *cavernous sinus*.

9. Identify the trigeminal nerve at the superior border of the petrous temporal bone. Follow it forward to locate the *trigeminal ganglion* on the anterior surface of the petrous bone near its apex (**Fig. 13.2**).

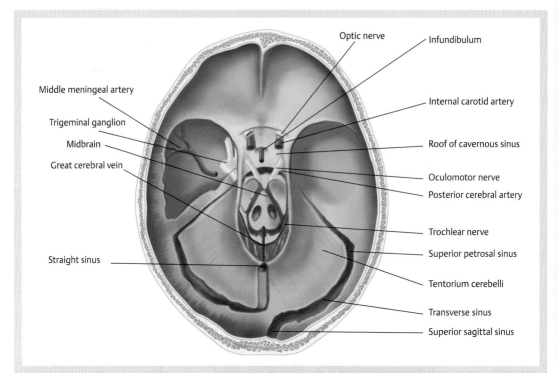

Fig. 13.2 Interior of the cranium after removal of the cerebrum. The transverse, straight, and superior petrosal sinuses have been opened, and the dura mater has been removed from the floor of the left middle cranial fossa to expose the middle meningeal artery.

10. Now trace the three divisions of the trigeminal nerve arising from the ganglion. The ophthalmic division passes through the lateral wall of the cavernous sinus.

11. Identify the *maxillary division* and follow it forward to the foramen rotundum. It runs through the lateral wall of the cavernous sinus.

12. Identify the *mandibular division* and follow it forward to the foramen ovale.

13. In the area of the cavernous sinus, deep to the nerves, clean the *internal carotid artery*. It makes an S-shaped band in the cavernous sinus and comes out close to the optic nerve.

C. Posterior cranial fossa.

1. This fossa lodges the brainstem and cerebellum.

2. Detach the dura from the posterior cranial fossa. Begin at the superior border of the petrous bone and reach till the internal occipital protuberance and internal occipital crest.

3. In the midline, on clivus, note the presence of the basilar plexus of vein.

4. Follow the *transverse sinus* from the internal occipital protuberance to the petrous bone. See its continuity with the *sigmoid sinus*. Trace the sigmoid sinus till it opens in the jugular foramen to become continuous with the *internal jugular vein*. Also, trace the *inferior petrosal sinus*.

5. Identify the facial and vestibulocochlear nerve as they enter the internal acoustic meatus.

6. Similarly, locate the glossopharyngeal, vagus, and accessory nerves entering the jugular foramen (refer to **Fig. 13.1**).

7. Identify the hypoglossal nerve as it enters the hypoglossal canal.

Middle Meningeal Artery

Middle meningeal artery is a branch of the first part of maxillary artery. It arises in the infratemporal fossa (refer to **Fig. 9.2b**).

The artery enters the middle cranial fossa through the foramen spinosum. It runs forward and laterally on the squamous part of the temporal bone for about 2 cm, over the floor of the middle cranial fossa. In the middle cranial fossa, it passes between two layers of dura (endosteal and meningeal layer) along with the meningeal vein. The vein lies superficial to the artery.

It divides into *frontal (anterior)* and *parietal (posterior)* branches (**Fig. 13.3**). *Frontal branch* runs forward and upward, first on the greater wing of the sphenoid and then on the anteroinferior angle of the parietal bone. Here it lies on the *pterion* in a groove. It then runs along the parietal bone about 1 cm behind the corona suture and divides into many branches that run predominantly upward and backward. *Parietal branch* first runs upward and backward on the squamous part of the temporal bone and then on the parietal bone, toward lambda.

It supplies blood to the skull bones, dura, trigeminal ganglion, and structures of the middle ear.

The artery is accompanied by the middle meningeal vein, which drains either in the cavernous sinus or in the sphenoparietal sinus or in the pterygoid plexus (through the foramen ovale).

Hypophysis Cerebri

This small master endocrine gland is suspended from the base of the brain through infundibular stalk. It is present in the middle cranial fossa and is situated on the pituitary fossa (sella turcica) of the sphenoid bone. The inner layer of the dura mater forms a diaphragm. This fold of the dura mater is known as the diaphragma sellae. It is perforated in the middle to give passage to the infundibular stalk. The gland is oval in shape and measures about 12 × 8 mm in size and weighs less than 1 g.

In the sagittal section, its subdivisions, that is, the anterior (adenohypophysis) and posterior (neurohypophysis) lobes are visible. The anterior lobe consists of anterior (pars distalis), intermediate (pars intermedia), and pars tuberalis. The pars anterior and pars intermedia are separated by a cleft. The neurohypophysis consists of pars posterior, infundibular stalk, and median eminence of tuber cinereum (**Fig. 13.4**).

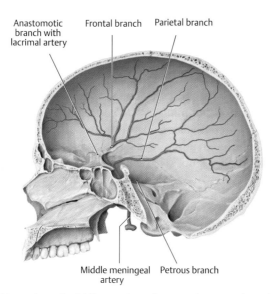

Fig. 13.3 Course and branches of middle meningeal artery. (From: Schuenke M, Schulte E, Schumacher U. THIEME Atlas of Anatomy. Head, Neck, and Neuroanatomy. Illustrations by Voll M and Wesker K. © Thieme 2020.)

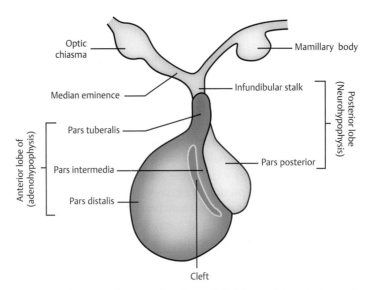

Fig. 13.4 Schematic drawing showing subdivisions of the pituitary gland as seen in the median (sagittal) section.

The anterior and intermediate lobes are made up of glandular cells (adenohypophysis) which secrete several hormones. The glandular cells are classified as acidophils, basophils, and chromophobes (growth hormone, adrenocorticotropic hormone, luteotropic hormone, thyroid-stimulating hormone, follicle-stimulating hormone, luteinizing hormone, etc.). The posterior lobe (pars nervosa) is made up of unmyelinated nerve fibers. These fibers are axons of supraoptic and paraventricular nuclei of hypothalamus. These nuclei are concerned with the production of antidiuretic hormone and oxytocin.

Relations: Superiorly, it is related to the diaphragma sellae, anterior and posterior intercavernous sinuses, optic chiasma, and tuber cinereum. Inferiorly, it is related to the sphenoidal air sinus and the inferior intercavernous sinus. On each side, the gland is related to the cavernous sinus and its contents. Posteriorly, it is related to the dorsum sellae.

Blood supply: The anterior and posterior parts of the pituitary gland are supplied by the superior and inferior hypophyseal arteries. Both are branches of the internal carotid artery.

Superior hypophyseal arteries: These are about 15 to 20 small twigs which supply the median eminence and infundibulum. Here, they end in the capillary plexuses from which hypophyseal portal vessels arise. These portal vessels descend in the anterior lobe where they once again break into sinusoids (capillary plexus). These plexuses drain through the hypophyseal veins in the neighboring sinuses. This arrangement of vessels is known as the *hypothalamo-hypophyseal portal system*. Through this portal system, *releasing and inhibitory factors* are brought from the hypothalamus to the anterior pituitary. Thus, the hypothalamus controls the secretion of the anterior pituitary.

Inferior hypophyseal arteries: Inferior hypophyseal set of small arteries arise from the internal carotid artery as it lies in the cavernous sinus. These branches are mainly distributed to the posterior pituitary but they also supply a few branches to the anterior pituitary.

Cavernous Sinus

Cavernous sinuses are paired dural venous sinuses which are located on either side of the body of the sphenoid bone in the middle cranial fossa (**Figs. 13.5, 13.6**, and **9.7**). The lumen of the sinus contains the network of communicating spaces, hence the name *cavernous*. Venous blood flows slowly through these spaces.

Each sinus extends anteriorly from the medial end of the superior orbital fissure to the apex of the petrous temporal bone, posteriorly. It is about 2 cm long and 1 cm wide.

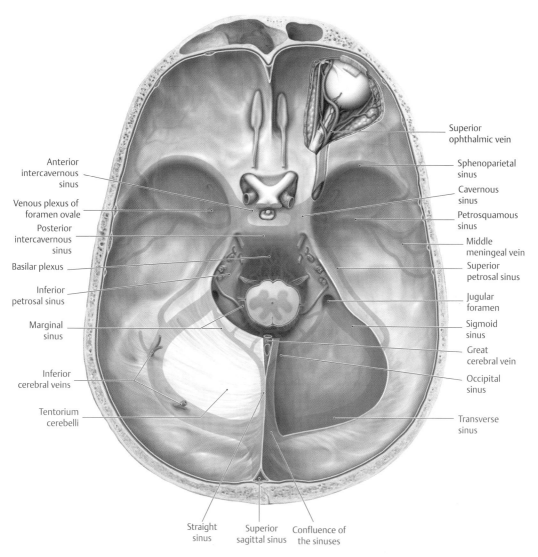

Fig. 13.5 Intracranial dural venous sinuses. (From: Schuenke M, Schulte E, Schumacher U. THIEME Atlas of Anatomy. Head, Neck, and Neuroanatomy. Illustrations by Voll M and Wesker K. © Thieme 2020.)

The cavity of sinus is formed due to the splitting of meningeal and endosteal layers of the dura. It has a medial wall, a lateral wall, a narrow roof, and a floor. The medial wall and floor are lined by the endosteal layer of the dura, while the lateral wall and roof are formed by the meningeal layer of the dura.

Tributaries of sinus: The following veins drain their blood into the cavernous sinus:

1. Superior ophthalmic vein, sometimes a branch of the inferior ophthalmic vein.

2. Central vein of the retina.

3. Superficial middle cerebral vein and inferior cerebral veins.

4. Tributary of the middle meningeal vein.

5. Sphenoparietal sinus.

Draining channels:

1. Superior petrosal sinus drains into the transverse sinus (**Figs. 13.5** and **9.7**).

2. Inferior petrosal sinus drains into the internal jugular vein.

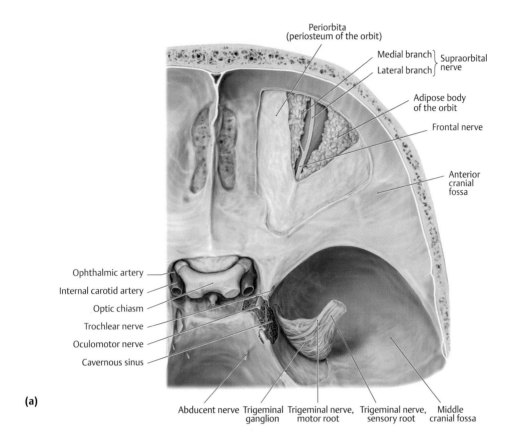

(a)

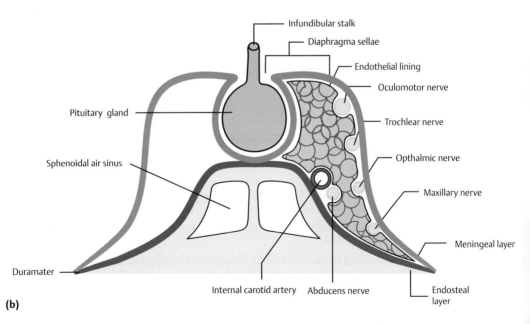

(b)

Fig. 13.6 **(a)** Relations of the cranial nerves to cavernous sinus that enter the orbit and location of trigeminal ganglion (anterior and middle cranial fossae on the right side, superior view). **(b)** Relations and contents of cavernous sinus in coronal section. (Figure a: From: Schuenke M, Schulte E, Schumacher U. THIEME Atlas of Anatomy. Head, Neck, and Neuroanatomy. Illustrations by Voll M and Wesker K. © Thieme 2020.)

Communicating channels:

1. Communicates with the cavernous sinus of the opposite side via anterior, posterior, and inferior intercavernous sinuses.

2. Communicates with the pterygoid venous plexus via emissary veins which may pass through the foramen ovale, emissary sphenoidal, and foramen lacerum (refer to **Fig. 9.7**).

3. Communicates with the facial vein via superior ophthalmic vein (refer to **Figs. 3.8** and **14.8**).

Contents: Like any other blood vessel, sinus is lined by the endothelial cells; therefore, its lumen contains only venous blood. Thus, the internal carotid artery and abducens nerve, which appears to be within the sinus, are actually outside the lumen and are placed closed to its medial wall.

The contents of its lateral wall, from above downwards, are oculomotor, trochlear, ophthalmic and maxillary nerves (**Fig. 13.6a** and **Fig. 13.6b**).

Relations:

1. *Superiorly*: The cavernous sinus is related to the optic tract, internal carotid artery, and anterior perforated substance.

2. *Inferiorly*: The sinus is related to the greater wing of the sphenoid bone.

3. *Medially*: The sinus is related to the pituitary gland and sphenoidal air sinus.

4. *Laterally*: The sinus is related to the temporal lobe of the cerebrum.

Trigeminal Ganglion

The trigeminal ganglion is a crescent-shaped structure. It lies in the depression (*trigeminal impression*) over the anterior part of the petrous temporal bone, near to its apex. It lies in a recess formed by the dura mater called the *trigeminal cave*. From its convex anterior border arise the *ophthalmic*, *maxillary*, and *mandibular nerves*. The concave posterior border is continuous with the sensory root, which lies on the superior border of the petrous temporal bone but inferior to the superior petrosal sinus. Sensory root also crosses the internal carotid artery as it lies in the carotid canal. The superomedial part of the ganglion is related to the posterior end of the cavernous sinus. Inferiorly, the ganglion is related to the motor root of the trigeminal nerve and greater petrosal nerve (**Fig. 13.6a**).

Tentorium Cerebelli

It is a horizontal fold of the dura mater which roofs the posterior cranial fossa like a tent (**Fig. 13.2** and refer to **Fig. 12.4**). It separates the occipital lobes of the cerebrum (which is placed superior to it) from the cerebellum (which is placed inferior to it in the posterior cranial fossa).

It has two borders, that is, *attached* and *free borders (margins)*.

Attached margin: From the anterior to the posterior border, it is attached to the superior border of the petrous temporal bone and lips of the transverse sulcus, up to the internal occipital protuberance.

Free margin: It is U-shaped and is known as the tentorial notch. If we trace the free margin anteriorly, it is attached to the anterior clinoid processes in the middle cranial fossa.

Contents: On each side, it contains the superior petrosal sinus and the transverse sinus. In the midline, it contains the straight sinus.

Functions: It plays an important role in supporting the brain tissue. Tentorium cerebelli divides the cranial cavity into supratentorial and infratentorial compartments and, thus, separates the cerebrum from the cerebellum parts of the brain. It restricts the displacement of some parts of the brain during forceful movements of the head.

Transverse Sinus

This is present on each side of the attached margin of the tentorium cerebelli (**Figs. 13.2** and **13.5**). This sinus extends from the internal occipital protuberance to the base of the petrous temporal bone. The right transverse sinus is formed by the continuation of the superior sagittal sinus, while the left transverse sinus is formed by the continuation of the straight sinus. The transverse sinuses receive blood from the veins of the occipital lobe of the cerebrum and cerebellum and ultimately drain into the right and left sigmoid sinuses.

Sigmoid Sinus

This is situated behind the base of the petrous temporal bone. This S-shaped sinus is the continuation of the transverse sinus (**Fig. 13.5**). It passes through the jugular foramen to form the internal jugular vein.

Structures Passing through the Foramen Magnum

This largest foramen of the skull is located in the midline of the occipital bone. It gives passage to the following structures (refer to **Fig. 13.1**):

1. Membrana tectoria, cruciate ligament, and apical ligament of dens.

2. Medulla covered with all three meninges, that is, pia, arachnoid, and dura.

3. Right and left vertebral arteries, one anterior spinal and two posterior spinal arteries.

4. Spinal root of the accessory nerve.

▌ Clinical Notes

1. *Middle meningeal artery*: Injury to the middle meningeal artery is very common as it lies just deep to the cranial bones. It is torn easily in fractures of the temporal region due to a blow on the side of the skull. Its frontal branch, which lies deep to the pterion, is commonly injured as it passes through a groove on the bone. This results in *extradural hemorrhage* which soon presses on the motor area of the cerebral cortex leading to *paralysis* of the opposite side of the body.

2. *Hypophysis cerebri*: Pituitary gland tumor causes symptoms due to pressure on related structures, such as optic chiasma, nerves of cavernous sinus, etc. Tumor of various cells of adenohypophysis leads to disturbance of the endocrine functions, that is, acromegaly or gigantism as in case of adenoma of acidophils.

3. *Cavernous sinus*: Thrombosis of cavernous sinus occurs due to infection in the dangerous areas of the face, nasal cavity, or paranasal air sinuses. The thrombosis leads to pain in the eye, swelling of the eyelid, and protrusion of the eyeball due to blockage of venous drainage.

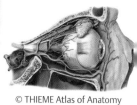
Learning Objectives

At the end of the dissection of the orbit, you should be able to identify the following:

- Walls of the bony orbit, superior orbital fissure, and optic canal.
- Lacrimal gland.
- Extraocular muscles.
- Ophthalmic nerve, oculomotor nerve, trochlear nerve, abducens nerve, and optic nerve.
- Ciliary ganglion and its connections.
- Ophthalmic artery, its course, and branches.
- Superior and inferior ophthalmic veins.

Introduction

The orbit is like a four-sided pyramidal cavity, which contains the eyeball, extraocular muscles, nerves, and vessels embedded in fat. It also contains the lacrimal gland and lacrimal sac. The eyeball is about 2.5 cm in diameter and occupies the anterior half of the orbit. The lacrimal gland is present anteriorly, close to the anterior border of the roof. The posterior part of the orbit contains six extraocular muscles, which move the eyeball. The optic nerve begins from the posterior aspect of the eyeball and leaves the orbital cavity through the optic canal. The orbit contains many cranial nerves, that is, oculomotor, trochlear, abducens, and branches of the ophthalmic nerve. Blood to the contents of the orbit is supplied by the ophthalmic artery, which is a branch of the internal carotid artery. The superior and inferior ophthalmic veins drain the blood from the orbit.

Surface Landmarks

With the help of a dry skull, review the bony features of the orbit (refer to **Fig. 1.8**). Identify its base and apex and study the bones forming its medial and lateral walls, roof, and floor. Similarly, review the bones forming the four borders of the orbital opening. Locate the lacrimal fossa for the lacrimal gland. Identify the opening of the optic canal, superior and inferior orbital fissures. On the medial wall, find the openings of the anterior and posterior ethmoidal foramina and on the floor see the infraorbital groove.

Also, realize that the medial wall of the orbit is related to the ethmoidal air sinuses, the roof of the orbit forms the floor of the anterior cranial fossa, and its floor is related to the maxillary air sinus.

Dissection and Identification

The contents of the orbital cavity are dissected and displayed by using the superior approach, that is, by breaking the orbital plate of the bone which forms the roof of the orbit. To visualize the inferior oblique muscle, we shall dissect using the anterior approach. We have already dissected the anterior part of the lacrimal gland (refer to Chapter 4). We shall now use the combination of both the superior and anterior approaches to see the complete lacrimal gland.

A. Dissection to expose the periorbita (periosteum of the orbit) (Videos 14.1 and 14.2).

1. We have already removed the dura mater from the floor of the anterior cranial fossa. With the help of a small hammer, gently break the orbital plate forming the floor of the anterior cranial fossa. Lift the pieces of the broken bone with the help of toothed forceps to expose the orbital periosteum (periorbita), which lines the roof of the orbit (**Fig. 14.1**).

2. Medially, the orbital plate also forms the lateral part of the ethmoid air sinuses. Thus, on the medial side, few ethmoidal air sinuses will be exposed.

3. Posteriorly, break the lesser wing of the sphenoid carefully so that the structures passing through the superior orbital fissure are not damaged. Preserve the bone forming the margin of the optic canal.

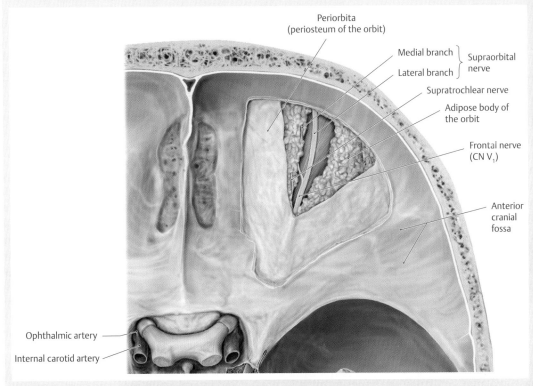

Fig. 14.1 Dissection of the orbit. The bony roof is removed to expose the periorbita. The triangular flap of the periorbita is removed to expose the frontal nerve and its branches. (From: Schuenke M, Schulte E, Schumacher U. THIEME Atlas of Anatomy. Head, Neck, and Neuroanatomy. Illustrations by Voll M and Wesker K. © Thieme 2020.)

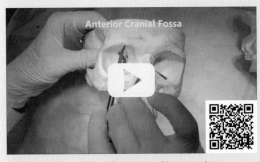

Video 14.1 Salient features of bony orbit.

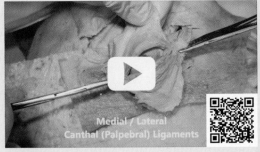

Video 14.2 Ocular muscles, lacrimal gland, and optic nerve.

4. The dissection so far will expose the orbital periosteum, which completely surrounds the contents of the orbit. You may see the frontal nerve passing deep to the periosteum. Give an anteroposterior incision in the periosteum along the midline, and a second incision transversely near the anterior margin of the orbit. Reflect the periosteum toward periphery.

B. Dissection to expose the nerves, vessels, and muscles after removal of periosteum of the orbit.

1. Clean and follow the frontal nerve anteriorly and see it dividing into supraorbital and supratrochlear branches. This nerve lies above the levator palpebrae superioris (LPS) muscle (**Fig. 14.2**).

2. Find a very thin nerve in the upper medial side of the orbit, that is, the trochlear nerve. It passes through the superior orbital fissure medial to the frontal nerve. When traced forward and medially the nerve goes to supply the superior oblique muscle. Follow the tendon of the superior oblique muscle anteriorly; it passes over a pulley at the superomedial angle of the orbit, then turns to go posterolaterally beneath the LPS and superior rectus (SR) muscles.

3. Near the lateral wall of the orbit, clean the fat and find the lacrimal nerve and lacrimal artery. The nerve passes through the superior orbital fissure lateral to the frontal nerve. Trace the nerve and artery anteriorly to the lacrimal gland (refer to **Fig. 14.2**).

4. Deep to the lacrimal nerve and lacrimal artery, clean the fat to find the lateral rectus muscle. Find the abducens nerve on the medial surface of the muscle belly (**Fig. 14.3**).

5. Now divide the frontal nerve near the middle of the orbit and reflect it to clean the LPS. This muscle is inserted to the upper eyelid which elevates it. Give a cut in the LPS and reflect it to

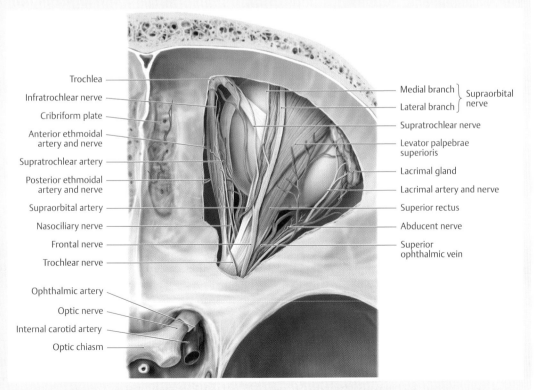

Fig. 14.2   Contents of the orbit seen after removing the roof of the periorbita and adipose tissue. (From: Baker EW. Anatomy for Dental Medicine. Illustrations by Markus Voll and Karl Wesker. © Thieme 2015.)

clean and expose the SR muscle which lies just beneath the LPS. It is attached to the superior aspect of the eyeball. Cut the SR near the eyeball and reflect it posteriorly. Note the superior division of the oculomotor nerve lying beneath the SR that supplies the RS and LPS.

C. Dissection to expose the optic nerves and structures crossing it superficially (Video 14.3).

1. After reflecting the SR, clean the fat (retrobulbar pad of fat) posterior to the eyeball to expose the optic nerve. Identify the structures crossing the optic nerve, from anterior to posterior, ophthalmic vein, ophthalmic artery, and nasociliary nerve (**Fig. 14.3**).

2. Clean all these structures and follow their branches. Nasociliary nerve gives few branches which run along the optic nerve to the eyeball. These are long ciliary nerves. Follow the nasociliary nerve anteriorly and find the posterior and anterior ethmoidal nerves which pass through the posterior and anterior ethmoidal foramina.

D. Exposure of ciliary ganglion and common tendinous ring.

1. *With the help of your teacher*, locate the very delicate short ciliary nerves as they surround the optic nerve while going toward the eyeball (**Fig. 14.3**). Your teacher will help you locate the pinhead ciliary ganglion by tracing one of the short ciliary nerves backward. Short ciliary nerves come out of the ciliary ganglion and innervate the smooth muscles of the iris and ciliary body. Ciliary ganglion is a parasympathetic ganglion located between the optic nerve and the lateral rectus, about 1 cm in front of the apex of the orbit (refer to **Fig. 14.3**). Learn about the ganglion from the textbook.

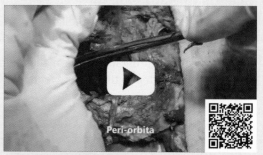

Video 14.3   Orbit: extraocular eye muscles and neurovascular structures.

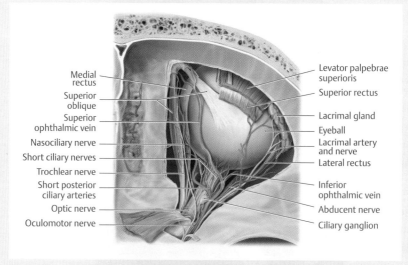

Fig. 14.3   Dissection of the orbit showing the ciliary ganglion and structures crossing the optic nerve. (From: Schuenke M, Schulte E, Schumacher U. THIEME Atlas of Anatomy. Head, Neck, and Neuroanatomy. Illustrations by Voll M and Wesker K. © Thieme 2020.)

2. Identify the branches of the ophthalmic artery.

3. Trace the optic nerve posteriorly as it comes out of the optic canal. Divide the optic nerve close to the canal and reflect it forward with the eyeball. Clean the inferior rectus and medial rectus muscles. Follow all the recti backward and note their origin from the common tendinous ring.

E. Dissection of lacrimal gland and exposure of attachment of tendons of recti on sclera.

1. At the superolateral angle of the orbit near the roof, dissect the area to find the lacrimal gland in the lacrimal fossa (refer to **Fig. 14.3**). We have already seen its anterior part from the anterior side while dissecting the lacrimal apparatus (refer to **Chapter 4**).

2. Give a horizontal cut in the orbital septum near the inferior orbital margin and expose with blunt dissection the inferior oblique muscle (**Fig. 14.4**).

3. Pull this muscle forward and locate the inferior division of the oculomotor nerve innervating it. Also, locate the nerve supply of the medial and inferior rectus muscles (**Fig. 14.4a**).

4. To expose the attachment of tendons of four recti on sclera, give a circular incision on the conjunctiva and facial sheath covering the sclera, close to the sclerocorneal junction. Reflect the conjunctiva and bulbar fascia backward on the eyeball. This will expose the attachments of the flat tendons on the sclera a few millimeters behind the cornea. The tendons are flat and closely attached on the sclera; therefore, pass a probe between the sclera and tendon to lift them. In case you are not able to see the attachments satisfactorily, dissect the eye outside the orbital cavity. For this, you will have to divide the inferior oblique, inferior rectus, medial rectus, and tendon of superior oblique muscles. Pull the eyeball forward and remove it from the orbital cavity. Now trace the insertion of all the extraocular muscles on the sclera.

5. Give a cut in the bulbar fascia and pass a probe between the bulbar fascia and sclera to see the space between the two.

6. Keep the eyeball in a preservative solution for dissection later.

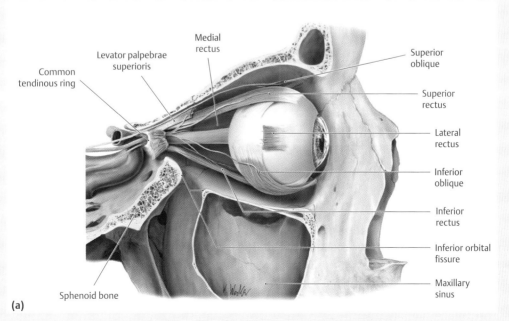

Fig. 14.4   Extraocular muscle of the right eye: **(a)** lateral view. *(Continued)*

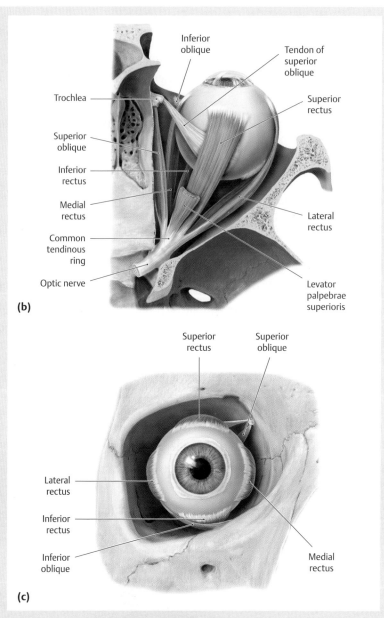

Fig. 14.4 *(Continued)* **(b)** Superior view. Extraocular muscle of the right eye: **(c)** anterior view. (From: Schuenke M, Schulte E, Schumacher U. THIEME Atlas of Anatomy. Head, Neck, and Neuroanatomy. Illustrations by Voll M and Wesker K. © Thieme 2020.)

Lacrimal Gland

The lacrimal gland is about the size and shape of an almond. It is located in a shallow orbital fossa in the anterolateral part of the roof of the orbit. The lacrimal gland consists of orbital and palpebral parts. The palpebral part extends in the upper eyelid inferior to the LPS, while the orbital part is situated deep in the lacrimal fossa superior to the LPS. Both the parts are continuous with each other at the lateral border of the LPS. The gland drains in the superior conjunctival fornix by about 15 ducts. All the ducts of the gland originate only through the palpebral part.

The secretomotor fibers of gland are supplied by the parasympathetic nerve derived from the greater petrosal branch of the facial nerve after relay in pterygopalatine ganglion. The general sensations are carried by the lacrimal nerve, a branch of the ophthalmic division of cranial nerve V. Blood is supplied by the lacrimal branch of the ophthalmic artery.

Extraocular Muscles

The extraocular muscles (**Table 14.1**) are four recti (superior, inferior, medial, and lateral), two oblique muscles (superior and inferior), and LPS. The origin, insertion, nerve supply, and actions of these muscles are given in **Table 14.1** and their actions are shown in **Fig. 14.5**.

Table 14.1   Extraocular muscles

Muscle	Origin	Insertion	Nerve supply	Action
Medial rectus	Common tendinous ring which encloses a part of the superior orbital fissure	On the sclera about 6 mm behind the limbus (sclerocorneal junction)	Inferior division of the oculomotor nerve (third nerve)	Adduction (medial deviation)
Lateral rectus	Common tendinous ring which encloses a part of the superior orbital fissure	On the sclera about 7 mm behind the limbus	Abducens nerve	Abduction
Superior rectus	Common tendinous ring which encloses a part of the superior orbital fissure	On the sclera about 8 mm behind the limbus	Superior division of the oculomotor nerve (third nerve)	Adduction, elevation, and intorsion
Inferior rectus	Common tendinous ring which encloses a part of the superior orbital fissure	On the sclera about 7 mm behind the limbus	Inferior division of the oculomotor nerve (third nerve)	Adduction, depression, and extorsion
Superior oblique	Medial and superior to the optic canal opening, from the body of the sphenoid	Upper lateral quadrant of the eyeball behind the equator	Trochlear nerve	Abduction, depression, and intorsion
Inferior oblique	From the floor of the orbit lateral to the opening of the nasolacrimal canal	Lateral part of the sclera deep to the lateral rectus muscle, behind the equator	Inferior division of the oculomotor nerve	Abduction, elevation, and extorsion
Levator palpebrae superioris	Above the opening of the optic canal, from the lesser wing of the sphenoid	Tarsal plate and skin of the eyelid	Superior division of the oculomotor nerve	Elevation of the upper eyelid

Summary of the action of muscles (**Fig. 14.5**):
- Adduction: MR/SR/IR.
- Abduction: LR/SO/IO.
- Depression: IR/SO.
- Elevation: SR/IO.
- Intorsion (medial rotation): SR/SO.
- Extorsion (lateral rotation): IR/IO.

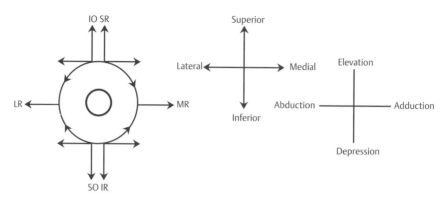

Fig. 14.5 Schematic diagram to show the actions of extraocular muscles. IO, inferior oblique; IR, inferior rectus; LR, lateral rectus; MR, medial rectus; SO, superior oblique; SR, superior rectus.

Nerves of the Orbit

The following nerves and ganglions are present in the orbit (**Fig. 14.6**):

1. Optic nerve.

2. Lacrimal, frontal, and nasociliary nerves.

3. Oculomotor, trochlear, and abducens nerve.

4. Ciliary ganglion.

Optic Nerve

Optic nerve (second cranial nerve) is the sensory nerve which originates in the retina and carries visual sensations to the brain. The nerve comes out of the sclera a short distance medial to the center of its posterior surface and runs posteromedially to the optic canal. Throughout its course in the orbit and the optic canal, it is surrounded by the three meninges—pia, arachnoid, and dura. Thus, the subarachnoid and subdural spaces reach up to the posterior surface of the eyeball.

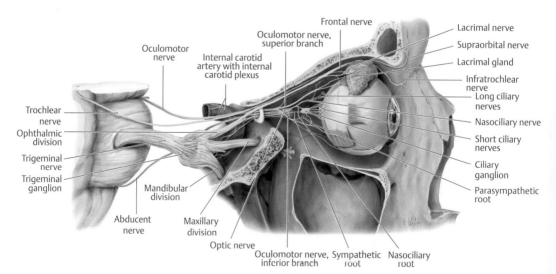

Fig. 14.6 Nerves of the orbit (right orbit, lateral view). (From: Schuenke M, Schulte E, Schumacher U. THIEME Atlas of Anatomy. Head, Neck, and Neuroanatomy. Illustrations by Voll M and Wesker K. © Thieme 2020.)

In the orbit, it is crossed by the superior ophthalmic vein, ophthalmic artery, and nasociliary nerve (refer to **Fig. 14.3**). The ciliary nerve and vessels surround the optic nerve near the eyeball.

Lacrimal Nerve

It is a branch of the ophthalmic nerve which enters the orbit through the lateral part of the superior orbital fissure. It runs above the lateral rectus muscle and innervates the sensory fibers to the lacrimal gland. It also receives the postganglionic parasympathetic fibers from the zygomatic nerve, which controls the secretion from the lacrimal gland (refer to **Fig. 14.3**). It also gives a palpebral branch to the lower eyelid.

Frontal Nerve

It is the direct continuation of the ophthalmic nerve. After entering the orbit through the superior orbital fissure, frontal nerve lies on the LPS deep to the periosteum. It divides into the supraorbital and supratrochlear branches in the orbit (refer to **Fig. 14.2**).

Supratrochlear nerve is the medial branch which runs toward the pulley of the superior oblique muscle. It leaves the orbit to run in the forehead. It supplies the sensory branches to the conjunctiva, upper eyelid, and skin of the forehead.

Supraorbital branch may further divide into medial and lateral branches that pass through the supraorbital notch or the foramen to the forehead (refer to **Fig. 14.2**). It innervates the skin of the forehead and scalp up to the vertex.

Nasociliary Nerve

It enters the orbit through the superior orbital fissure (within the common tendinous ring). It crosses the optic nerve from the lateral to the medial side. It lies close to the medial wall of the orbit between the superior oblique and medial rectus muscle. It ends by dividing into anterior ethmoidal and infratrochlear nerves. It gives a communicating branch to the ciliary ganglion and posterior ethmoidal and long ciliary branches (refer to **Fig. 14.3**).

Two *long ciliary nerves* pass to the eyeball on the medial side of the optic nerve. These fibers are sensory to the eyeball.

The *posterior ethmoidal nerve* passes through the posterior ethmoidal foramen in the medial wall of the orbit. It supplies the mucous membrane of the ethmoidal and sphenoidal air sinuses.

Infratrochlear nerve passes below the trochlea and innervates the eyelids and skin of the nose.

Anterior ethmoidal nerve leaves the orbit by the anterior ethmoidal foramen and after passing through the ethmoid sinus and anterior cranial fossa comes to the nasal cavity. It innervates the mucous membrane of the ethmoidal air sinuses, dura mater of the anterior cranial fossa, mucous membrane of the nose, and skin of the nose.

Oculomotor Nerve

It is the third cranial nerve which is predominantly a motor nerve. The two divisions of the oculomotor nerve (superior and inferior or upper and lower) enter the orbit through the superior orbital fissure (refer to **Fig. 14.6**) passing between the two heads of the lateral rectus muscle.

The *superior division* runs upward and passes through the SR to the LPS. The *inferior division* runs downward and innervates the medial rectus, inferior rectus, and inferior oblique muscles (refer to **Fig. 14.4a**). The nerve to the inferior oblique gives a communicating branch to the ciliary ganglion (**Fig. 14.6**). This communicating twig brings the parasympathetic fibers to the ciliary ganglion.

Trochlear Nerve

This is the fourth cranial nerve which innervates a single muscle, that is, the superior oblique. After entering through the superior orbital fissure, it runs medially to the superior oblique muscle (refer to **Fig. 14.2**).

Abducens Nerve

This nerve is the sixth cranial nerve. It lies between the two heads of the lateral rectus and runs forward on the medial surface of the lateral rectus to innervate it (refer to **Fig. 14.3**).

Ciliary Ganglion

This pinhead-sized ganglion is the collection of *postganglionic parasympathetic neurons* (refer to **Figs. 14.3** and **14.6**). It is located at the apex of the orbit in fatty tissues between the optic nerve and lateral rectus muscle. Thus, medially it is related to the optic nerve and laterally to the lateral rectus muscle. It has three different types of connections:

Parasympathetic: Preganglionic parasympathetic fibers arise from the Edinger–Westphal nucleus and after coming through the oculomotor nerve relay in the ciliary ganglion. The postganglionic fibers from this ganglion then pass as short ciliary nerves to the eyeball to innervate the sphincter pupillae and ciliary body.

Sensory: A branch from the nasociliary passes through the ganglion without relay and carries general sensation from the eye.

Sympathetic fibers: Postganglionic sympathetic fibers arise from the *superior cervical sympathetic ganglion* and pass through the ophthalmic artery to the ciliary ganglion. These fibers pass through the ganglion (without relay) to the dilator pupillae muscle through the short ciliary nerves.

About 6 to 10 *short ciliary nerves* take origin from the ganglion and pass along the optic nerve toward the eye. After further branching, they pierce the sclera around the entrance of the optic nerve (**Fig. 14.6**).

Arteries of the Orbit

The orbit contains two arteries which supply blood to the orbital structures and neighboring areas. These are:

1. *Ophthalmic artery*: Branch of the internal carotid artery (**Fig. 14.7**).
2. *Infraorbital artery*: Branch of the maxillary artery.

Ophthalmic Artery

The ophthalmic artery enters the orbit through the optic canal after arising from the internal carotid artery in the middle cranial fossa. In the optic canal, it runs inferolateral to the nerve within the meninges of the optic nerve. It then pierces the arachnoid and dural sheath to lie lateral to the nerve. Then it winds around the optic nerve and crosses it dorsally from the lateral to the medial side (**Fig. 14.7**). Now it runs along the medial orbital wall. Following are the branches of the ophthalmic artery:

Central artery of the retina: This artery runs within the optic nerve to reach the retina. It supplies blood to the retina. This is an end artery and any blockage results in blindness of the affected area of the retina.

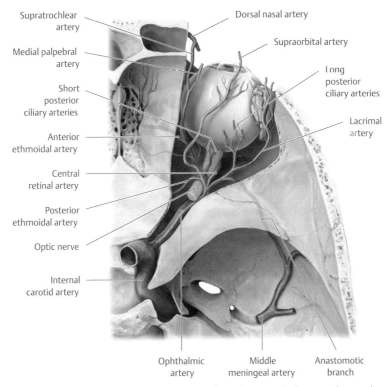

Fig. 14.7 Ophthalmic artery. (From: Schuenke M, Schulte E, Schumacher U. THIEME Atlas of Anatomy. Head, Neck, and Neuroanatomy. Illustrations by Voll M and Wesker K. © Thieme 2020.)

Lacrimal artery: This runs along the upper border of the lateral rectus and supplies blood to the lacrimal gland, conjunctiva, and eyelid.

Posterior ethmoidal: This enters the ethmoid air cells through the posterior ethmoidal foramen in the medial wall of the orbit. From here it reaches the anterior cranial fossa and then through the cribriform plate to the nasal cavity. It supplies blood to the ethmoidal air sinus, dura of anterior cranial fossa, and nasal mucosa.

Anterior ethmoidal: This enters the cranial cavity through the anterior ethmoidal foramen and ultimately comes out on the dorsum of the nose. It supplies blood to the ethmoidal sinuses, meninges, nasal mucosa, and skin of dorsum of the nose.

Short ciliary arteries: These are many in number and after their origin they enter the sclera near the optic nerve. These supply blood to the choroid and ciliary processes.

Supraorbital and supratrochlear: These branches come out of the orbit through the notch or foramen at the supraorbital margin. They supply blood to the skin and muscles of the forehead.

Dorsal nasal: It comes out of the orbit between the trochlea and medial palpebral ligament. It supplies blood to the skin of dorsum of the nose and lacrimal sac.

Medial palpebral arteries: They supply blood to the upper and lower eyelids.

Infraorbital Artery

This is the branch from the third part of the maxillary artery. After passing through the infraorbital fissure, it lies in the infraorbital groove, at the floor of the orbit. It emerges from the infraorbital foramen on the face.

Within the orbit it gives *anterosuperior alveolar* branches which supply the maxillary (upper) canine and incisors teeth. It also gives blood to the maxillary air sinus. In the orbit, it also gives a few unnamed branches which innervate a few infraorbital muscles and lacrimal sac. On the face, it supplies the skin of the lower eyelid, side of the nose, and cheeks.

Veins of the Orbit

Contents of the orbit and forehead are drained by two ophthalmic veins, that is, superior and inferior ophthalmic veins (**Fig. 14.8**). These veins drain into the cavernous sinus and have communication with other veins, plexus, and sinuses.

Structures Passing through the Superior Orbital Fissure

The superior orbital fissure is a gap between the greater and lesser wings of the sphenoid. Medially, it is bounded by the body of the sphenoid. It communicates with the middle cranial fossa (posteriorly) and orbit (anteriorly). At the fibrotendinous ring (which gives origin to the extraocular muscles), it is divided into upper lateral, middle, and lower medial parts. The following structures pass through its various parts (**Fig. 14.9**):

Upper lateral part: Recurrent meningeal branch of the ophthalmic artery, lacrimal, frontal, and trochlear nerves, and superior ophthalmic vein.

Middle part: The upper and lower divisions of the oculomotor, nasociliary, and abducens nerves.

Lower medial part: The inferior ophthalmic vein.

Structures Passing through the Inferior Orbital Fissure

It lies between the posterior wall of the maxilla and greater wing of the sphenoid. It communicates anterosuperiorly with the orbit, posterolaterally with the infratemporal fossa, and medially with the pterygopalatine fossa.

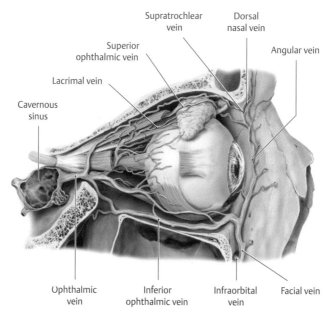

Fig. 14.8   Veins of the orbit (right orbit, lateral view). (From: Schuenke M, Schulte E, Schumacher U. THIEME Atlas of Anatomy. Head, Neck, and Neuroanatomy. Illustrations by Voll M and Wesker K. © Thieme 2020.)

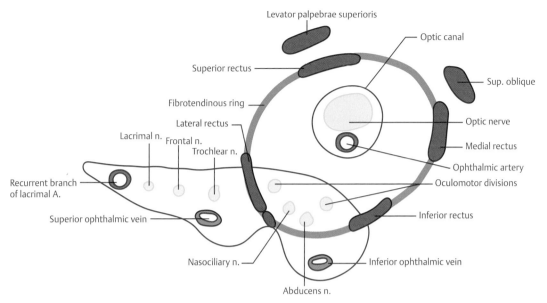

Fig. 14.9   Structures passing through the superior orbital fissure as seen through right orbit.

It gives passage to the maxillary nerve which becomes continuous as the infraorbital nerve, zygomatic nerve, infratemporal artery, and vein. It also gives passage to the communicating channel between the inferior ophthalmic vein and pterygoid plexus of veins.

Structures Passing through the Optic Canal

The structures passing through the optic canal are as follows (**Fig. 14.9**):

1. Optic nerve.

2. Ophthalmic artery.

Both these structures are surrounded by the meninges.

▌ Clinical Notes
Extraocular Muscles' Paralysis due to Lesion of the Cranial Nerves

1. The lesion of the oculomotor nerve produces paralysis of the muscles and the upper eyelid supplied by it.

   a. *Ptosis* due to paralysis of the upper eyelid. The eyelid cannot be elevated.

   b. Lateral squint due to unopposed action of the lateral rectus (and almost complete ophthalmoplegia).

   c. Dilation of the pupil and loss of accommodation reflex.

2. The lesion of the trochlear nerve produces diplopia, while the lesion of the abducens nerve produces medial squint and diplopia.

3. If sympathetic innervation of the eyeball is involved, it will cause *Horner syndrome*. It is characterized by:

   a. Slight partial drooping of the upper eyelid (due to paralysis of the Müller muscle [smooth muscle component of LPS]).

b. Constriction of the pupil (miosis) due to unopposed action of the parasympathetic supply.

c. Dry face (anhidrosis) due to loss of sweating on the affected side.

d. Flushed hot face due to vasoconstriction on the affected side.

e. Enophthalmos, that is, sunken eyeball.

4. The central artery of the retina is an end artery. Blockage of the central artery of the retina leads to blindness as it is the only artery supplying the retina.

5. The medial wall and floor of the orbit are thin; hence, cancer and infections from the ethmoidal and maxillary sinus may spread to the orbit.

15 Deep Dissection of the Neck—I: Thyroid Gland

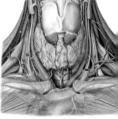

© THIEME Atlas of Anatomy

Introduction

The deep part of the cervical region is clinically very important as it contains many important structures such as the larynx and trachea, pharynx and esophagus, and glands, such as thyroid and parathyroid. The thyroid and parathyroid glands are located deep to the infrahyoid muscles, while the larynx and trachea are located posterior to these glands. On either side, the thyroid gland lies close to the carotid sheath, which contains the carotid artery, internal jugular vein, and vagus nerve. Thyroid gland is richly supplied with vessels, which also form its immediate relation.

Surface Landmarks

1. Once again, review the bony features of the hyoid bone, sternum, and the medial end of the clavicle.

2. On a living person, in the midline from above downward, palpate the hyoid bone, laryngeal prominence of the thyroid cartilage, cricoid cartilage, isthmus of the thyroid gland, and trachea just above the sternal notch.

3. Also, palpate the sternoclavicular joint. Note the origin of the sternal head of the sternomastoid muscle.

Dissection and Identification

We have already studied the infrahyoid group of muscles and sternocleidomastoid muscle and their nerve supply while dissecting the triangles of the neck (refer to **Chapter 7**).

A. Dissection to expose the thyroid gland.

1. Displace the sternomastoid muscle laterally and transect the superior belly of the omohyoid near its attachment to the hyoid bone and reflect it downward.

2. Similarly, cut the sternohyoid and sternothyroid muscles from above and reflect them downward toward the sternum.

3. Transect the thyrohyoid muscle from below and reflect it upward toward the hyoid bone.

4. Look for the superior root of the ansa cervicalis deep to the sternomastoid muscle.

5. Clean the fat and connective tissues from an area just above the sternal notch. You shall find the *inferior thyroid veins* on the anterior surface of the *trachea* (**Fig. 15.1**). Find the upper end of the lobes of the atrophied thymus, the major part of which lies in the thoracic cavity.

B. Exposure of recurrent laryngeal nerve, thoracic duct, superior laryngeal nerve and blood vessels of thyroid gland (Video 15.1).

1. After cleaning the trachea, lift the lower part of the gland gently to clean the lateral aspect of the trachea and esophagus. With the help of a forceps, clean the space between the trachea and esophagus; you shall find the recurrent laryngeal nerve. This nerve is going upward to supply the larynx.

2. Similarly, on the left side find the thoracic duct coming from behind the esophagus.

3. Now remove the fascia from the right and left lobes of the thyroid. Two lobes are connected by the isthmus which crosses the anterior aspect of the second and third tracheal rings. Sometimes, a pyramidal lobe is present on the isthmus of the gland (**Fig. 15.1**).

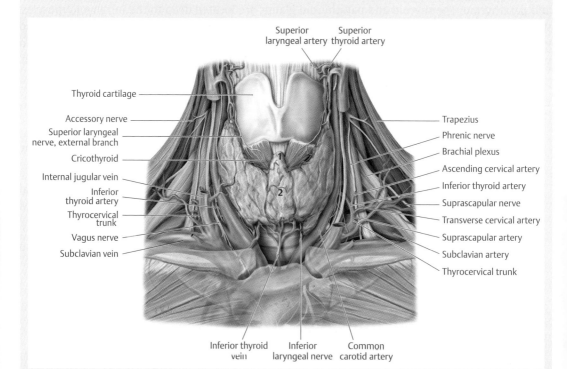

Fig. 15.1 Deep dissection of the neck showing the thyroid gland and associated nerves and vessels. 1, Pyramidal lobe; 2, isthmus. (From: Schuenke M, Schulte E, Schumacher U. THIEME Atlas of Anatomy. Head, Neck, and Neuroanatomy. Illustrations by Voll M and Wesker K. © Thieme 2020.)

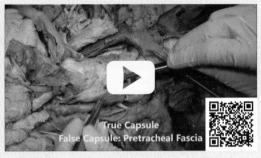

Video 15.1 Thyroid gland and its relations.

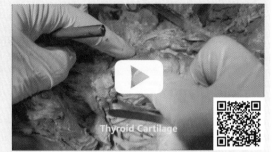

Video 15.2 Larynx and trachea.

4. Now expose the blood vessels of the gland.

5. Identify the superior thyroid, inferior thyroid, thyroid ima, and superior laryngeal arteries and superior, middle, and inferior thyroid veins (**Figs. 15.1** and **15.2**).

6. Identify the superior laryngeal, external laryngeal, internal laryngeal, and recurrent laryngeal nerves.

7. Give a midline cut in the isthmus of the gland and reflect the cut ends laterally on either side to expose the tracheal rings. Now pull the lobes further laterally, on either side, to expose the groove between the trachea and esophagus containing the recurrent laryngeal nerve. The nerve passes immediately posterior to the lobe of the thyroid gland.

C. Dissection of parathyroid gland (Video 15.2).

1. On one side (either left or right side), cut all the blood vessels (entering or leaving) the lobe.

2. With the help of blunt dissection, free the lobe from the connective tissues and remove it.

3. Identify two parathyroid glands on the posterior surface of this lobe, with the help of the hand lens. These are yellowish-brown tiny structures embedded in the capsule of the thyroid gland.

4. Examine the trachea and esophagus in midline from the larynx to the root of the neck, as they disappear behind the sternum.

Note: The thymus is present in a child till the age of puberty. At puberty, it gets atrophied and is replaced by fibrofatty tissues. It consists of two lobes and lies anterior to the pericardium in the thorax. It also covers great vessels at the root of the neck and thus may extend in the lower part of the neck. Thymus is an important lymphoid organ in which occurs the differentiation of T lymphocytes.

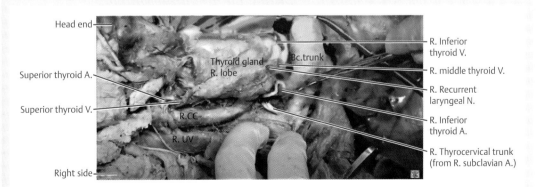

Fig. 15.2 Inferior thyroid artery.

Glands of the Region

The thyroid and parathyroid are two endocrine glands of this region, which are interposed between the infrahyoid muscles and larynx and trachea.

Thyroid Gland

Thyroid is an endocrine gland. It is located in the neck deep to the infrahyoid muscles and superficial to the larynx and trachea. It extends from the oblique line of the thyroid cartilage to the sixth tracheal ring. Thus, it lies opposite to the level from the fifth cervical vertebra to the first thoracic vertebra.

The pretracheal layer of the deep cervical fascia forms a sheath to enclose the gland. Sometimes, this sheath is known as the false capsule of the gland as the true capsule of the gland is formed by the condensation of the fibrous connective tissue on the surface of the gland. Between true and false capsules lie the arteries and veins. The pretracheal layer (false capsule) of the gland is thickened where it is attached to the oblique line of the thyroid cartilage and to the arch of the cricoid cartilage. This thickening is known as *ligament of Berry*. Because of this reason the gland moves with the movements of the larynx, as in the case of swallowing.

The gland consists of right and left lateral lobes, which are joined together by a narrow isthmus (**Fig. 15.3**). The isthmus lies in front of the second and third tracheal rings. Each lobe is conical in shape and triangular on section. Apex of the gland lies at the oblique line undercover of the sternothyroid muscle. Thus, each lobe has a superficial surface, a medial and a posterior surface. The superficial surface of the lobe is covered by the sternohyoid, sternothyroid, omohyoid muscles, and sternomastoid. Sternomastoid lies superficial to these infrahyoid muscles. The medial surface of the lobe is related superiorly to the inferior constrictor and cricothyroid muscles with the external laryngeal nerve. Below, the medial surface is related to the trachea and esophagus with the recurrent laryngeal nerve. Posterior surface is related to the structures of the carotid sheath, inferior thyroid artery, and parathyroid glands (**Fig. 15.4**).

Pyramidal lobe is an elongated conical mass of the glandular tissue. It is occasionally present on the isthmus of the gland. The pyramidal lobe extends toward the hyoid bone as a fibrous strand (levator glandulae thyroideae), which is the remnant of the thyroglossal duct.

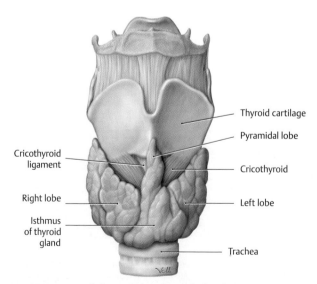

Fig. 15.3 Parts/lobes of the thyroid gland. (From: Schuenke M, Schulte E, Schumacher U. THIEME Atlas of Anatomy. Head, Neck, and Neuroanatomy. Illustrations by Voll M and Wesker K. © Thieme 2020.)

Arteries of Thyroid Gland

Thyroid gland is usually supplied by two arteries, that is, superior thyroid and inferior thyroid arteries (**Fig. 15.5**). An occasional small artery (thyroid ima) which arises from the brachiocephalic trunk may also supply the isthmic part of the gland. The superior thyroid is a branch from the external carotid artery. After reaching the apex of the gland, it divides into anterior and posterior branches. Anterior branch anastomoses with the artery of opposite side at the upper border of isthmus in midline. The posterior branch runs down on the back of the lobe. The inferior thyroid artery is the branch from the thyrocervical trunk and supplies the major part of the gland (lower two-thirds of the lateral lobe).

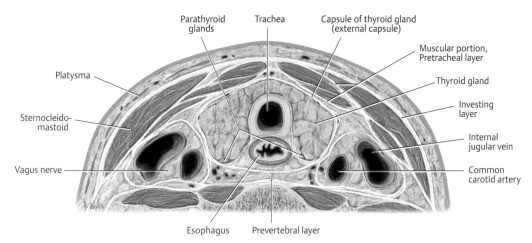

Fig. 15.4 Relationship of the thyroid gland with the trachea, esophagus, and neurovascular structures. (From: Schuenke M, Schulte E, Schumacher U. THIEME Atlas of Anatomy. Head, Neck, and Neuroanatomy. Illustrations by Voll M and Wesker K. © Thieme 2020.)

Veins of Thyroid Gland

The veins of the thyroid form a venous plexus just beneath the true capsule of the gland. From this plexus veins arise. The venous drainage of the thyroid is through three pairs of veins, that is, superior, middle and inferior thyroid veins (**Fig. 15.6**). The superior and middle thyroid veins drain to the internal jugular vein, while the inferior vein drains to the brachiocephalic vein.

Nerves of Thyroid Gland

The sympathetic innervation of the gland comes from the middle and inferior cervical sympathetic ganglia. These fibers supply the vessels of the gland. The parasympathetic innervation probably comes from the vagus through the recurrent laryngeal nerve (**Fig. 15.5**).

Lymphatic Drainage of Thyroid Gland

Lymphatic drainage of the gland mostly goes to the small nodes on the surface of the gland or on the trachea. From here, lymph is drained to the deep cervical groups of the lymph nodes.

Parathyroid Glands

These are small endocrine glands present on the posterior surface of the thyroid gland (**Figs. 15.4** and **15.8**). Usually, they are four (two pairs) in number, one pair in each lobe. Each measures about 6 × 4 × 2 mm and are embedded in the capsule of the thyroid gland. Superior parathyroid is present about the middle of the posterior surface, while inferior parathyroid is variable in position and may be present close to the inferior end.

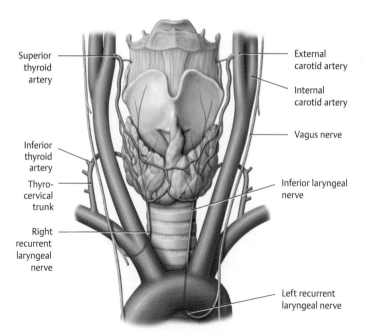

Fig. 15.5   Arteries supplying the thyroid gland. (From: Schuenke M, Schulte E, Schumacher U. THIEME Atlas of Anatomy. Head, Neck, and Neuroanatomy. Illustrations by Voll M and Wesker K. © Thieme 2020.)

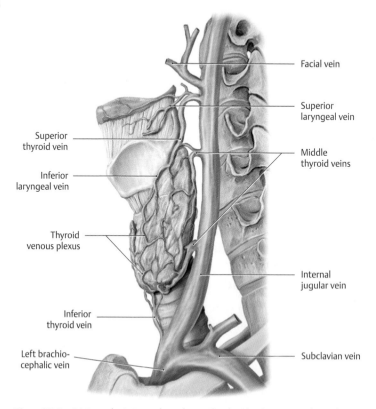

Fig. 15.6   Veins draining the thyroid gland. (From: Schuenke M, Schulte E, Schumacher U. THIEME Atlas of Anatomy. Head, Neck, and Neuroanatomy. Illustrations by Voll M and Wesker K. © Thieme 2020.)

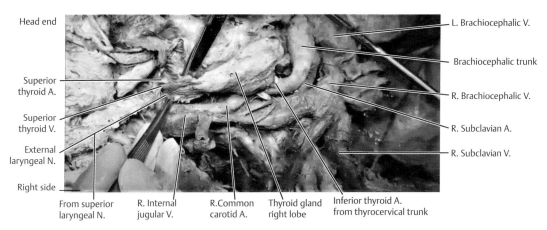

Head end
L. Brachiocephalic V.
Brachiocephalic trunk
Superior thyroid A.
R. Brachiocephalic V.
Superior thyroid V.
R. Subclavian A.
External laryngeal N.
R. Subclavian V.
Right side

From superior laryngeal N. | R. Internal jugular V. | R.Common carotid A. | Thyroid gland right lobe | Inferior thyroid A. from thyrocervical trunk

Fig. 15.7   Thyroid gland and associated neurovasculature structures.

The upper parathyroid is supplied by the superior and inferior thyroid arteries. The inferior parathyroid is supplied by the inferior thyroid artery. The tracheal arteries may also supply both the parathyroids. The gland secretes the parathyroid hormone, which regulates the calcium metabolism.

Cervical Part of the Trachea and Esophagus

The trachea is placed anterior to the esophagus. Both these structures begin at the level of the cricoid cartilage anterior to the sixth cervical vertebra. Both of them descend into the thorax by passing posteriorly to the sternum.

Trachea: The cervical part of the trachea is about 7 cm in length. It is a tubular structure with flattened posterior wall. Its lumen is always kept open by the C-shaped cartilaginous incomplete rings. Posteriorly, these rings are deficient; therefore, its posterior wall is flattened.

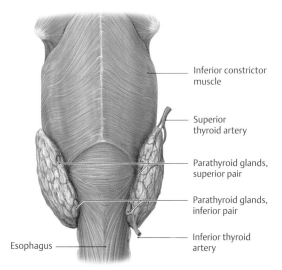

Inferior constrictor muscle

Superior thyroid artery

Parathyroid glands, superior pair

Parathyroid glands, inferior pair

Esophagus

Inferior thyroid artery

Fig. 15.8   Thyroid and parathyroid glands (posterior view). (From: Schuenke M, Schulte E, Schumacher U. THIEME Atlas of Anatomy. Head, Neck, and Neuroanatomy. Illustrations by Voll M and Wesker K. © Thieme 2020.)

Anteriorly, the cervical trachea is in relation with the isthmus of the thyroid gland, anastomosis of the two superior thyroid arteries, inferior thyroid veins, anterior jugular vein, and jugular arch. All these structures are covered by the infrahyoid muscles.

Laterally, the trachea is in relation with the medial surface of the thyroid gland, inferior thyroid artery, and common carotid artery within the carotid sheath.

Posteriorly, the trachea is in relation with the esophagus and is in contact with the recurrent laryngeal nerve (**Fig. 15.4**).

It is supplied by the branches of the inferior thyroid artery and drains to the inferior thyroid vein. The trachea is innervated by both the sympathetic (middle cervical ganglion) and parasympathetic (vagus) nerves.

Esophagus: The cervical part of the esophagus, similar to the trachea, extends from the lower end of the pharynx, which lies at the level of the sixth cervical vertebra and cricoid cartilage to the level of the sternal notch.

Anteriorly, the esophagus is related to the trachea and recurrent laryngeal nerve.

Posteriorly, it is related to the vertebral column, longus colli muscles, and prevertebral fascia. The thoracic duct is on the left side near the lower end of the cervical part of the esophagus.

Laterally, it is related to the lobes of the thyroid and carotid sheath.

Blood for the cervical part of the esophagus comes from the inferior thyroid artery and it drains in the inferior thyroid vein.

▊ Clinical Notes
Thyroid Gland

1. *Direction of enlargement of the gland*: The pretracheal fascia, posterior and inferior to the thyroid gland, is very thin. The sternothyroid muscle after covering the thyroid is attached to the thyroid cartilage. Therefore, the gland can only enlarge in backward or downward directions.

2. *Anatomical considerations during thyroid surgery*: During the surgical removal of the thyroid gland (thyroidectomy) ligation of thyroid arteries and veins is compulsory. The thyroid is richly supplied with blood and there is the presence of venous plexus just beneath the true capsule. Any injury to the vessel would lead to severe bleeding. The main trunks of the artery and veins are safely ligated outside the true capsule (i.e., between true and false capsules). An injury to the true capsule will lead to severe bleeding. Also, arteries of the thyroid are closely related to the nerves of the larynx; therefore, before cutting the vessels these nerves should be preserved.

3. *Ligation of the superior thyroid artery*: The external laryngeal nerve and superior thyroid artery run close to each other before the artery lies close to the apex of the lateral lobe (**Fig. 15.9**).

   Therefore, to avoid injury to the nerve, the artery is ligated very close to the gland and then cut. The external laryngeal nerve is concerned with the pitch of the voice.

4. *Ligation of the inferior thyroid artery*: The inferior thyroid artery is closely related to the recurrent laryngeal nerve very close to the gland (**Fig. 15.9**). Hence, this artery is ligated away from the gland before cutting. Injury to the recurrent laryngeal nerve leads to huskiness of the voice.

5. *Thyroglossal cyst or sinus*: It may be seen as a swelling in midline along the course of the duct, usually below the hyoid bone. This can be removed surgically.

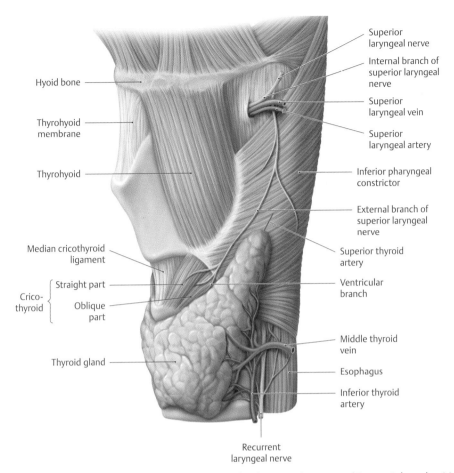

Fig. 15.9 Relationship of the arteries with the laryngeal nerves. (From: Schuenke M, Schulte E, Schumacher U. THIEME Atlas of Anatomy. Head, Neck, and Neuroanatomy. Illustrations by Voll M and Wesker K. © Thieme 2020.)

6. *Preservation of the parathyroid glands at the time of thyroidectomy*: Thyroid gland is removed only after leaving its small posterior part, which contains the parathyroid. Its accidental removal with the thyroid leads to hypoparathyroidism.

Trachea

Tracheotomy: In this surgical procedure, an artificial opening is made surgically, below or above the isthmus of the thyroid gland. It is a life-saving procedure after laryngeal obstruction. While performing the tracheotomy below the isthmus (low tracheotomy), care should be taken of the vessels in front of the trachea.

16 Deep Dissection of the Neck—II: Structures under Cover of the Sternocleidomastoid and Posterior Belly of Digastric

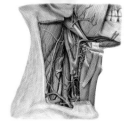

© THIEME Atlas of Anatomy

Learning Objectives

At the end of the deep dissection of the neck (structures under cover of the sternocleido-mastoid and posterior belly of the digastric muscle), you should be able to identify the following:

- Accessory nerve as it is crossed by the deep surface of the sternomastoid muscle.
- Hypoglossal nerve as it lies deep to the posterior belly of the digastric muscle.
- Occipital and posterior auricular arteries.
- Superior and inferior roots of the ansa cervicalis.
- External and internal branches of the superior laryngeal nerves.
- Contents of the carotid sheath—common and internal carotid artery, internal jugular vein, and vagus nerve.
- Bifurcation of the common carotid artery into external and internal carotids/carotid body.

Introduction

We have already seen the superficial contents of the digastric and carotid triangles. However, many structures were not seen clearly and completely as they were hidden under the cover of the posterior belly of the digastric and sternomastoid muscles. In this dissection, we shall reflect the sternomastoid and posterior belly of the digastric muscle to see many deeper structures which are situated deep to the *upper and middle* parts of the sternomastoid. Structures deep to the lower part of the sternomastoid are present at the *root of the neck*. Structures at the *root of the neck* will be studied in the next dissection (Chapter 18). Similarly, structures at the *base of the skull* (i.e., cranial nerves IX, X, XI, and XII, internal carotid and upper end of internal jugular veins, stylo-pharyngeus, superior constrictor, and styloglossus muscles) will be dissected later.

In the upper part, sternomastoid muscle lies on the posterior belly of the digastric, levator scapu-lae, and splenius capitis muscles. In the upper part, it also covers the cervical plexus and is in relation to the deep cervical group of the lymph nodes.

The middle part of the muscle lies on the carotid sheath, ansa cervicalis, the bifurcation of the common carotid artery and commencement of the external and internal carotid arteries, and brachial plexus. The sympathetic trunk lies posterior to the carotid sheath.

Surface Landmarks

On a dry skull, see the site of attachment of the posterior belly of the digastric muscle at the mastoid groove. Also, review the attachments of greater cornu of the hyoid bone. Review the two heads of origin (from clavicle and sternum) and insertion (on the mastoid process) of the sterno-mastoid muscle in a living person.

Dissection and Identification

A. Exposure of structures under cover of sternomastoid.

1. Give a cut in the clavicular and sternal heads of origin of the sternomastoid muscle, about an inch above their origin. Reflect the sternomastoid muscle by carefully dissecting it from its covering of the investing layer of the deep fascia. Reflect it upward till the mastoid process.

2. Remove the three tributaries of the internal jugular vein (common facial vein, superior and middle thyroid veins) from the field as they may interfere with the dissection (**Fig. 16.1**).

3. Identify the accessory nerve as it lies deep to its undersurface below the mastoid process. Trace the accessory nerve superiorly as far as possible. We shall see its exit from the jugular foramen in a later dissection (**Fig. 16.2**).

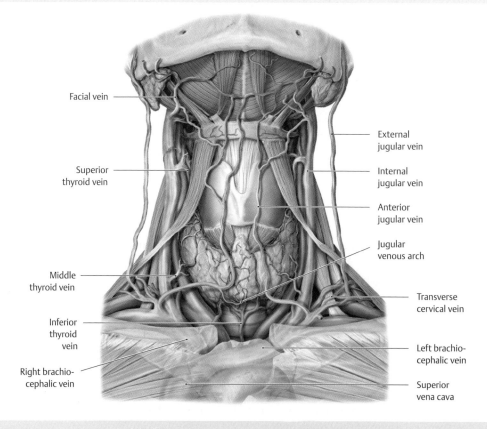

Fig. 16.1 Cervical veins (anterior view). (From: Schuenke M, Schulte E, Schumacher U. THIEME Atlas of Anatomy. Head, Neck, and Neuroanatomy. Illustrations by Voll M and Wesker K. © Thieme 2020.)

4. Identify the branches of the cervical plexus at the posterior border of the sternomastoid muscle and trace these branches toward the cervical vertebral column.

5. Now identify the upper and lower border of the posterior belly of the digastric muscle. Look for the occipital branch of the external carotid artery on its inferior border and posterior auricular artery on its superior border.

6. If you can save these two arteries, it is good, otherwise detach the digastric muscle from its attachment on the mastoid groove and reflect it downward toward the intermediate tendon along with both the arteries.

7. Look for many large lymph nodes lying on the surface of the carotid sheath. The jugulodigastric and jugulo-omohyoid groups are in relation to the posterior belly of the digastric and inferior belly of the omohyoid, respectively.

B. Dissection of hypoglossal nerve, ansa cervicalis, carotid sheath (Video 16.1).

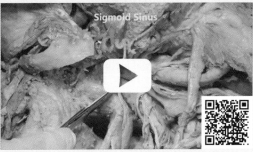

1. Just above the tip of the greater cornu of hyoid bone, find the hypoglossal nerve. Also, trace the nerve to the thyrohyoid muscle as it is given when the hypoglossal nerve lies on hyoglossus muscle (**Fig. 16.4**).

Video 16.1   Cranial nerves X, XI, XII and ansa cervicalis in neck.

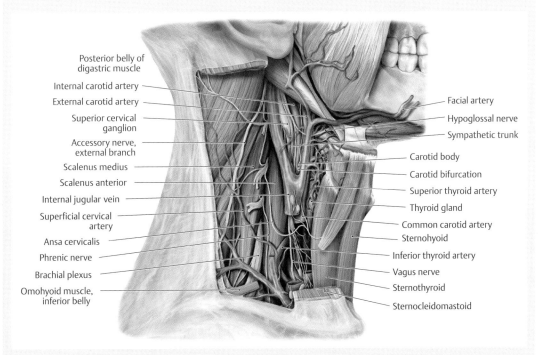

Fig. 16.2   Deep dissection of the neck showing structures under cover of sternocleidomastoid. (From: Schuenke M, Schulte E, Schumacher U. THIEME Atlas of Anatomy. Head, Neck, and Neuroanatomy. Illustrations by Voll M and Wesker K. © Thieme 2020.)

2. Follow the hypoglossal nerve backward to locate the superior root of the ansa cervicalis, which travels along with the hypoglossal nerve. More laterally on the carotid sheath, find the inferior root of the ansa cervicalis. See the loop formed by joining both the roots (**Figs. 16.2–16.4**).

3. We have already exposed the contents of the carotid sheath in the carotid triangle. Extend the incision on the sheath upward as far as possible and downward up to the root of the neck. Use blunt dissection to separate the internal jugular vein from the common carotid and internal carotid artery. We have already seen three important tributaries (common facial vein, superior and inferior thyroid veins) of the internal jugular vein.

4. Once again, review the bifurcation of the common carotid artery at the level of the upper border of the thyroid cartilage. Identify the carotid body and carotid sinus at the bifurcation of the common carotid artery.

5. The branches of the external carotid artery have already been explained in the carotid triangle and posterior auricular branch at the superior border of the digastric muscle before detaching it from its attachment on the mastoid. We have also seen its two terminal branches in relation to the parotid gland.

6. At the posterior border of the thyrohyoid muscle, search for the internal laryngeal nerve and superior laryngeal artery piercing the thyrohyoid membrane.

C. Dissection of cricothyroid muscle, external laryngeal nerve, and sympathetic trunk

1. Deep to the lateral lobe of the thyroid gland, search for the cricothyroid muscle and inferior constrictor of the pharynx. On their surface, find the external laryngeal nerve which innervates the cricothyroid muscle (**Fig. 15.9**). Now follow both the external and internal laryngeal nerves backward and upward; they will join together to form the superior laryngeal nerve. Superior laryngeal nerve is a branch of the vagus, which lies below the base of the skull, at a higher level. We shall dissect it later.

2. Pull the carotid arteries anteromedially and find the sympathetic trunk posterior to the carotid sheath.

Muscles

(Note: In this dissection, we have seen that there lie many muscles deep to the sternomastoid, that is, posterior belly of the digastric, stylohyoid, splenius capitis, and levator scapulae. We have studied these muscles in Chapters 6 and 7. Similarly, in this area of dissection we have also exposed constrictors of the pharynx and cricothyroid muscle. We shall study these muscles later when we dissect the pharynx and larynx.)

Carotid Sheath

The major part of the carotid sheath is under the cover of the sternomastoid muscle. The carotid sheath is the facial sheath which encloses the internal jugular vein, carotid arteries (common carotid and internal carotid), and vagus nerve. The internal jugular vein lies lateral to the artery. Within the sheath, up to the level of the upper border of the thyroid cartilage, common carotid artery lies medial to the internal jugular vein. At this level, the artery divides into external and internal carotid. Above this level, the internal carotid artery lies medial to the internal jugular vein, while the external jugular artery comes out of the carotid sheath.

On the anterior surface of the carotid sheath, there are lymph nodes and roots of the ansa cervicalis, while posteromedially to the carotid sheath lies the sympathetic trunk.

Arteries

(We have already studied the terminal branches of the external carotid [maxillary and superficial temporal] during the dissection of the parotid gland and all others [except the posterior auricular] during the dissection of the carotid triangle.)

Posterior auricular: It arises from the external carotid artery above the level of posterior belly of the digastric muscle and runs upward and posteriorly to ends near the base of the mastoid process. Its branches are parotid, auricular, occipital, and stylomastoid arteries.

Carotid sinus: It is a dilatation at the upper end of the common carotid artery and at the beginning of the internal carotid artery. The sinus is innervated by the branches of the glossopharyngeal nerve. It acts as a blood pressure receptor. Increase in blood pressure leads to the stimulation of the glossopharyngeal nerve which reflexly stimulates the vagus nerve, leading to a fall in blood pressure and slowing of the heart rate.

Carotid body: It is a small mass of cells which acts as chemoreceptor monitoring the concentration of oxygen within the arterial blood. The carotid body is present posterior to the bifurcation of the common carotid artery. Fall in the oxygen level of blood leads to the stimulation of the carotid body which reflexly produces the rise in blood pressure, heart rate, and changes in depth and rate of respiration.

Veins

Four tributaries of the internal jugular vein are seen deep to the sternomastoid.

Lingual vein: It is formed at the posterior border of the hyoglossus muscle. It crosses the carotid arteries and ends in the internal jugular vein. Sometimes, it may also join the facial vein.

Common facial vein: The facial vein first crosses the posterior belly of the digastric and then unites with the anterior branch of the retromandibular vein to form the common facial vein. After crossing the carotid arteries, it joins the internal jugular vein (refer to **Fig. 16.1**).

Superior and middle thyroid veins: The superior thyroid vein may join the facial vein; otherwise, both superior and middle veins open in the internal jugular vein.

(We shall study the internal jugular vein after it is completely dissected at the root of the neck and the base of the skull.)

Nerves

Ansa Cervicalis

Ansa cervicalis is a nerve loop which lies in the carotid triangle in front of the carotid sheath (common carotid artery). It is formed by two roots (refer to **Figs. 16.2–16.4**):

1. *Superior root*: It arises from the hypoglossal nerve. However, in the true sense, it is not the branch of the hypoglossal nerve but is made up of fibers arising from the first cervical (C1) spinal nerve. These fibers of the spinal nerve run with the hypoglossal nerve for some distance and form the superior root and also supply motor fibers to the thyrohyoid and geniohyoid muscles.

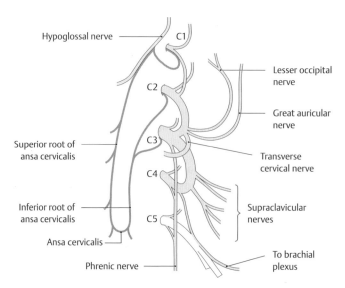

Fig. 16.3 Cervical plexus and ansa cervicalis. (From: Schuenke M, Schulte E, Schumacher U. THIEME Atlas of Anatomy. Head, Neck, and Neuroanatomy. Illustrations by Voll M and Wesker K. © Thieme 2020.)

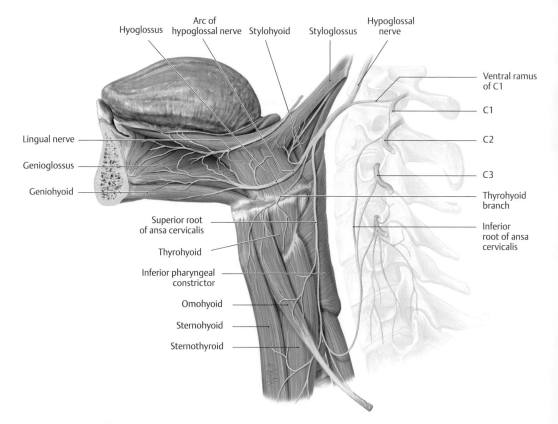

Fig. 16.4 Hypoglossal nerve (CN XII) and ansa cervicalis (left lateral view). (From: Schuenke M, Schulte E, Schumacher U. THIEME Atlas of Anatomy. Head, Neck, and Neuroanatomy. Illustrations by Voll M and Wesker K. © Thieme 2020.)

2. *Inferior root*: It arises from the ventral rami of C2 and C3 spinal nerves. It descends superficially into the internal jugular vein and then joins the superior root at the level of common carotid artery.

Branches arising from the ansa cervicalis supply motor fibers to the infrahyoid group of muscles, that is, the superior belly of the omohyoid, sternohyoid, and sternothyroid, and the inferior belly of the omohyoid.

Lymph Nodes

Deep cervical groups of lymph nodes are vertically arranged around the carotid sheath from the base of the skull to the root of the neck, deep to the sternocleidomastoid muscle (refer to **Figs. 7.6** and **11.8**). They drain to the superficial groups of the cervical lymph nodes and deeper tissues of the head and neck. They are divided into jugulodigastric (upper) and jugulo-omohyoid (lower) deep cervical groups.

Jugulodigastric (upper or superior) nodes: These lymph nodes are present on the carotid sheath where it is crossed by the posterior belly of the digastric muscle. They drain the cranial cavity, infratemporal fossa, parotid and submandibular nodes, tonsil, pharynx and root of tongue, etc. These nodes drain to the inferior deep cervical group of the nodes.

Jugulo-omohyoid (lower or inferior) nodes: These lymph nodes are present on the carotid sheath where it is crossed by the omohyoid muscle. They drain the superior deep cervical group, thyroid gland, lower larynx, cervical trachea, and esophagus. This group also drains the tip of the tongue.

Deep cervical groups of the lymph nodes are linked by the afferent and efferent vessels. All lymph from the head and neck region passes through the deep cervical groups of the lymph nodes. These groups finally drain the lymph in the jugular lymph trunk at the root of the neck. This lymph trunk drains to the thoracic duct on the left side and at the junction of the internal jugular vein and sub-clavian vein on the right side.

■ Clinical Notes

Cervical groups of the lymph nodes are of great clinical significance because they get enlarged during malignancy and tubercular infections. In malignancy, the nodes may adhere or infiltrate the internal jugular vein.

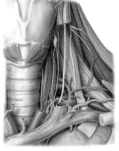

© THIEME Atlas of Anatomy

Learning Objectives

At the end of the deep dissection of the root of the neck, you should be able to identify the following:

- The subclavian vein joining the internal jugular vein to form the brachiocephalic vein on the right and left sides.
- Opening of the right lymphatic and thoracic ducts at the junction of the subclavian and internal jugular vein on the right and left sides, respectively.
- The vagus and phrenic nerves as they lie anterior to the subclavian artery.
- The subclavian artery and its branches.
- The scalene muscles.
- The cervical pleura.
- The root and trunks of the brachial plexus.
- The right and left recurrent laryngeal nerves in the groove between the esophagus and trachea.
- The cervical sympathetic trunk.

Introduction

The root of the neck is an important anatomical region as it contains structures passing between the head and thorax and also between the upper limb and thorax. These structures pass through *superior thoracic aperture*, which is sometimes also known as the *thoracic outlet*. The aperture is bounded anteriorly by the manubrium sterni, on the sides by the first rib and posteriorly by the first thoracic vertebra. The aperture is inclined anteriorly; therefore, the cervical pleural sac with the apex of the lung projects from the aperture into the root of the neck.

The subclavian and internal jugular veins join to form the brachiocephalic vein on either side of the root of the neck. Internal carotid artery and internal jugular vein run upward along with the vagus nerve in the carotid sheath. The subclavian artery and its branches are important constituents at the root of the neck. The phrenic nerve is anterior to the scalenus anterior muscle. This muscle divides the subclavian artery into three parts. The roots and trunks of the brachial plexus lie posterior to the scalenus anterior muscle. Deep to the internal jugular vein lie the cervical sympathetic trunk and the inferior cervical sympathetic ganglion. The trachea and esophagus lie in the midline with the left recurrent laryngeal in the groove between the two. The right recurrent laryngeal nerve winds around the right subclavian artery to lie in the groove between the esophagus and trachea on the right side.

Surface Landmarks

1. On an articulated skeleton, see the boundaries of the superior thoracic aperture.

2. Note that the aperture is inclined anteriorly.

3. Also, note the superior border of the manubrium sterni and sternoclavicular joint.

4. Learn the bony features of the cervical vertebrae. Look for the anterior and posterior tubercles of the transverse processes (refer to **Fig. 1.13a**).

5. See the scalene tubercle on the first rib and grooves for the subclavian vein and subclavian artery.

Dissection and Identification

A. Dissection to expose the junction of internal jugular and subclavian vein (formation of brachiocephalic vein), thoracic duct, and right lymphatic duct.

1. At the root of the neck, we have already reflected the sternomastoid, sternohyoid, and sterno-thyroid muscles (**Fig. 17.1**).

2. Clean the inferior belly of the omohyoid muscle. Cut the fascial sling, which binds the inter-mediate tendon to the clavicle. Reflect the inferior belly of the omohyoid downward.

3. With the help of a saw, give a cut in the middle of the clavicle. Disarticulate the medial end of the clavicle at the sternoclavicular joint and remove the medial half of the clavicle. This will help dissect the structures at the root of the neck (thoracic outlet).

4. With a blunt dissection, clean the lower end of the internal jugular vein and subclavian vein. Follow the formation of the brachiocephalic vein and trace it downward till it disappears in the thorax (**Fig. 17.2**). See the external jugular vein joining the subclavian vein. If possible, lift the brachiocephalic vein and see the vertebral vein joining the posterior surface of the brachiocephalic vein.

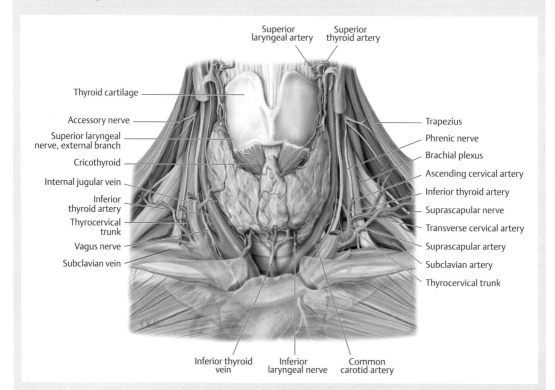

Fig. 17.1 Structures and their relationship at the root of the neck. (From: Schuenke M, Schulte E, Schumacher U. THIEME Atlas of Anatomy. Head, Neck, and Neuroanatomy. Illustrations by Voll M and Wesker K. © Thieme 2020.)

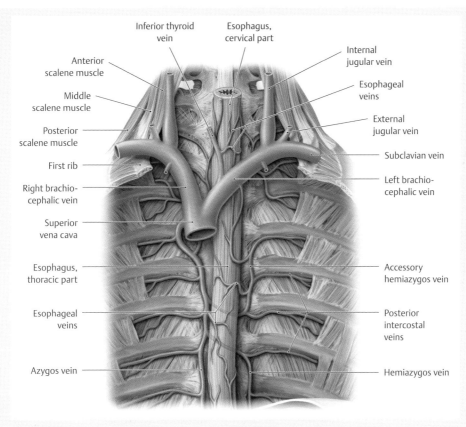

Fig. 17.2   Formation of brachiocephalic veins. (From: Schuenke M, Schulte E, Schumacher U. THIEME Atlas of Anatomy. Internal Organs. Illustrations by Voll M and Wesker K. © Thieme 2020.)

5. On the left side, find the thoracic duct at the junction of the left subclavian and left internal jugular vein (**Fig. 17.3**). Follow the thoracic duct upward as it crosses the first part of the left subclavian artery to **go deep toward** the esophagus.

6. On the right side, find the right lymphatic duct in the same position, that is, at the junction of the right subclavian and right internal jugular veins.

B. Dissection to subclavian artery, scalenus anterior muscle, vagus, recurrent laryngeal and phrenic nerves (Videos 17.1 and 17.2).

1. Now give a cut in the subclavian vein at the level where it lies on the first rib. Reflect the vein toward the medial side to expose the subclavian artery.

2. Dissect a part of the right brachiocephalic trunk as it lies on the root of the neck.

3. See that the right subclavian artery is taking origin from the brachiocephalic trunk at the root of the neck (**Fig. 17.4**), while the left subclavian artery is coming out at the outlet of the thorax, as it arises from the arch of the aorta in the thoracic cavity.

4. With the help of blunt dissection, clean the anterior surface of the scalenus anterior muscle, transverse cervical and suprascapular arteries, vagus, and phrenic nerves, which are related to its anterior surface (refer to **Fig. 17.3**). Follow this muscle inferiorly at its attachment to the first rib. Anterior to this attachment lies the subclavian vein and posterior to it lies the subclavian artery.

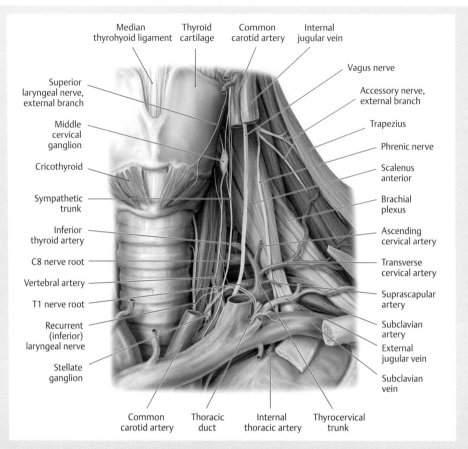

Fig. 17.3 Deep dissection of the root of the neck (right side). (From: Schuenke M, Schulte E, Schumacher U. THIEME Atlas of Anatomy. Head, Neck, and Neuroanatomy. Illustrations by Voll M and Wesker K. © Thieme 2020.)

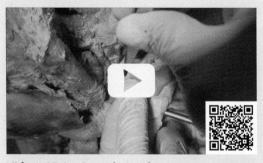

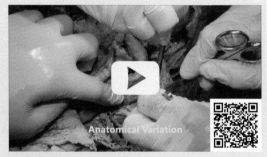

Video 17.1 Carotid, jugular, vagus, recurrent laryngeal nerve.

Video 17.2 Scalene triangle.

5. The subclavian artery is divided into three parts (first, second, and third) by its relationship with the scalenus anterior muscle (refer to **Fig. 17.4**).

6. Clean the vagus nerve as it crosses the first part of the subclavian artery. On the right side, it gives origin to the right recurrent laryngeal nerve. Follow the right recurrent laryngeal nerve winding around the subclavian artery to the groove between the trachea and esophagus. On the left side, follow the left recurrent laryngeal nerve.

7. Clean the phrenic nerve as it crosses the first part of the subclavian artery. On the left, see the thoracic duct crossing the first part of the subclavian artery.

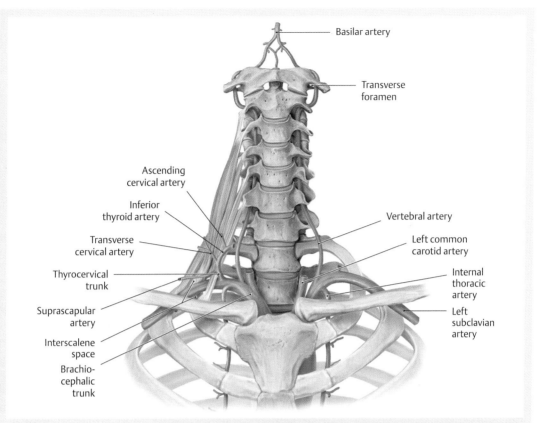

Fig. 17.4   Arteries at the root of the neck. (From: Schuenke M, Schulte E, Schumacher U. THIEME Atlas of Anatomy. Head, Neck, and Neuroanatomy. Illustrations by Voll M and Wesker K. © Thieme 2020.)

8. Clean the cervical pleura posterior to the first part of the subclavian artery (**Fig. 17.5**).

9. With the help of blunt dissection, clean the branches of the subclavian artery (i.e., vertebral, internal thoracic, thyrocervical trunk, costocervical trunk, and dorsal scapular artery) and follow each of them as far as possible (refer to **Fig. 17.4**).

Video 17.3   Subclavian vessels, brachial plexus, and scalene triangle.

10. Clean the vertebral artery and vein above the first part of the subclavian artery, as they lie between the longus colli and anterior scalene muscle (**Table 17.1** and **Fig. 17.3**). The vertebral artery passes anterior to the transverse process of the seventh cervical vertebra and disappears in the transverse process of the sixth.

C. Dissection to expose sympathetic trunk, inferior and middle cervical ganglia, and roots and trunks of cervical plexus (Video 17.3).

1. Expose the ventral rami of the seventh and eighth cervical nerves, posterior to the vertebral artery.

2. Pull the common carotid artery laterally and look for the sympathetic trunk posterior to it. Trace the trunk inferiorly and find the cervicothoracic ganglion (inferior cervical ganglion) near the neck of the first rib (at the superior thoracic aperture) (refer to **Fig. 17.3**).

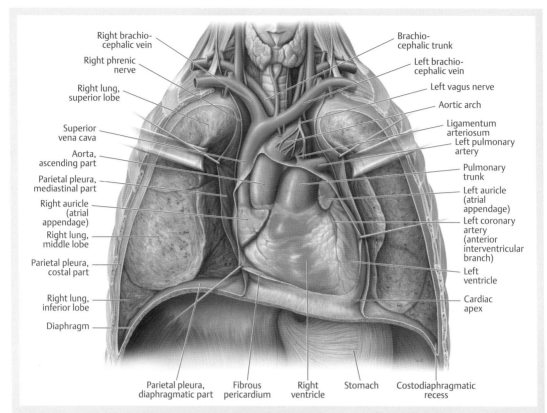

Fig. 17.5 Dissection of the root of the neck extended into the thoracic cavity. (From: Schuenke M, Schulte E, Schumacher U. THIEME Atlas of Anatomy. Internal Organs. Illustrations by Voll M and Wesker K. © Thieme 2020.)

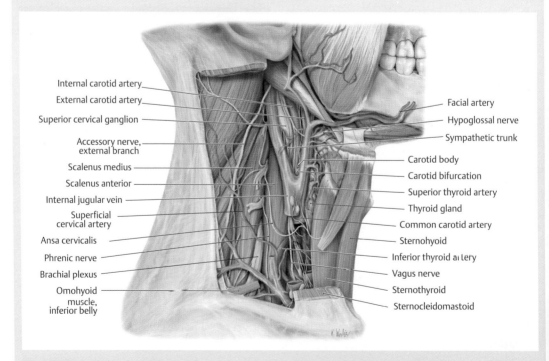

Fig. 17.6 Muscles forming the floor of posterior triangle exposed. (From: Schuenke M, Schulte E, Schumacher U. THIEME Atlas of Anatomy. Head, Neck, and Neuroanatomy. Illustrations by Voll M and Wesker K. © Thieme 2020.)

3. Trace the trunk superiorly and find the middle cervical ganglion close to the transverse process of the sixth cervical vertebra.

4. Clean the gap between the anterior and middle scalene muscles. Find the roots and trunks of the brachial plexus above the third part of the subclavian artery (refer to **Fig. 17.3** and **Table 17.2**).

5. Once again, review the muscles forming the floor of the posterior triangle of the neck, that is, the splenius capitis, levator scapulae, anterior, middle, and posterior scalene muscles (**Fig. 17.6**).

Muscles

Scalene Muscles

These muscles are present at the side of the neck (lateral vertebral muscles) and extend between the cervical transverse processes and the first two ribs (**Fig. 17.7**).

Table 17.1   Scalene muscles

Muscle	Origin	Insertion	Nerve supply	Action
Scalenus anterior	From the anterior tubercles of the typical cervical vertebrae (C3–C6)	On the scalene tubercle on the inner border of the first rib	From the ventral rami of C4, C5, and C6 spinal nerves	Flexion of the cervical column when both muscles contract together from below Elevation of the ribs when they act from above as in inspiration Lateral flexion of the cervical vertebrae when acting unilaterally
Scalenus medius	Transverse process of the C2 and posterior tubercles of the transverse process of C3–C7 vertebrae	On the rough area of the first rib between its tubercle and the groove for the subclavian artery	From the ventral rami of C3–C8 spinal nerves	Lateral flexion of the neck to the same side. It also elevates the first rib in inspiration
Scalenus posterior	From the posterior tubercles of transverse processes of C4–C6 vertebrae	On the outer surface of the second rib	By the ventral rami of the lower five spinal nerves	Lateral flexion of the neck and elevation of the second rib

Relations of the Scalenus Anterior Muscle

The anterior scalenus muscle is the *key muscle at the root of the neck* (**Fig. 17.3**).

Anteriorly: It is crossed by the phrenic nerve, internal jugular vein (as it lies within the carotid sheath), subclavian vein, clavicle, and clavicular head of the sternomastoid. It is also crossed anteriorly by the inferior belly of the omohyoid, transverse cervical, and suprascapular arteries.

Posteriorly: It is crossed by the scalenus medius, roots of the brachial plexus, subclavian artery, costocervical trunk (from the second part of the subclavian artery), suprapleural membrane, and cervical pleura.

Medially: It is crossed by the thyrocervical trunk, vertebral artery, thoracic duct on the left side, and lymphatic trunk on the right side.

Laterally: It is crossed by the trunks of the brachial plexus and the subclavian artery lies close to its lateral border.

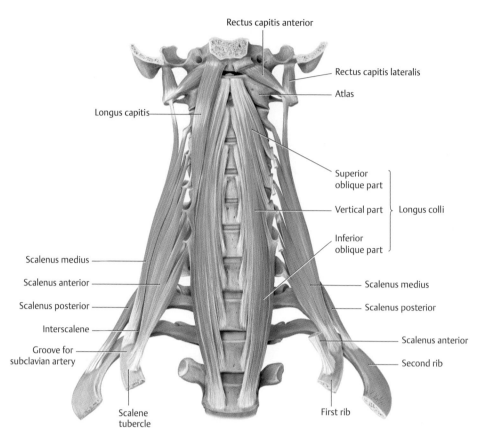

Fig. 17.7 Pre- and paravertebral muscles of the neck. (From: Schuenke M, Schulte E, Schumacher U. THIEME Atlas of Anatomy. Head, Neck, and Neuroanatomy. Illustrations by Voll M and Wesker K. © Thieme 2020.)

Arteries

Common Carotid Artery

In the neck, both the common carotid arteries lie behind the sternoclavicular joint. Though the left common carotid arises from the arch of the aorta in the thorax, the right arises from the brachiocephalic trunk posterior to the right sternoclavicular joint.

The course of both the common carotid arteries from the sternoclavicular joint to the upper border of the thyroid cartilage is the same **(Fig. 17.1).** They run upward with a slight posterolateral inclination. At the level of the upper border of the thyroid cartilage, it terminates by dividing into internal and external carotid arteries.

Throughout its course, the artery is enclosed in the carotid sheath. The internal jugular vein lies anterolateral to it and the vagus nerve posterolateral. Posteriorly, the artery is related to the cervical transverse processes, prevertebral muscles, and sympathetic trunk. Anteriorly, the artery is covered by the sternomastoid and infrahyoid muscles. The thyroid gland and ansa cervicalis also overlap the internal carotid artery. Medially, the artery is in relation with the esophagus and trachea with the recurrent laryngeal nerve between them. At the upper level, it is related medially to the larynx and pharynx. No branch arises from the common carotid artery.

Subclavian Artery

The subclavian artery is the artery of the upper limb and also supplies blood to the neck and brain. On the right side, the subclavian artery arises from the brachiocephalic trunk behind the sternoclavicular joint. On the left side, the artery arises from the arch of the aorta in the thorax. On each side, the artery arches upward and crosses the dome of the cervical pleura and first rib and behind the scalenus anterior muscle. At the outer border of the first rib, it becomes the axillary artery (refer to **Fig. 17.4**).

Parts of the Artery

For the purpose of description, the artery is divided into three parts: the *first part* extends from behind the sternoclavicular joint to the medial border of the scalenus anterior muscle. The *second part* lies behind the muscle and the *third part* extends from the lateral border of the scalenus anterior muscle to the outer border of the first rib.

1. *Relations of the first part: Anteriorly*, the first part of the artery is related to the internal jugular vein, vertebral vein, vagus nerve, phrenic nerve on the left side, and ansa subclavia. On the *posterior aspect* of the first part of the artery lies the cervical pleura and suprapleural membrane. The right recurrent laryngeal nerve winds around the first part.

2. *Relations of the second part: Anteriorly*, the second part is in relation with the scalenus anterior muscle and structures lying on the muscle. *Posteriorly*, it is in relation with the cervical pleura, lower trunk of the brachial plexus, and scalenus medius muscle.

3. *Relations of the third part: Anteriorly*, it is related to the external jugular vein with its tributaries, nerve to the subclavius, suprascapular artery, and clavicle. *Posteriorly*, it is related to the scalenus medius and lower trunk of the brachial plexus.

Branches of the Artery

For branches of subclavian artery, refer to **Fig. 17.4** and **Table 17.2**.

Table 17.2   Branches of the subclavian artery

Parts	Branches	Short description
First part	1. Vertebral	It supplies the brain. It originates from the first part and ascends between the longus colli and the medial border of the scalenus anterior. It passes through the foramen transversarium of the sixth cervical vertebra. It is usually described to have four parts. It terminates in the posterior cranial cavity by joining its fellow to form the basilar artery at the lower border of the pons.
	2. Internal thoracic	It arises close to the medial border of the scalenus anterior muscle. It runs downward, forward, and medially on the cervical pleura posterior to the first costal cartilage. In the thorax, it divides into two terminal branches: the superior epigastric and musculophrenic arteries.
	3. Thyrocervical trunk	It arises close to the medial margin of the scalenus muscle and immediately divides into three branches.
	• Inferior thyroid	After origin from the thyrocervical trunk close to the medial border of the scalenus anterior, it curves backward over the dome of the pleura. It supplies the lobe of the thyroid gland.

(Continued)

Table 17.2 *(Continued)* Branches of the subclavian artery

Parts	Branches	Short description
	• Suprascapular	After origin from the thyrocervical trunk, it runs transversely in front of the scalenus anterior and crosses the phrenic nerve. It reaches the posterior triangle.
	• Transverse cervical	After origin, it runs transversely and crosses the scalenus anterior and phrenic nerve. It reaches the posterior triangle.
Second part	Costocervical trunk 1. Deep cervical It passes backward to reach the deep muscles of the back of the neck	It arises from the back of the second part of the artery. It runs backward over the dome of the cervical pleura to reach the neck of the first rib, where it divides into two branches.
	2. Highest intercostal	After reaching the neck of the first rib, it descends downward to the first intercostal space to divide into the first and second posterior intercostal arteries
Third part	Dorsal scapular (occasional branch)	When present, it may replace the transverse cervical artery.

Veins

Subclavian Vein

The subclavian vein lies on the first rib in front of the insertion of the scalenus anterior muscle and on the cervical pleura, behind the clavicle. The subclavian vein is a continuation of the axillary vein and begins at the outer border of the first rib. It joins the internal jugular to form the brachiocephalic vein. Its tributary is the external jugular vein. Sometimes, the dorsal scapular and anterior jugular veins may directly open in it instead of opening in the external jugular vein (refer to **Fig. 17.2**).

Brachiocephalic Vein

The right and left brachiocephalic veins begin by the union of the internal jugular vein and the subclavian vein between the cervical pleura and the medial part of the clavicle. Soon after their formation, they go into the thorax where the right and left veins join to form the superior vena cava. The left vein is larger and crosses the median plane posterior to the manubrium to join the right vein. The right vein descends medially behind the first costal cartilage to join the left vein.

Tributaries of each brachiocephalic vein are vertebral vein, highest intercostal vein, and few lymph trunks. The left vein receives the thoracic duct.

Thoracic Duct

Thoracic duct is a thin-walled, slender vessel which drains the lymph into the venous system. It drains the lymph from both sides of the body below the diaphragm and from the left side of the body above the diaphragm. It ascends from the thorax along the left margin of the esophagus. At the level of C7 vertebra, it arches laterally to end at the junction of the subclavian and internal jugular veins to drain the lymph in the brachiocephalic vein (refer to **Fig. 17.3**).

At the root of the neck, the thoracic duct lies posterior to the carotid sheath. From the medial to lateral, it crosses many structures posteriorly—left sympathetic chain, vertebral artery and vein, inferior thyroid artery, transverse cervical artery, suprascapular artery, phrenic nerve, and the first part of the subclavian artery.

Cervical Pleura

The cervical pleura forms the dome of the pleural sac which encloses the apex of the lung. On either side, it bulges upward in the root of the neck through the superior thoracic aperture (outlet of the thorax). Due to the inclined plane of the thoracic aperture, the cervical pleura projects in the neck about 5 cm in front of the first costal cartilage, while posteriorly till the level of the neck of the first cervical rib.

The dome of the cervical pleura is covered by the suprapleural membrane, which arises from the transverse process of the seventh cervical vertebra and spreads over the pleura to be attached to the inner margin of the first rib. The great vessels of the head and neck and upper limb lie anterior to it (refer to **Fig. 17.5**). On its posterior aspect lies the sympathetic trunk. Laterally, it is related to the lower trunk of the brachial plexus and scalenus anterior muscle. Medially, the pleura is related to the esophagus and vertebral bodies.

Nerves

Phrenic Nerve

The phrenic nerve supplies the diaphragm; therefore, it is an important nerve of respiration. It arises from the ventral rami of the C3, C4, and C5 spinal nerves. It begins at the lateral border of the scalenus anterior muscle at the level of the upper border of the thyroid cartilage. The nerve runs obliquely toward the medial side on the anterior aspect of the scalenus anterior muscle (refer to **Fig. 17.3**). On the left side, it crosses the medial border of the muscle to lie in front of the first part of the subclavian artery. While on the right side, it does not cross the first part of the subclavian artery but remains in front of the scalenus muscle as it crosses the second part of the subclavian artery.

Recurrent Laryngeal Nerves

The right recurrent laryngeal nerve arises at the root of the neck from the vagus nerve, where the vagus crosses the first part of the subclavian artery. It hooks below the subclavian artery and ascends in the groove between the esophagus and trachea. The left recurrent laryngeal nerve arises in the thorax as the vagus crosses the arch of the aorta. It also ascends in the groove between the esophagus and trachea on the left side, at the root of the neck (refer to **Figs. 18.2** and **18.5**).

Both the right and left nerves then pass deep to the lobe of the thyroid gland, among the branches of the inferior thyroid artery. Thereafter, each nerve enters the larynx deep to the inferior constrictor muscle of the pharynx (refer to **Fig. 15.9**).

Branches: Each recurrent laryngeal nerve gives the following branches:

1. All the intrinsic muscles of the larynx except the cricothyroid.

2. The mucous membrane of the larynx below the vocal fold.

3. The trachea, inferior part of the pharynx, and esophagus.

4. The cardiac branch to the heart.

Brachial Plexus

The brachial plexus lies in the root of the neck between the scalenus anterior and medius muscle, behind the clavicle, and in the axilla (**Fig. 17.1**). It mainly supplies the upper limb and consists of four parts, that is, *roots*, *trunk*, *division*, and *cords*. Roots and trunks lie in the root of the neck, divisions are behind the clavicle, and cords and their branches are in the axilla.

Roots: The roots are derived from the ventral rami of the lower four (C5–C8) cervical and first thoracic spinal nerves.

Trunks: The upper trunk is formed by the union of the ventral rami of C5 and C6 nerves. The middle trunk is formed by the C7 ventral ramus. The lower trunk is formed by the union of the ventral rami of C8 and T1 nerves.

Divisions: Each trunk divides into anterior and posterior divisions.

Cords: The three posterior divisions unite to form the posterior cord (root value C5–T1), upper two anterior divisions unite to form the lateral cord (root value C5, C6, and C7), while the lower anterior division forms the medial cord (root value C8 and T1).

Branches of the brachial plexus arising in the neck: The branches to scalene muscle and longus cervicis contribute to the *phrenic nerve* from C5 (supplies diaphragm), the *dorsal scapular* (supplies the levator scapulae, rhomboids major and minor), *suprascapular* (supplies the supraspinatus and infraspinatus muscles), *long thoracic nerve* (supplies the serratus anterior muscle), and nerve to the *subclavius* muscle (supplies the subclavius muscle).

Lymph Nodes and Lymph Trunks

Jugulo-omohyoid or inferior deep cervical group of lymph nodes are present on the carotid sheath close to the intermediate tendon and inferior belly of the omohyoid muscle (**Fig. 11.9**).

There are three lymph trunks on the right side at the root of the neck, that is, the right subclavian trunk, right jugular trunk, and right bronchomediastinal trunk. The subclavian trunk drains the superior extremity and ends in the subclavian vein, the right jugular trunk drains the head and neck and ends in the internal jugular vein, and the bronchomediastinal trunk drains the brachiocephalic trunk. Mostly, the right subclavian and jugular trunk join and form the right lymphatic trunk.

▎Clinical Notes

Cervical rib: The subclavian artery and brachial plexus, at the root of the neck, pass through a narrow space (triangle). This triangle is bounded anteriorly by the scalenus anterior, posteriorly by the medius, and below by the first rib. If there is a presence of the *cervical rib*, it raises the base of the triangle, thus displacing and compressing the brachial plexus and subclavian artery upward.

Scalene syndrome: Due to the spasm of the scalene muscles, the first rib is elevated. This causes the displacement and compression of the brachial plexus and subclavian artery (refer to **Fig. 17.3**). This phenomenon is known as the scalene syndrome.

The cervical rib and scalene syndrome both result in similar neurological and vascular symptoms:

1. *Vascular symptoms*: In severe cases, ischemia occurs in the limb, leading to gangrene of the fingers.

2. *Neurological symptoms*: As C8 and T1 (lower trunk of the brachial plexus) are compressed, tingling pain occurs along the inner border of the forearm and hand. This also leads to weakness and wastage of the intrinsic muscles of the hand.

Deep Dissection of the Neck—IV: Upper Part of the Cervical Vessels and Nerves

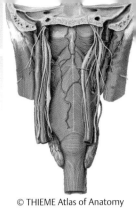

© THIEME Atlas of Anatomy

Introduction

During the previous dissection of the neck, we could not expose the superior part of the internal carotid artery and internal jugular vein. We could also not see the upper part of the last four cranial nerves, that is, the glossopharyngeal, vagus, accessory, and hypoglossal nerves, as they are located deep at the base of the skull. To visualize these deeply situated nerves and vessels and also to expose the cervical viscera (larynx and pharynx) from the posterior side, we shall remove the skull from the vertebral column by giving a wedge-shaped cut in the occipital bone.

After the disarticulation of the head from the vertebral column, we shall be able to study the internal carotid artery in the upper part of the neck and its disappearance in the carotid canal; upper part of the internal jugular vein as it begins below the jugular fossa; and the last four cranial nerves coming out of the jugular foramen and hypoglossal canal. All these structures are closed together and enclosed in a dense mass of connective tissue. We shall now also follow the cervical part of the sympathetic trunk.

Surface Landmarks

1. On the base of a dried skull, identify the jugular foramen, carotid canal, and hypoglossal canal, both on the external and internal surfaces (refer to Figs. **1.5** and **1.7**).

2. Review the structures passing through these foramina and canals (**Fig. 18.1**).

3. On a dried skull, review the parts of the occipital bone (i.e., basilar, condylar, and squamous).

4. Review the bony features of the occipital condyle, pharyngeal tubercle, and superior articular facet of the atlas (refer to **Fig. 1.5**).

5. Review the structures passing through the foramen magnum (refer to **Fig. 13.1**).

Dissection and Identification

A. Dissection to disarticulate the head from the cervical vertebral column (the sternomastoid and posterior belly of the digastric muscles have already been reflected).

1. Separate the cervical viscera from the vertebral column by passing fingers through the retropharyngeal space. For this, pass your fingers behind the carotid sheath and cervical viscera on both sides. Move your fingers medially till they touch in the midline. Now move your fingers upward toward the base of the skull and inferiorly toward the superior aperture of the thorax.

2. Two oblique cuts are to be given in the occipital bone (as shown in **Fig. 18.1**). These cuts should be parallel to the upper border of the petrous temporal bone and should pass just posterior to the hypoglossal canal. Both these cuts will reach anteriorly into the anterior part of the foramen magnum. Externally, the posterior end of the cut should pass posteriorly to the mastoid process and the anterior end of the cut will pass through the atlanto-occipital joint.

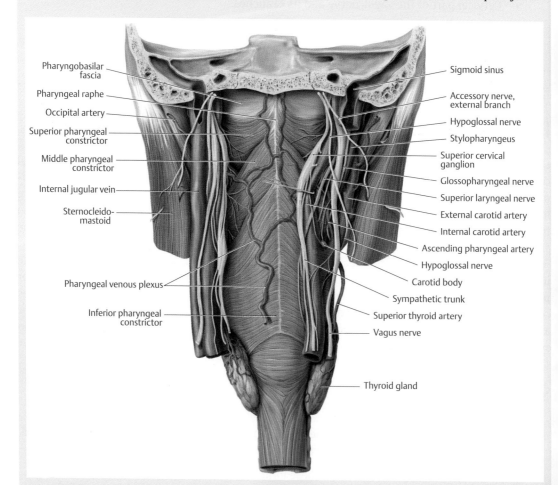

Fig. 18.1   The cervical viscera and parapharyngeal space (posterior view). (From: Schuenke M, Schulte E, Schumacher U. THIEME Atlas of Anatomy. Head, Neck, and Neuroanatomy. Illustrations by Voll M and Wesker K. © Thieme 2020.)

3. Give a cut between the anterior ends of the two oblique cuts (at the basilar part of the occipital bone) so that the apical ligament, longitudinal band of the cruciate ligament, and membrana tectoria (these ligaments attach the basilar part of bone to the vertebral column) are cut.

4. Pull the head anteriorly to release it from the vertebral column. You may have to use the chisel to pry it forward. The atlanto-occipital joint will have to be broken to complete this step.

5. Cut the rectus capitis anterior and longus capitis muscles at the base of the skull.

B. Dissection of sympathetic trunk, vagus, glossopharyngeal, accessory, and hypoglossal nerves (Video 18.1).

1. Identify the superior cervical sympathetic ganglion and sympathetic trunk on the right and left sides lying on the anterior surface of the cervical vertebral column (**Fig. 18.1**). (Note: sometimes both the sympathetic trunks may go with the disarticulated head.) Identify the carotid nerve, which passes from the superior ganglion to the internal carotid artery. On one side, you may cut the carotid nerve and leave the sympathetic trunk attached to the vertebral column. On the other side, leave the carotid nerve intact and reflect the sympathetic trunk and superior cervical ganglion on the cervical viscera, with the specimen of the disarticulated head (**Fig. 18.1**).

2. With the help of blunt dissection, find the upper part of the cervical nerves and vessels at the base of the skull on the back of the specimen of the disarticulated head. Find the internal laryngeal nerve at the thyrohyoid membrane and trace it upward to the superior laryngeal nerve medial to both the external and internal carotid arteries. Follow the superior laryngeal nerve to the vagus (**Fig. 18.2**). Now find the pharyngeal branch of the vagus and trace it downward to the pharynx.

3. With the help of blunt dissection, expose the glossopharyngeal, accessory, and hypoglossal nerves (refer to **Fig. 18.1**) and follow them distally. Now identify the stylopharyngeus muscle as it enters the pharynx between the superior and middle constrictor muscles. Follow this muscle backward as it is attached to the styloid process. The glossopharyngeal nerve will curve around and then run on the surface of this muscle to go to the pharynx (**Fig. 18.3**).

4. Find the hypoglossal nerve as it winds around the origin of the occipital artery. Trace it forward to find the superior root of the ansa cervicalis. Follow the hypoglossal nerve backward to find its union with the branch from C1 (**Fig. 18.4**).

5. Identify the cervical sympathetic trunk and superior cervical ganglion (refer to **Fig. 18.1**) and try to find its branches to the external carotid and internal carotid arteries. Also, find the branches to the cranial nerves. Also, try to find the delicate grey rami which communicates to the upper four cervical ventral rami. Find the middle and inferior cervical sympathetic ganglia (**Fig. 18.5**).

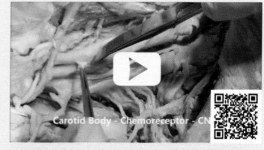

Video 18.1   Last four cranial nerves: Glossopharyngeal, vagus, hypoglossal, and accessory nerves in neck.

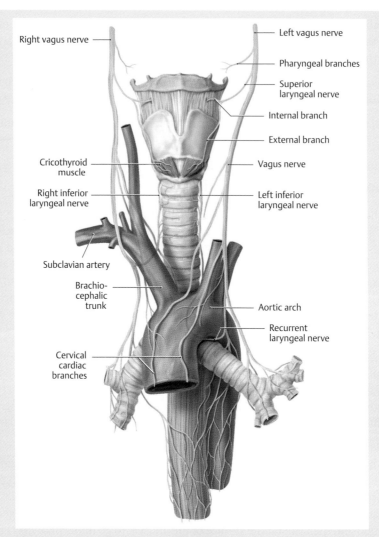

Fig. 18.2 Branches of the vagus nerve (CN X) in the neck. (From: Schuenke M, Schulte E, Schumacher U. THIEME Atlas of Anatomy. Head, Neck, and Neuroanatomy. Illustrations by Voll M and Wesker K. © Thieme 2020.)

C. Dissection of internal carotid artery and internal jugular vein (Video 18.2).

1. At the base of the skull, follow the internal carotid artery as it lies deep to the styloid process and structures attached to it. Before it enters the carotid canal, it lies anterior to the internal jugular vein (refer to **Fig. 18.1**).

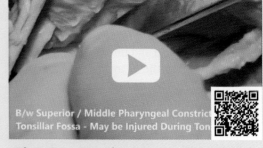

Video 18.2 Carotid arteries.

2. Note the upper end of the internal jugular vein, at the base of the skull. It dilates into the jugular fossa to form the jugular bulb. The internal jugular vein lies posterolateral to the internal carotid artery. In between the artery and vein lie the glossopharyngeal, vagus, accessory, and hypoglossal nerves (refer to **Figs. 18.1** and **18.5**).

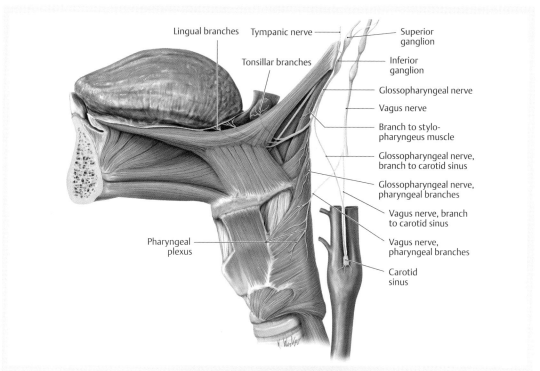

Fig. 18.3 Branches of the vagus and glossopharyngeal nerves beyond the skull base (left lateral view). (From: Schuenke M, Schulte E, Schumacher U. THIEME Atlas of Anatomy. Head, Neck, and Neuroanatomy. Illustrations by Voll M and Wesker K. © Thieme 2020.)

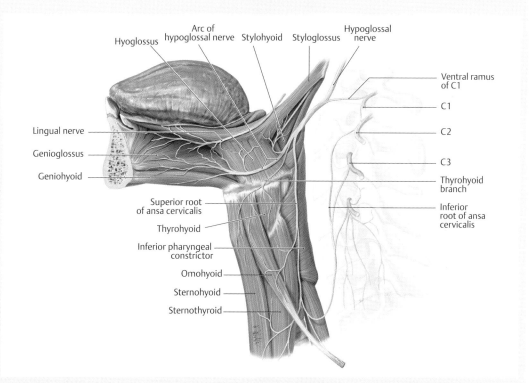

Fig. 18.4 Hypoglossal nerve (CN XII) and ansa cervicalis (left lateral view). (From: Schuenke M, Schulte E, Schumacher U. THIEME Atlas of Anatomy. Head, Neck, and Neuroanatomy. Illustrations by Voll M and Wesker K. © Thieme 2020.)

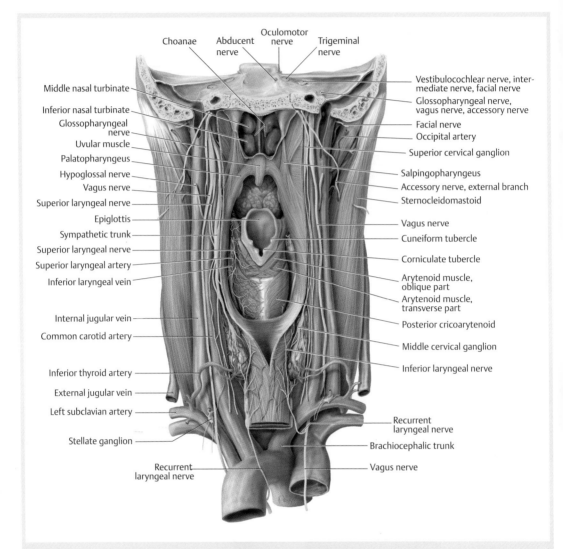

Fig. 18.5 Parapharyngeal space with posterior pharyngeal wall slit open. (From: Schuenke M, Schulte E, Schumacher U. THIEME Atlas of Anatomy. Head, Neck, and Neuroanatomy. Illustrations by Voll M and Wesker K. © Thieme 2020.)

Vessels

Cervical Part of the Internal Carotid Artery

The internal carotid artery begins at the bifurcation of the common carotid artery at the level of the upper border of the thyroid cartilage (**Fig. 18.6**). The cervical part ends as it passes through the carotid canal (in front of the jugular foramen) to become the petrous part.

The cervical part of the internal carotid artery is superficial as it lies in the carotid triangle; then it passes deeper as it ascends upward. It lies within the carotid sheath with the internal jugular vein and the vagus nerve (refer to **Fig. 18.1**).

Posterior relations: It lies on the transverse process of the upper three cervical vertebrae and longus capitis muscle. The internal jugular vein is also posterior to the upper part of the artery and intervening between the artery and vein are the last four cranial nerves.

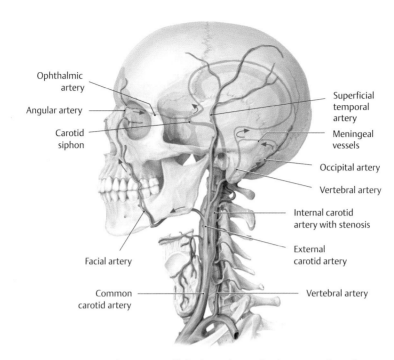

Fig. 18.6 Carotid arteries (left lateral view). (From: Schuenke M, Schulte E, Schumacher U. THIEME Atlas of Anatomy. Head, Neck, and Neuroanatomy. Illustrations by Voll M and Wesker K. © Thieme 2020.)

Anterior relations: Sternomastoid, posterior belly of the digastric and stylohyoid, hypoglossal nerve. At the higher level, it lies posterior to the styloid process and structures attached to it and the glossopharyngeal nerve.

Medial relations: Superior and middle constrictor of the pharynx and ascending pharyngeal artery.

Lateral relations: The internal jugular vein and vagus nerve.

The internal carotid artery has no branch in the neck.

Internal Jugular Vein

The internal jugular vein is the largest vein of the neck. It begins below the jugular foramen where it presents a dilatation known as the superior bulb (**Fig. 18.1**). It terminates behind the sternal end of the clavicle in a swelling called the inferior bulb. Below the inferior bulb, a valve is present to prevent the reflux of blood into the neck. Here, it joins with the subclavian vein to form the brachiocephalic vein (**Fig. 18.7**).

The vein descends vertically within the carotid sheath, first with the internal carotid artery and then with the common carotid artery and vagus nerve (refer to **Fig. 18.5**).

Relations

Posterior relations: The vein lies on the following structures from above downward: the rectus capitis lateralis, transverse process of the atlas, levator scapulae, scalenus medius and cervical plexus, scalenus anterior and phrenic nerve, thyrocervical trunk, vertebral artery, and first part of the subclavian artery.

Anterolateral relations: The following structures are related anterior to the internal jugular vein from above downward: the internal carotid artery, spinal accessory nerve, styloid process, and

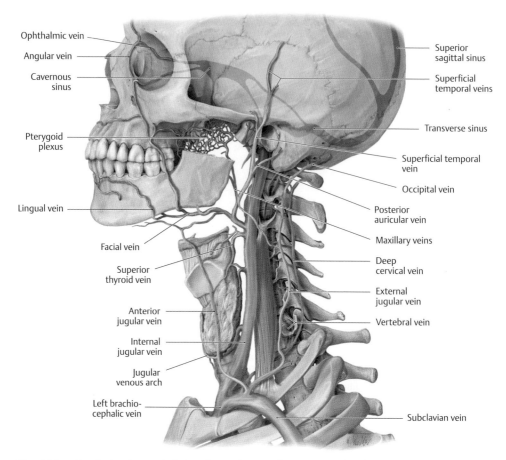

Fig. 18.7 Cervical veins and their relationship to the veins of the skull and dural sinuses (left lateral view). (From: Schuenke M, Schulte E, Schumacher U. THIEME Atlas of Anatomy. Head, Neck, and Neuroanatomy. Illustrations by Voll M and Wesker K. © Thieme 2020.)

structures attached to the styloid process. Then it is related to the posterior belly of the digastric, posterior auricular artery and occipital artery, deep cervical lymph nodes and inferior root of the ansa cervicalis, and infrahyoid muscles overlapped by the sternomastoid muscle.

Medial relation: The vein is situated medially to the internal carotid artery above the level of the upper border of the thyroid cartilage and to the common carotid below this level. Posteromedially, it is related to the vagus nerve. The glossopharyngeal, accessory, and hypoglossal nerves are situated anteromedially to the internal jugular vein.

Tributaries: From above downward following are the tributaries: inferior petrosal sinus, common facial vein, lingual vein, pharyngeal venous plexus, superior thyroid vein, and middle thyroid vein (**Fig. 18.7**).

Nerves

Glossopharyngeal Nerve

The glossopharyngeal nerve is the ninth cranial nerve. It is a mixed nerve, that is, motor and sensory. It is sensory to the tongue and pharynx and motor to the stylopharyngeus muscle (refer to **Fig. 18.3**).

Course

The nerve arises by three or four rootlets from the posterolateral sulcus of the medulla. It passes through the jugular foramen. Just below the foramen, it has two ganglia (superior and inferior ganglion). It lies between the internal jugular vein and internal carotid artery. It lies deep to the styloid process and structures attached to it. It curves around the stylopharyngeus muscle to lie on its lateral side. Then it passes deep to the hyoglossus muscle and enters the pharynx between the middle and superior constrictor muscles.

Branches

1. *Tympanic branch*: It enters the middle ear cavity where it forms the tympanic plexus. Branches from the plexus supply many structures such as the mucous membrane of the middle ear cavity, mastoid antrum and mastoid air cells, tympanic membrane, and auditory tube. A branch from this plexus forms the lesser petrosal nerve (which contains the secretomotor fibers for the parotid gland and arising from the inferior salivatory nucleus). The lesser petrosal nerve passes through the foramen ovale to end in the otic ganglion. The postganglionic fibers from the otic ganglion supply the secretomotor fibers to the parotid gland.

2. *Nerve to stylopharyngeus*: It is the only motor branch (**Fig. 18.3**).

3. *Carotid sinus nerve*: It innervates the carotid body and carotid sinus.

4. *Pharyngeal branch*: It takes part in the formation of pharyngeal plexus.

5. *Tonsillar branch*: It is sensory nerve to the palatine tonsil.

6. *Lingual branches*: These are the branches to the posterior one-third of the tongue to carry general sensation and for sensation of taste.

Cervical Part of the Vagus Nerve

The vagus nerve is the tenth cranial nerve. It is a mixed nerve, that is, sensory and motor. It is the longest cranial nerve, which runs from the cranial cavity to the abdomen, and innervates the structures of the head, neck, thorax, and abdomen.

The nerve takes its origin by 8 to 10 rootlets from the posterolateral sulcus of the medulla located between the olive and inferior cerebellar peduncle. These rootlets join to form the nerve which passes through the middle part of the jugular foramen along with the accessory nerve. At this point, it presents two swellings, the superior and inferior ganglia (refer to **Figs. 18.1–18.3** and **18.5**).

In the neck, the vagus nerve runs vertically downward within the carotid sheath between the internal jugular vein and first to the internal carotid and then to the common carotid artery. At the root of the neck, the right vagus nerve passes in front of the first part of the right subclavian artery to enter the thorax, while the left vagus nerve passes between the left common carotid and left subclavian arteries (refer to **Fig. 18.1**).

Branches

1. *Auricular branch*: It is a sensory branch which takes origin from the superior ganglion and is distributed to the skin of the pinna, external acoustic meatus, and tympanic membrane.

2. *Meningeal branch*: This sensory branch takes origin from the superior ganglion and goes back to the posterior cranial fossa through the jugular foramen. It supplies the dura mater of the posterior cranial fossa.

3. *Pharyngeal branch*: This branch takes its origin from the inferior ganglion and is motor to the muscles of the pharynx and soft palate. It passes between the external and internal carotid arteries to the pharyngeal plexus (**Fig. 18.2**).

4. *Superior laryngeal nerve*: After taking origin from the inferior ganglion, it divides into two branches, that is, the internal laryngeal and external laryngeal. The internal laryngeal supplies sensory fibers to the mucous membrane of the larynx above the vocal cord, while the external laryngeal supplies the cricothyroid muscle.

5. *Carotid branch*: It supplies fibers to the carotid body and carotid sinus.

6. *Cardiac branches*: These branches are given by the cervical trunk of the vagus nerve to end in the deep cardiac plexus in the thorax.

7. *Recurrent laryngeal nerve*: The right recurrent laryngeal nerve arises as the vagus crosses the first part of the subclavian artery. The left recurrent laryngeal nerve is given by the vagus in the thorax as it lies on the arch of the aorta.

Accessory Nerve

The accessory nerve is the 11th cranial nerve. It is purely motor. It has two roots, that is, the cranial and spinal roots. The cranial root supplies most of the muscles of the palate, pharynx, and larynx, while the spinal root supplies the sternomastoid (**Fig. 18.5**) and trapezius muscles.

The fibers of the cranial root arise by four or five rootlets from the medulla below the origin of the vagus. The fibers of the spinal root arise from the side of the spinal cord, midway between the dorsal and ventral spinal roots of the upper cervical spinal nerves (C1–C5). The spinal root ascends through the foramen magnum and runs toward the jugular foramen (**Fig. 18.8**). In the jugular foramen, the cranial and spinal roots of the accessory nerve unite with each other and again separate. The cranial root finally fuses with the vagus nerve and is distributed through it to the muscles of the palate, pharynx, and larynx.

The spinal root after separating from the cranial root leaves the skull by passing through the jugular foramen. The spinal root descends between the internal jugular vein and internal carotid artery. Then it crosses the transverse process of the atlas vertebra to lie deep to the styloid process and posterior belly of the digastric muscle. It then passes through the sternomastoid muscle and emerges through its posterior border to lie in the posterior triangle.

Branches

Cranial root: Through the vagus nerve it innervates the muscles of the larynx, pharynx, and soft palate.

Spinal root: It gives branches to the sternomastoid and trapezius muscles.

Hypoglossal Nerve

It is the 12th cranial nerve and motor to the muscles of the tongue except the palatoglossus muscle. It arises by many rootlets from the anterolateral sulcus (between the pyramid and olive) of the medulla. The nerve leaves the cranial cavity through the hypoglossal canal.

At the base of the skull, the nerve lies behind other cranial nerves, that is, the glossopharyngeal, vagus, and accessory nerves (refer to **Fig. 18.4**). Soon, it is joined by a branch from C1 ventral ramus. The nerve now lies between the internal carotid artery and internal jugular vein. The nerve then lies deep to the stylohyoid muscle and posterior belly of the digastric. At the origin of the occipital artery, it curves forward and crosses the internal and external carotid arteries and the loop of the lingual artery to lie on the hyoglossus muscle. Here, it enters the substance of the tongue to supply its muscles.

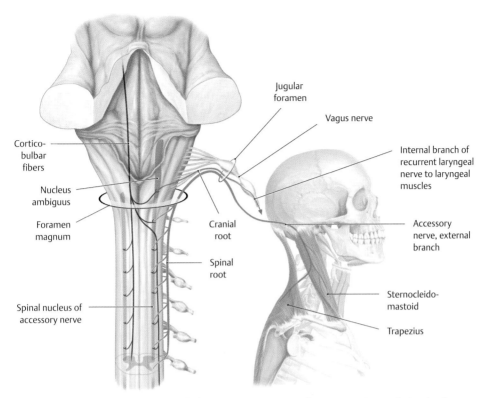

Fig. 18.8 Nucleus and course of the accessory nerve (posterior view of the brainstem, with the cerebellum removed). Fibers of cranial root are distributed through vagus nerve. (From: Schuenke M, Schulte E, Schumacher U. THIEME Atlas of Anatomy. Head, Neck, and Neuroanatomy. Illustrations by Voll M and Wesker K. © Thieme 2020.)

Branches

1. *Muscular branches to the tongue*: These are the branches to the extrinsic and intrinsic muscles of the tongue except the palatoglossus, which is supplied by the cranial accessory.

2. *Through its communication with C1*: The C1 branch, which travels with the hypoglossal nerve, gives branches to the superior root of the *ansa cervicalis, geniohyoid*, and *thyrohyoid* muscles. It also gives a *meningeal branch* for dura mater of the posterior cranial fossa.

Cervical Part of the Sympathetic Trunk

The cervical part of the sympathetic trunk extends from the base of the skull to the neck of the first rib. Below the superior thoracic aperture, it enters the thoracic cavity.

In the neck, it runs vertically on the longus colli and longus capitis muscles in front of the transverse processes of the cervical vertebrae. It is related anteriorly to the prevertebral fascia and carotid sheath. It is embedded in the posterior wall of the carotid sheath.

The cervical part of the sympathetic trunk has three ganglia (**Figs. 18.1** and **18.5**). These are superior, middle, and inferior ganglia. The superior ganglion is the largest (about 3 cm long), fusiform in shape, and located in front of the C2 and C3 vertebrae. It represents the four fused ganglia (C1–C4). Its upper end tapers into its internal carotid branch. The middle cervical ganglion is the smallest cervical ganglion and lies in front of the transverse process of C6 vertebra behind or in front of the inferior thyroid artery. It represents two fused ganglia (C5 and C6) in one. The inferior cervical ganglion is situated between the transverse process of C7 vertebra and neck of the first rib. It represents the fused C7 and C8 ganglia. Sometimes, the inferior cervical ganglion may fuse with the thoracic first ganglion to form the stellate or cervicothoracic ganglion.

Branches

Superior cervical ganglion:

1. Grey rami communicates to C1, C2, C3, and C4 spinal nerves.

2. Cardiac branch to the carotid body and branch to the pharyngeal plexus.

3. To plexus on the internal and external carotid arteries.

4. Communicating branches to CN IX, X, and XI.

Middle cervical ganglion:

1. Grey rami communicate to C5 and C6.

2. Cardiac branch to the heart.

3. To plexus of the inferior thyroid artery.

4. Ansa subclavia connects it to the inferior cervical ganglion by looping the first part of the subclavian artery. This loop gives communicating twig to the phrenic nerve and fibers to the subclavian artery.

Inferior cervical ganglion:

1. Grey rami communicate to C7, C8 (and T1) spinal nerves.

2. Cardiac branch to the heart.

3. To plexus on the vertebral and subclavian artery.

▌Clinical Notes

Internal Jugular Vein

1. The internal jugular vein is used to record the venous pressure.

2. The deep cervical groups of lymph nodes (jugulo-omohyoid and jugulodigastric) are located on its surface.

3. The internal jugular vein gets dilated due to the congestive cardiac failure.

Glossopharyngeal Nerve

Complete section of the glossopharyngeal nerve results in sensory loss in the pharynx, weakness of pharynx (due to paralysis of the stylopharyngeus muscle), loss of taste and general sensations from the posterior one-third of the tongue, and loss of salivary secretion from the parotid gland from the injured side.

Vagus Nerve

1. In the bilateral paralysis of the vagus nerve, there is regurgitation through nose due to paralysis of the soft palate.

2. If the external laryngeal nerve is damaged, the cricothyroid muscle is paralyzed. This leads to a change in the quality of voice as tension in the vocal cord is abolished.

3. Injury to the recurrent laryngeal nerve leads to hoarseness of the voice.

Accessory Nerve

1. Due to injury to the spinal part of the nerve both the sternomastoid and trapezius muscles are paralyzed. The face is turned toward the side of the injury due to unopposed action of the sternomastoid of opposite side. There is inability to surge the shoulder on the side of the injury due to paralysis of the trapezius.

2. The cranial part is damaged along with the injury to the vagus nerve.

Hypoglossal Nerve

In case of injury to the hypoglossal nerve, when the tongue is protruded it will deviate to the side of the injury. This is because of unopposed action of the genioglossus muscle of the healthy side.

Cervical Sympathetic Trunk

Any injury to the cervical sympathetic trunk at or above the T1 level, on one side, will result in a condition known as *Horner syndrome*. This occurs because of the interruption in the sympathetic nerve supply to the head and neck on that side. It is characterized by the following:

1. *Constriction of the pupil* due to unopposed action of the parasympathetic supply.

2. *Partial ptosis* due to paralysis of the smooth muscles of the upper eyelid.

3. *Anhydrosis* due to interruption in the sympathetic innervation to the sweat glands on that side of the face.

4. *Enophthalmos (retraction of the eyeball).*

19 Dissection of the Prevertebral Region and Cervical Plexus

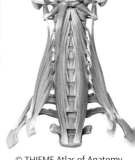

© THIEME Atlas of Anatomy

Learning Objectives

At the end of the deep dissection of the prevertebral region, you should be able to identify the following:

- Prevertebral fascia and prevertebral muscles on the ventral aspect of the cervical vertebral column.
- Formation of the cervical plexus and its branches.
- Second part of the vertebral artery and vein.

Introduction

The prevertebral muscles are covered by the prevertebral cervical fascia. These muscles are present on the anterior aspect of the cervical vertebral column. These muscles are responsible for the flexion of the neck and head. This part of the vertebral artery runs through the foramina transversaria (C6 to C1). The second part of the artery is surrounded by the plexus of veins. The cervical plexus is formed by communication between the ventral rami of the upper four cervical nerves.

Surface Landmarks

1. Review an area surrounding the foramen magnum and jugular foramen on the external surface of the base of the skull.

2. Examine the body, transverse process, and foramina transversaria of the cervical vertebrae.

Dissection and Identification

A. Dissection of the prevertebral muscles.

1. After the disarticulation of the head from the vertebral column, pull down the head, larynx, pharynx, esophagus, and trachea downward toward the thorax so that the prevertebral muscles are exposed.

2. Look for the prevertebral fascia on the anterior surface of the cervical vertebral column. Trace it upward toward the base of the skull and downward toward the superior thoracic aperture. It covers the prevertebral muscles near the median plane and scalene muscles laterally.

3. Identify the cut ends of the rectus capitis anterior and rectus capitis lateral muscles. These muscles were cut during the disarticulation of the head from the vertebral column.

4. Identify the longus capitis, longus colli, and scalenus anterior, middle, and posterior muscles (refer to **Fig. 19.1**).

5. Detach the origin of the scalenus anterior muscle to expose the anterior and posterior inter-transverse muscles, which extend between the corresponding cervical transverse processes.

B. Exposure of ventral rami of cervical nerves, cervical plexus, and vertebral artery (Video 19.1).

1. Note the ventral rami of the cervical nerves as they come out between the anterior and posterior intertransverse muscles (except C1 ramus), which comes out between the rectus capitis anterior and rectus capitis lateralis (**Fig. 19.1**).

2. Trace the ventral rami of the first five cervical nerves and note the formation of the cervical plexus (**Fig. 19.2**).

3. Follow the formation of the phrenic nerve.

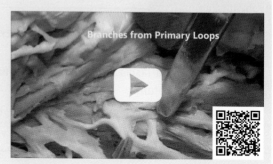

Video 19.1 Cervical plexus.

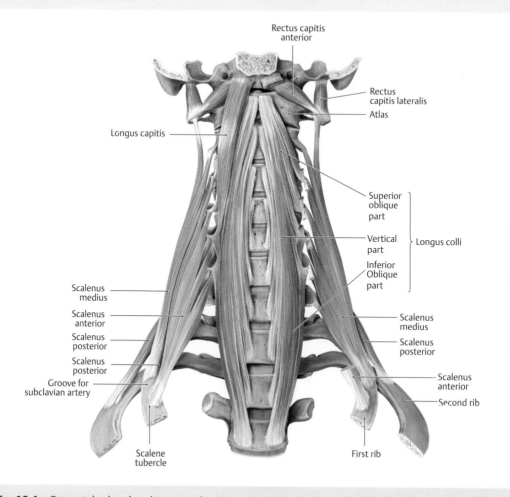

Fig. 19.1 Prevertebral and scalene muscles (anterior view). (From: Schuenke M, Schulte E, Schumacher U. THIEME Atlas of Anatomy. Head, Neck, and Neuroanatomy. Illustrations by Voll M and Wesker K. © Thieme 2020.)

4. Remove the anterior intertransverse muscles to expose the second part of the vertebral artery in the intertransverse spaces (**Fig. 19.3**). We may also remove the anterior tubercles and costal processes of the C3 to C6 vertebrae. This will expose the vertebral artery.

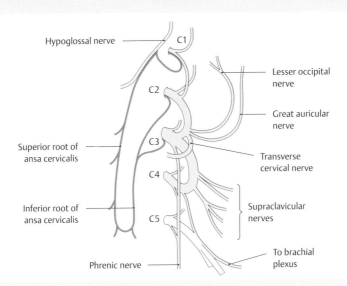

Fig. 19.2   Cervical plexus (viewed from the left side). (From: Schuenke M, Schulte E, Schumacher U. THIEME Atlas of Anatomy. Head, Neck, and Neuroanatomy. Illustrations by Voll M and Wesker K. © Thieme 2020.)

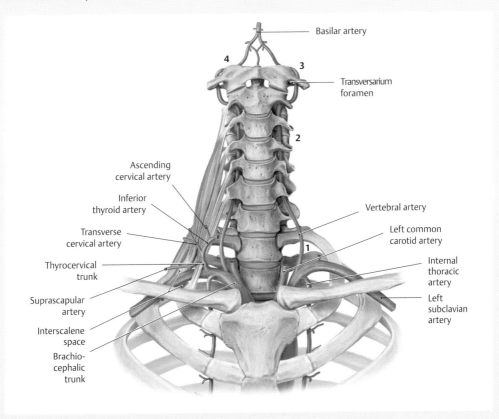

Fig. 19.3   Origin, course, and parts (1, 2, 3, and 4) of the vertebral artery. (From: Schuenke M, Schulte E, Schumacher U. THIEME Atlas of Anatomy. Head, Neck, and Neuroanatomy. Illustrations by Voll M and Wesker K. © Thieme 2020.)

Muscles

We have already dissected the anterior, middle, and posterior scalene muscles while dissecting the structures at the root of the neck. We shall now study the prevertebral muscles (the rectus capitis anterior and rectus capitis lateralis, longus capitis, and longus colli) and intertransverse muscles (**Table 19.1**).

Table 19.1   Prevertebral muscles and intertransverse muscles

Muscle	Origin	Insertion	Nerve supply	Action
Rectus capitis anterior	Anterior surface of the lateral mass of the atlas vertebra	Anterior to the occipital condyle, at the base of the skull	Ventral ramus of C1	Stabilizes the skull on the vertebral column
Rectus capitis lateralis	Superior surface of the transverse processes of the atlas	Jugular process of the occipital bone	Ventral ramus of C1	Stabilizes the skull on the vertebral column
Longus capitis	From the anterior tubercles of the transverse processes of the C3 to C6 vertebrae	Base of the skull in front of the rectus capitis anterior	Ventral rami of C1 to C3	Flexes the head over the neck
Longus colli	From the anterior tubercles of the C1 to the T3 vertebrae	Bodies of intervening vertebrae and transverse processes of the C3 to C6 vertebrae	Ventral rami of C3 to C6	Flexes the neck and head over the neck
Anterior and posterior inter transverse muscles	From anterior and posterior tubercles of the cervical transverse processes	To corresponding tubercles of the adjacent cervical vertebrae	Ventral rami of the corresponding cervical nerves	Lateral flexion of the neck

Artery

Vertebral Artery

The vertebral artery is the largest branch of the first part of the subclavian artery. It begins at the root of the neck and runs vertically upward, passing through the foramen traversia of C6 to C1 to enter cranial cavity where it terminates by joining its fellow of the opposite side to form the basilar artery in the posterior cranial fossa. The course of the artery for descriptive purpose is divided into four parts (**Fig. 19.3**) as discussed next.

Parts

First part: It begins at its origin from the first part of the subclavian artery to the foramen transversarium of the C6 vertebra. Here, it lies between the scalenus anterior and longus colli muscles, deep to the common carotid artery and vertebral vein. It is crossed by the inferior thyroid artery and thoracic duct (on the left side).

Second part: It lies in the foramina transversaria of the C6 to C1 vertebrae and it is surrounded by the sympathetic plexus and venous plexus. In the intertransverse spaces, the artery is related to the anterior and posterior intertransverse muscles, which extend between the corresponding cervical transverse processes. The artery lies anterior to the ventral rami of the cervical nerves. After coming out through the foramen transversarium of the atlas, it winds around the lateral mass of the atlas. It then lies on the groove on the upper surface of the posterior arch of the atlas.

Third part: It lies in the suboccipital triangle. After coming out through the foramen transversarium of the atlas, it winds around the lateral mass of the atlas. It then lies on the groove on the upper surface of the posterior arch of the atlas. It leaves the triangle by passing anterior to the posterior atlanto-occipital membrane.

Fourth part: It enters the cranial cavity through the foramen magnum after piercing the dura and arachnoid mater. It joins its fellow at the lower border of the pons to form the basilar artery.

Branches

1. In the neck, it gives *spinal branches* to the vertebral canal. They supply the spinal cord and vertebrae.

2. The *muscular branches* are given in the suboccipital triangle.

3. The *posterior spinal artery* and *anterior spinal artery* are given in the cranial cavity. These branches supply the cervical spinal cord.

4. The *posterior inferior cerebellar artery* is also given in the cranial cavity. It supplies blood to the cerebellum.

Vein

Vertebral Vein

A venous plexus is formed around the third part of the vertebral artery in the suboccipital triangle. This plexus communicates with the internal vertebral venous plexus. The plexus around the vertebral artery runs with its second part through the foramina transversaria. Below the C6 transverse process, it forms one or two veins called vertebral vein(s) which after crossing the subclavian artery open on the posterior surface of the brachiocephalic vein.

Nerves

We have already dissected the phrenic nerve and brachial plexus along with the structures at the root of the neck. We shall now study the cervical plexus.

Cervical Plexus

The cervical plexus is formed by the ventral rami of the C1 to C4 cervical nerves. Except the ventral ramus of C1, all the others divide in ascending and descending branches which join each other to form the cervical plexus (**Fig. 19.2**).

Branches

Cutaneous Branches

1. These are the lesser occipital (C2), transverse cervical (C2 and C3), great auricular (C2 and C3), and supraclavicular (C3 and C4).

Muscular Branches

1. The branches to the *prevertebral group of muscles* (rectus capitis lateralis, rectus capitis anterior, longus capitis, and longus colli).

2. The branches to the *muscles of the posterior triangle*—sternomastoid and trapezius (C2 to C4, sensory fibers only); levator scapulae and scalenus medius (C3 and C4).

3. The *phrenic nerve* is formed by the branches from the C3 to C5 roots.

4. The branches to the *infrahyoid muscles* through the ansa cervicalis (C1 to C3).

▌Clinical Notes

The second part of the vertebral artery may be pressed by the osteophytes in *cervical spondylosis* leading to inadequate blood supply to the brain. This may result in transient ischemia of the brain causing dizziness. Similarly, the third and fourth parts of the artery may be affected due to the formation of atheroma leading to the inadequate blood supply to the brain.

Pharynx, Palatine Tonsil, and Soft Palate

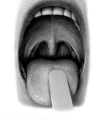

© THIEME Atlas of Anatomy

At the end of the dissection of the pharynx and soft palate, you should be able to identify the following:

- *External aspects of the pharynx.*
- Buccopharyngeal fascia covering the constrictor muscles of the pharynx.
- Superior, middle, and inferior constrictors of the pharynx.
- Levator palatine, tensor palatine, and stylopharyngeus muscles.
- Glossopharyngeal nerve, pharyngeal plexus of nerves and veins, superior laryngeal nerve and vessels, inferior laryngeal artery, and recurrent laryngeal nerve.
- *Internal aspects of the pharynx* (in the midsagittal section of the head and neck).
- Nasopharynx, oropharynx, and laryngopharynx.
- Opening of the auditory tube, salpingopharyngeal fold, and pharyngeal tonsil.
- Oropharynx, palatoglossal fold, palatopharyngeal fold, and palatine tonsil.
- Laryngopharynx, piriform recess.
- Musculature of the soft palate.
- Pharyngeal muscles from the medial side.

Introduction

The pharynx is a muscular tube which extends from the base of the skull to the vertebral level C6 (inferior border of the cricoid cartilage). The wall of the pharynx consists of five layers from the outer to the inner side: buccopharyngeal fascia, muscular layer, pharyngobasilar fascia, submucosa, and mucous membrane. The muscles of the pharynx consist of three constrictors (superior, middle, and inferior) and the stylopharyngeus and palatopharyngeus.

The cavity of the pharynx is divided into nasal, oral, and laryngeal parts as it lies posterior to the nasal cavities (nasopharynx), oral cavity (oropharynx), and larynx (laryngopharynx). The nasopharynx shows the opening of the auditory tube, salpingopharyngeal fold, and pharyngeal tonsil; the oropharynx shows the palatine tonsil; and the laryngopharynx shows the laryngeal inlet and piriform fossa.

The soft palate is present between the nasopharynx and oropharynx. It is made up of many small muscles, that is, the levator palati, tensor palati, palatoglossus, palatopharyngeus, and musculus uvulae (**Fig. 20.1**).

Surface Landmarks

The following bony structures give attachments to the muscles of the pharynx and soft palate:

1. View the external aspect of the base of the dried skull for the pharyngeal tubercle, hard palate, medial pterygoid plate, and pterygoid hamulus.

2. View the inner aspect of the mandible, hyoid bone, thyroid, and cricoid cartilages.

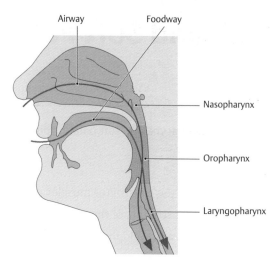

Fig. 20.1 Subdivisions of the pharynx, showing path of food and air. (From: Schuenke M, Schulte E, Schumacher U. THIEME Atlas of Anatomy. Head, Neck, and Neuroanatomy. Illustrations by Voll M and Wesker K. © Thieme 2020.)

For the bisection of the head, identify the following bony features on a dried skull:

1. Nasal bone and frontal bone on the skeleton of the face.

2. Crista galli and cribriform plate of the ethmoid bone, body of the sphenoid and basal part of the occipital bone, and foramen magnum.

3. Hard palate on the external surface of the base of the skull.

4. Medial pterygoid plate and pterygoid hamulus.

Dissection and Identification

*Students are advised to study the parts of the nasal cavity, oral cavity, larynx, and pharyngeal cavity from the textbook of gross anatomy before undertaking the dissection of the pharynx. You should also see these structures in the specimen of midsagittal section of the head and neck, available in your anatomy museum or dissection hall (**Fig. 20.2**).*

You should also learn from the textbook description about the lips, cheeks, vestibule of the mouth, gums and teeth, floor, and roof of the mouth cavity.

A. Dissection of the external surface of the pharynx from its posterior aspect.

1. Carefully clean the buccopharyngeal fascia from the posterior surface of the pharynx.

2. Identify the *pharyngeal raphe* in the midline (**Fig. 20.3**).

3. Trace the fibers of the *inferior constrictor muscle* from the oblique line of the thyroid cartilage and cricoid cartilage to the pharyngeal raphe. The fibers of muscle run posteromedially to gain attachment on the pharyngeal raphe (**Figs. 20.3** and **20.4**).

4. Just above the inferior pharyngeal constrictor, identify the *middle constrictor muscle* of the pharynx. It extends from the greater cornu of the hyoid bone to the pharyngeal raphe and its lower border lies deep to the middle constrictor (**Figs. 20.3** and **20.4**).

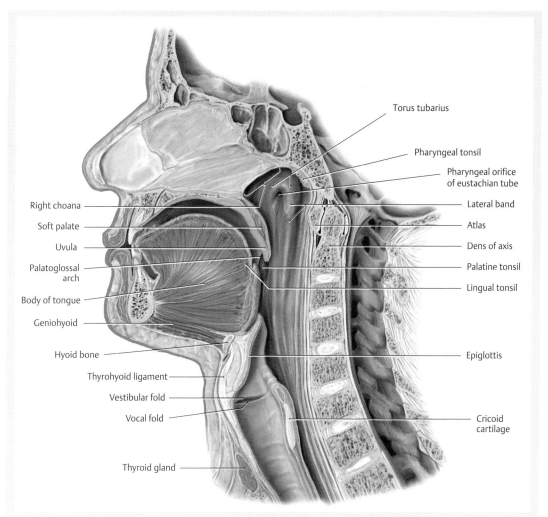

Fig. 20.2 Midsagittal section of head and neck. (From: Schuenke M, Schulte E, Schumacher U. THIEME Atlas of Anatomy. Head, Neck, and Neuroanatomy. Illustrations by Voll M and Wesker K. © Thieme 2020.)

5. Identify the *superior constrictor muscle* which takes origin from the *pterygomandibular raphe*. It is also attached to the pharyngeal raphe and pharyngeal tubercle at the base of the skull. The upper border of the muscle is free and crescentic. A gap is seen between the superior border of this muscle and base of the skull.

6. The *pharyngobasilar fascia* is seen at the superior border of the superior constrictor muscle in the gap. Above this, fascia is attached to the base of the skull (refer to **Fig. 20.3**).

7. Identify the *levator and tensor muscle of the palate* above the superior border of the superior constrictor and lateral to the pharyngobasilar fascia. Note the presence of the *auditory tube* between these two muscles.

8. On the lateral wall of the pharynx, search for the *stylopharyngeus muscle* between the superior and middle constrictor muscles (**Fig. 20.3**). It originates from the styloid process and gains insertion on the inner aspect of the pharyngeal wall. On the posterior and lateral surface of the stylopharyngeus muscle, the *glossopharyngeal nerve* is seen (**Fig. 20.4**).

9. A nerve plexus may be seen on the posterolateral aspect of the pharynx. This is known as the *pharyngeal plexus of nerves*. The plexus is contributed by the glossopharyngeal nerve, vagus nerve and sympathetic fibers. Similarly, a pharyngeal plexus of vein is also present on the posterior aspect of the pharynx (refer to **Fig. 18.1**).

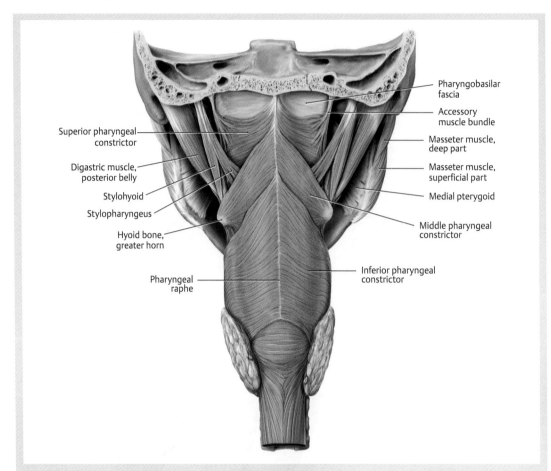

Fig. 20.3 Pharyngeal muscles (posterior view). (From: Schuenke M, Schulte E, Schumacher U. THIEME Atlas of Anatomy. Head, Neck, and Neuroanatomy. Illustrations by Voll M and Wesker K. © Thieme 2020.)

B. Exposure of cavity of the pharynx (Video 20.1).

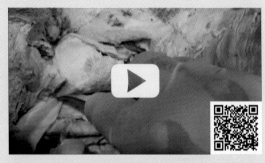

1. Now with the help of a scalpel give a midline cut on the posterior wall of the pharynx from the pharyngeal tubercle to the superior end of the esophagus. This will expose the three parts of the pharyngeal cavity (nasopharynx, oropharynx, and laryngopharynx). Now examine the structures of the pharyngeal cavity (**Fig. 20.5**).

Video 20.1 Laryngopharynx and piriform fossa.

2. Identify the posterior *and piriform fossa. aperture* and posterior end of the *nasal septum*. The nasal aperture is located above the soft palate. Identify the opening of the auditory tube and *salpingopharyngeal fold* in the lateral wall of the nasopharynx.

3. The oropharynx is to be identified between the soft palate and epiglottis. Identify the palatoglossus and palatopharyngeal folds. Between these folds lies the palatine tonsil (refer to **Fig. 20.2**).

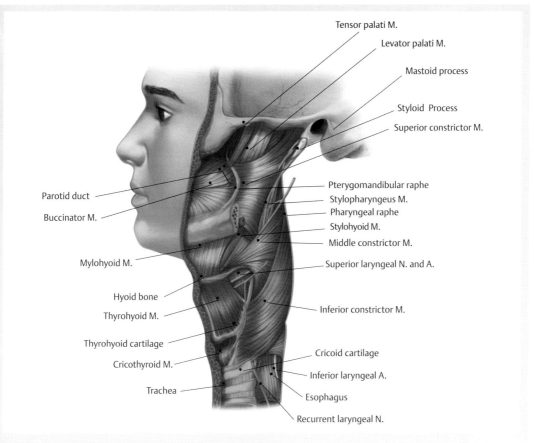

Fig. 20.4 Constrictors of the pharynx (lateral view).

4. In the laryngopharynx, identify the epiglottis, inlet of larynx, and piriform recess (refer to **Fig. 20.5**).

C. Dissection of the head, larynx, pharynx, trachea, and esophagus.

1. With the help of a saw, cut through the nasal and frontal bone, ethmoid bone, body of the sphenoid, dorsum sellae, and basilar part of the occipital bone up to the foramen magnum.

2. Extend this saw cut lower down, in the midline, through the nasal cavity, hard palate, tongue, pharynx, larynx, and up to the upper part of the trachea and esophagus.

3. The right and left halves of the head should be separated from each other (refer to **Fig. 20.2**).

D. Dissection of the soft palate, hard palate, and muscles of the pharynx.

1. On the cut hemisection of the head, remove the mucous membrane from both the surfaces of the soft palate.

2. Also, remove the mucosa from the *palatoglossus fold* and expose the *palatoglossus muscle* located deep to the mucous membrane. The muscle extends between the soft palate and lateral side of the tongue.

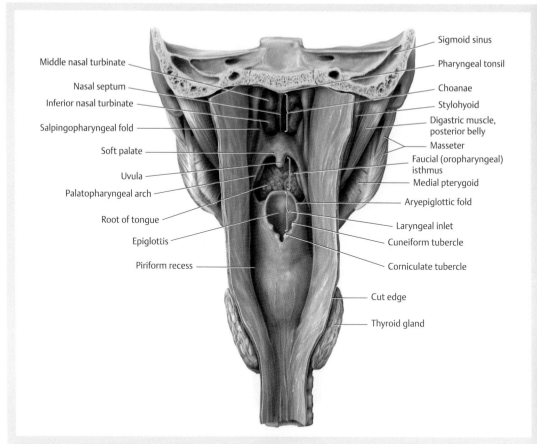

Fig. 20.5   Surface anatomy of pharyngeal mucosa lining nasopharyx, oropharynx, and laryngopharynx (posterior view). (From: Schuenke M, Schulte E, Schumacher U. THIEME Atlas of Anatomy. Head, Neck, and Neuroanatomy. Illustrations by Voll M and Wesker K. © Thieme 2020.)

3. Similarly, remove the mucosa from the *palatopharyngeal fold* and identify the *palatopharyngeus muscle*. This muscle is attached above to the palatine aponeurosis and below to the pharyngeal wall (**Fig. 20.6**).

4. Identify the salpingopharyngeus muscle after removing the mucosa from the salpingopharyngeal fold (**Fig. 20.6**).

5. Remove the remaining mucosa from the nasopharynx and oropharynx. Between the superior and middle constrictor, identify the stylopharyngeus muscle (refer to **Fig. 20.4**).

6. Remove the *pharyngobasilar fascia* which is located between the base of the skull and superior border of the superior constrictor muscle. Lateral to the pharyngobasilar fascia lie the *levator* and *tensor veli palatini muscles* (**Fig. 20.6**). The medial end of the auditory tube lies between these two muscles.

7. The levator veli palatini is attached above to the cartilage of the auditory tube and below to the *palatine aponeurosis*.

8. The tensor veli palatini muscle originates from the *scaphoid fossa*. Its tendon turns medially around the *hamulus of the medial pterygoid plate* and forms the *palatine aponeurosis* (**Figs. 20.5** and **20.6**).

9. Identify the pterygomandibular raphe passing from the hamulus to the mandible and follow the superior constrictor anteriorly to the raphe.

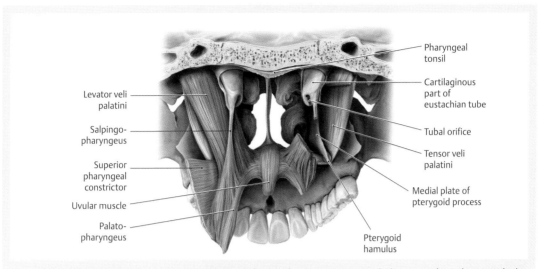

Levator veli palatini
Salpingo-pharyngeus
Superior pharyngeal constrictor
Uvular muscle
Palato-pharyngeus

Pharyngeal tonsil
Cartilaginous part of eustachian tube
Tubal orifice
Tensor veli palatini
Medial plate of pterygoid process
Pterygoid hamulus

Fig. 20.6 Muscles of the soft palate and eustachian tube (posterior view). (From: Schuenke M, Schulte E, Schumacher U. THIEME Atlas of Anatomy. Head, Neck, and Neuroanatomy. Illustrations by Voll M and Wesker K. © Thieme 2020.)

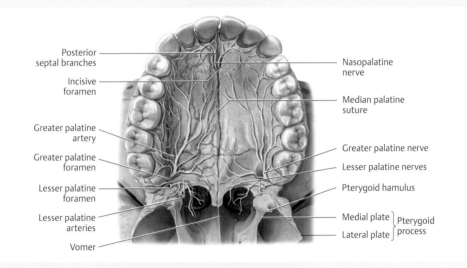

Posterior septal branches
Incisive foramen
Greater palatine artery
Greater palatine foramen
Lesser palatine foramen
Lesser palatine arteries
Vomer

Nasopalatine nerve
Median palatine suture
Greater palatine nerve
Lesser palatine nerves
Pterygoid hamulus
Medial plate ⎫ Pterygoid
Lateral plate ⎭ process

Fig. 20.7 Neurovascular structures of the hard palate (inferior view). (From: Schuenke M, Schulte E, Schumacher U. THIEME Atlas of Anatomy. Head, Neck, and Neuroanatomy. Illustrations by Voll M and Wesker K. © Thieme 2020.)

10. Now remove the mucosa from the hard palate and look for the *greater palatine nerve* and artery as they come out through the greater palatine foramen. Follow these nerve and vessels anteriorly toward the *incisive foramen*. The *nasopalatine nerve* comes on the hard palate through the incisive foramen (**Fig. 20.7**).

11. Find the lesser palatine nerve and artery which come out through the lesser palatine foramen and supply the soft palate.

12. Identify the palatine tonsil and remove it. The tonsillar bed lies on the superior constrictor muscle between the palatoglossus and palatopharyngeal folds (**Fig. 20.8**). The *glossopharyngeal nerve* lies on the tonsillar bed. Look for the branches of the artery supplying the tonsil.

13. Finally, clean the mucous membrane from the medial surface of the inferior constrictor, *piriform recess*, and upper part of the *esophagus* (**Fig. 20.5**).

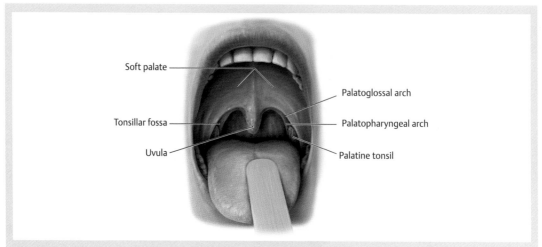

Fig. 20.8 Location of palatine tonsils. (From: Schuenke M, Schulte E, Schumacher U. THIEME Atlas of Anatomy. Head, Neck, and Neuroanatomy. Illustrations by Voll M and Wesker K. © Thieme 2020.)

Muscles

Muscles of the Pharynx

The muscles forming the pharynx (**Table 20.1**) are arranged in two directions, that is, semicircular and longitudinal. The three curved, semicircular muscles form the posterior wall and lie on the sides of the pharynx. These muscles are called the superior, middle, and inferior constrictors. They overlap each other from below upward (refer to **Figs. 20.3** and **20.4**). The longitudinal muscles (palatopharyngeus, salpingopharyngeus, and stylopharyngeus) form the inner layer and pass into the pharyngeal wall from above downward between the constrictors.

Table 20.1 Muscles of the pharynx

Muscle	Origin	Insertion	Nerve supply	Action
Superior constrictor	Posterior border of the medial pterygoid plate and its hamulus/pterygomandibular raphe/posterior end of the mylohyoid line and side of the tongue	To the median raphe and highest fibers are attached to the pharyngeal tubercle	From the pharyngeal plexus, this is formed by the pharyngeal branch of the vagus (containing fibers of the cranial accessory), and pharyngeal branch of the glossopharyngeal and sympathetic fibers form superior cervical sympathetic ganglion	The constrictors propel the bolus of food downward; longitudinal muscles lift the larynx during swallowing
Middle constrictor	Stylohyoid ligament and lesser and greater cornu of the hyoid bone	To the median pharyngeal raphe. The upper fibers overlap the superior constrictor and lower fibers are overlapped by the inferior constrictor	Pharyngeal plexus of the nerve	

(Continued)

Table 20.1   *(Continued)* Muscles of the pharynx

Muscle	Origin	Insertion	Nerve supply	Action
Inferior constrictor	From the oblique line of the thyroid cartilage and arch of the cricoid cartilage	To the median pharyngeal raphe and lower fibers form loop around the superior end of the esophagus	Pharyngeal plexus of the nerve External laryngeal and recurrent laryngeal nerves	
Palatopharyngeus	Posterior border of the hard palate and palatine aponeurosis	Posterior border of the thyroid cartilage and pharyngeal raphe	Pharyngeal plexus of the nerve	Pulls the wall of the pharynx superiorly, medially, and anteriorly during swallowing
Stylopharyngeus	From the base of the styloid process	Posterolateral border of the thyroid cartilage	Glossopharyngeal nerve	
Salpingopharyngeus	Cartilaginous part of the auditory tube	Musculature of the pharynx and posterolateral border of the thyroid cartilage	Pharyngeal plexus of the nerve	

Muscles of the Soft Palate (refer to Fig. 20.6; Table 20.2)

Table 20.2   Muscles of the soft palate

Muscle	Origin	Insertion	Nerve supply	Action
Tensor palate	Scaphoid fossa, auditory tube, and spine of the sphenoid	Crest on the inferior surface of the palatine bone as palatine aponeurosis	Mandibular nerve	Closing of the oropharynx from the nasopharynx during swallowing and speech Squeezing of bolus against the tongue Opening of the auditory tube to equalize pressure on two sides of the tympanic membrane
Levator palate	Petrous part of the temporal bone and auditory tube	On the upper surface of the palatine aponeurosis	Pharyngeal plexus (motor fibers from the cranial part of the accessory nerve)	Elevation of the soft palate
Palatoglossus	Inferior surface of the palatine aponeurosis	Side of the tongue	Pharyngeal plexus of the nerves	Elevation of the tongue
Musculus uvulae	Posterior border of the hard palate near midline	Mucous membrane of the uvula	Pharyngeal plexus of the nerves	Raises uvula in swallowing, also shortens it
Palatopharyngeus	Posterior border of the hard palate and palatine aponeurosis	Posterior border of the thyroid cartilage and pharyngeal raphe	Pharyngeal plexus of the nerves	Pulls the wall of the pharynx superiorly, medially, and anteriorly during swallowing

Arteries

Greater and Lesser Palatine Arteries, Ascending Palatine Artery

1. *Greater palatine artery* is a branch of the third part of the maxillary artery. It comes out on the oral surface of the hard palate after coursing through the greater palatine foramen. It lies in a groove on the alveolar border of the palate which extends till the incisive fossa. It runs upward in the incisive foramen to anastomose with the branch of the sphenopalatine artery.

2. *Lesser palatine arteries* consist of two or three branches which arise from the greater palatine artery as it passes through the greater palatine canal. These branches come out through the lesser palatine canals in the pyramidal process of the palatine bone. They supply the soft palate and tonsil (refer to **Fig. 20.7**).

3. *Ascending palatine artery* is a branch of the facial artery. It runs upward along the side of the pharynx. It supplies the soft palate and anastomoses with the greater palatine artery.

4. *Palatine branch of the ascending pharyngeal artery* also supplies the soft palate.

Tonsillar Branch of the Facial Artery

It ascends between the styloglossus and medial pterygoid muscle. It perforates the superior constrictor muscle to supply the tonsil and root of the tongue (refer to **Fig. 8.4**).

Pharyngeal Branches of the Ascending Pharyngeal Artery

The ascending pharyngeal artery is the first branch of the external carotid artery, which ascends between the internal carotid and pharynx. It gives many pharyngeal arteries and also supplies the soft palate and tonsil (refer to **Fig. 8.6**).

Vein

Pharyngeal plexus of vein lies in the connective tissue layer of the pharynx. It communicates with the pterygoid plexus of veins and drains into the internal jugular and facial vein (refer to **Figs. 18.1** and **18.7**).

Nerves

Pharyngeal Plexus of Nerves

All the muscles of the pharynx (except the stylopharyngeus) are innervated by the pharyngeal plexus of nerves. The pharyngeal plexus of nerves is formed by the following components:

Motor: The pharyngeal branch of the vagus carries fibers from the cranial part of the accessory nerve. It is motor to the muscles of the pharynx. The stylopharyngeus muscle is supplied by the glossopharyngeal nerve.

Sensory: The pharyngeal branch of the glossopharyngeal nerve is sensory to the mucous membrane of the pharynx.

Sympathetic: The pharyngeal branch of the superior cervical sympathetic ganglion innervates the vessels of the pharynx. This nerve is vasoconstrictor in function.

Greater and Lesser Palatine Nerves

1. The *greater palatine nerve* passes through the greater palatine canal. It runs on the hard palate close to the alveolar process toward the incisive fossa. It supplies the mucous membrane of the hard palate, part of the lateral wall of the nose, and maxillary air sinus.

2. The *lesser palatine nerves* come out through the lesser palatine foramina. They innervate the tonsil, uvula, and soft palate (refer to **Fig. 20.7**).

Lymphoid Tissues of the Pharynx

At the entrance of the pharynx, there are groups of lymphoid tissues. This forms a strong defense system to prevent spreading of infection from oral and nasal cavities to the lower respiratory and gastrointestinal tracts. These lymphoid tissues surround the beginning of the respiratory and gastrointestinal tracts in the form of a ring. This ring is called *Waldeyer ring* and is formed by many tonsils (a tonsil is a collection of lymphoid tissues):

1. *Anteriorly*: Lingual tonsil present on the posterior one-third of the dorsum of the tongue.

2. *Laterally*: Palatine tonsil.

3. *Posterolaterally*: Tubal tonsil.

4. *Posteriorly*: Adenoids or pharyngeal tonsils, which are collection of lymphoid tissues in the posterior wall of the nasopharynx.

Waldeyer ring of tonsils acts as the first line of defense against the ingested and inspired microorganisms.

Palatine Tonsil

Palatine tonsils are a part of the Waldeyer ring. These tonsils are situated on the right and left sides of the oropharynx wall. Each tonsil is located between the palatoglossal and palatopharyngeal folds above the posterior part of the tongue and below the soft palate (refer to **Figs. 20.8 and 21.1**).

The palatine tonsil is ovoid in shape and about 2 cm in dimension. It has two surfaces, that is, medial and lateral. It has anterior and posterior borders and upper and lower ends.

The lateral surface of the palatine tonsil has a fibrous capsule, which is formed by the pharyngobasilar fascia. The capsule is absent on the medial surface.

Relations

Medial: This surface is covered by the mucous membrane of the pharynx, which shows the presence of many tonsillar crypts.

Lateral: It is related to the superior constrictor muscle of the pharynx, ascending palatine and tonsillar branches of the facial artery, styloglossus and stylopharyngeus muscles. Sometimes, the styloid process and stylohyoid ligament may lie laterally to the tonsil, if the styloid process is too long.

Blood Supply

1. Tonsillar branch of the facial artery, ascending palatine branch of the facial artery.

2. Dorsal lingual branch of the lingual artery.

3. Ascending pharyngeal branch of the external carotid.

Veins

Blood drains to the peritonsillar venous plexus around the capsule. This plexus is also connected to the pharyngeal venous plexus. The main drainage of tonsil is to the lingual vein. Paratonsillar vein is a large vein, which after draining the soft palate goes to the pharyngeal venous plexus through the upper end of the tonsil.

Nerves

The tonsillar branch of the *glossopharyngeal* and *lesser palatine* nerves supplies the sensory fibers to the mucous membrane covering the medial surface of the tonsil.

Lymphatic Drainage

Lymphatics from the tonsil drain the lymph to the jugulodigastric group of lymph nodes (**Fig. 7.6**).

▌Clinical Notes

1. Foreign bodies may lodge in the piriform recess.

2. Paratonsillar vein may be the main source of bleeding after tonsillectomy.

3. Sometimes, the glossopharyngeal nerve may get injured during tonsillectomy as it is closely related to the lateral aspect of the tonsil.

4. Swelling of adenoids (pharyngeal tonsils) may interfere with nasal breathing.

5. Enlargement of the tubal tonsil may occlude the tympanic tube leading to deafness and middle ear infection.

6. Incomplete cleft palate may involve only uvula of the soft palate, soft palate only or soft palate, and a part of the hard palate.

7. Complete cleft palate may be unilateral or bilateral involving one side of the premaxilla or both sides of the premaxilla.

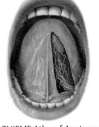

© THIEME Atlas of Anatomy

At the end of the dissection of the tongue, you should be able to identify the following:

- *Parts*: Root, body, and apex of the tongue.
- *On the dorsal aspect*: Median sulcus, foramen caecum, sulcus terminalis, lingual tonsils, and lingual papillae (circumvallate, fungiform, and filiform).
- *At the root*: Median and lateral glossoepiglottic folds and palatoglossal arch.
- *On the ventral aspect*: Sublingual folds, frenulum, and deep lingual vein.
- *Muscles*: Extrinsic muscles (hyoglossus, styloglossus, genioglossus, and palatoglossus) and intrinsic muscles (superior and inferior longitudinal, vertical, and transverse).
- *Nerves and vessels*: Lingual, glossopharyngeal, and hypoglossal nerves, lingual artery, and vein.

Introduction

Tongue is a mobile muscular organ located on the floor of the mouth. It is concerned with speech, swallowing, and taste. It has a root, body, and tip. The tip is directed anteriorly and comes in contact with the incisor teeth. The body has dorsal and ventral surfaces and is placed horizontally. The root (or the posterior part) of the tongue forms the anterior wall of the oral part of the pharynx. The dorsum (or the superior surface) of the tongue is divided into anterior (two-thirds) and posterior (one-third) parts by the presence of a V-shaped groove called sulcus terminalis (**Fig. 21.1**).

The ventral aspect (inferior surface) of the tongue is covered by the smooth thin mucous membrane. This surface presents a median fold of the mucosa called frenulum linguae, which stretches between the tongue and the floor of the mouth. This surface shows the opening of the submandibular salivary gland and we can also see the mucosal vein through the mucosa (**Fig. 21.2**).

The substance of the tongue is divided into two halves by the median fibrous septum. It consists of the extrinsic and intrinsic skeletal muscles, little fat, and mucous and serous glands.

Surface Landmarks

On your own tongue or on the tongue of your fellow colleague, look for the following structures:

1. On the dorsal aspect of the tongue, identify the apex, body, and root of the tongue. Look for the sulcus terminalis at the junction of the anterior two-thirds and posterior one-third.

2. Observe the circumvallate, filiform, and fungiform papillae, on the anterior two-thirds of the tongue, with the help of a hand lens.

3. On the posterior one-third of the dorsal surface, observe the lingual tonsils and look for the palatoglossal fold and median glossoepiglottic fold (refer to **Fig. 21.1**).

4. On the ventral surface of the tongue, observe the frenulum, sublingual papilla, deep lingual vein, and sublingual fold (refer to **Fig. 21.2**).

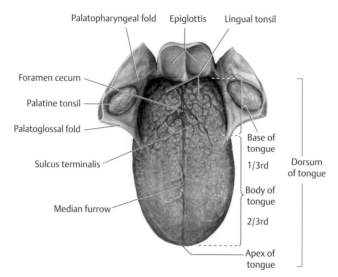

Fig. 21.1 Dorsum of the tongue, epiglottis, and palatine tonsils. (From: Schuenke M, Schulte E, Schumacher U. THIEME Atlas of Anatomy. Head, Neck, and Neuroanatomy. Illustrations by Voll M and Wesker K. © Thieme 2020.)

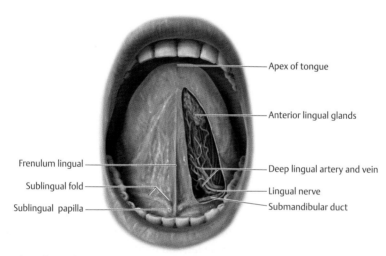

Fig. 21.2 Ventral surface of the tongue. (From: Schuenke M, Schulte E, Schumacher U. THIEME Atlas of Anatomy. Head, Neck, and Neuroanatomy. Illustrations by Voll M and Wesker K. © Thieme 2020.)

Dissection and Identification

After identifying the surface anatomy of the ventral and dorsal surfaces of the tongue, proceed for the dissection of the tongue.

A. Dissection of tongue on midsagittal section of head.

1. On the midsagittal section of the tongue, identify the cut surface of the hyoid bone and mandible (**Fig. 21.3**).

2. Identify the cut edge of the mylohyoid muscle and separate it from the geniohyoid muscle by sliding the handle of the scalpel backward and forward between the two muscles.

3. With the help of blunt dissection, follow the attachment of the geniohyoid muscle, which extends between the inferior genial tubercle of the mandible and the hyoid bone (**Fig. 21.4**).

4. Similarly, just above the geniohyoid, identify the genioglossus muscle and follow it from the superior genial tubercle of the mandible to the midsagittal section of the tongue.

5. The fibers of the genioglossus muscle are fan-shaped and are spread out in the tongue in a vertical plane. It extends from the tip almost to the hyoid bone into the paramedian part (refer to **Fig. 21.3**).

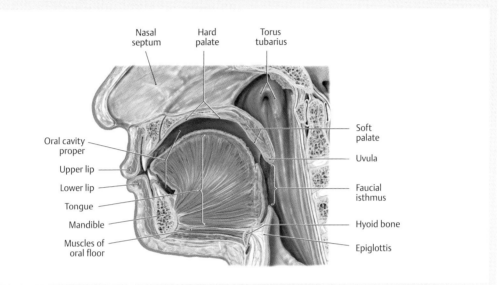

Fig. 21.3 Midsagittal section of the tongue. (From: Schuenke M, Schulte E, Schumacher U. THIEME Atlas of Anatomy. Head, Neck, and Neuroanatomy. Illustrations by Voll M and Wesker K. © Thieme 2020.)

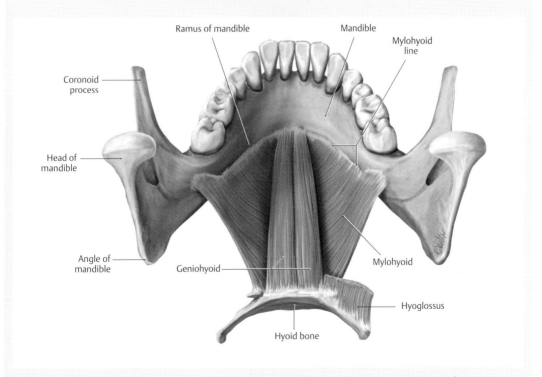

Fig. 21.4 Muscles of the floor of the oral cavity. (From: Schuenke M, Schulte E, Schumacher U. THIEME Atlas of Anatomy. Head, Neck, and Neuroanatomy. Illustrations by Voll M and Wesker K. © Thieme 2020.)

B. Exposure of sublingual gland and submandibular duct (Video 21.1).

1. Now you shall dissect the sublingual region. For this, on the outer surface (face) separate the buccinators, pterygomandibular raphe, and superior constrictor from their attachments to the mandible. Now pull the tongue laterally and give an incision on the mucous membrane along the medial surface of the mandible. Strip the mucous membrane from the floor of the mouth and the mandible to expose the sublingual gland which lies just beneath the mucous membrane above the mylohyoid muscle (**Fig. 21.5**).

2. Pull the sublingual gland laterally to find the submandibular duct. Dissect the submandibular duct anteriorly till it opens in the sublingual papilla (refer to **Fig. 21.2**).

3. Follow the submandibular duct posteriorly till it goes up to the deep part of the submandibular gland (refer to **Fig. 21.5**). The deep part of the gland lies between the mylohyoid and hyoglossus muscles.

C. Exposure of hyoglossus muscle and its relations.

1. Just posterior to the sublingual gland find the lingual nerve; this lies in close relation to the submandibular duct. Follow the lingual nerve backward on the surface of the hyoglossus and styloglossus muscles. Find a tiny submandibular ganglion hanging

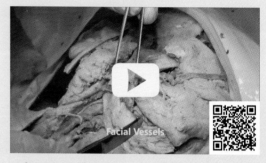

Video 21.1   Floor of the mouth.

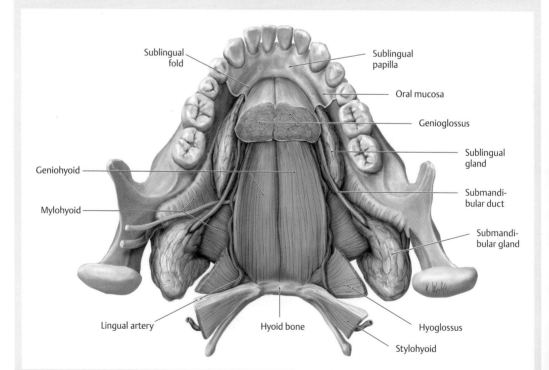

Fig. 21.5   Sublingual and submandibular salivary glands (superior view). (From: Schuenke M, Schulte E, Schumacher U. THIEME Atlas of Anatomy. Head, Neck, and Neuroanatomy. Illustrations by Voll M and Wesker K. © Thieme 2020.)

from the lingual nerve (**Fig. 21.6**). Note that the lingual nerve lies on the mandible posteroinferior to the last molar teeth.

2. Now turn the specimen to see the submandibular triangle. With the help of scissors, cut the origin of the mylohyoid muscle from the hyoid bone and reflect it toward the mandible. This will expose the hyoglossus muscle completely.

3. Follow the origin of the hyoglossus muscle from the hyoid bone and its superior attachment to the lateral side of the tongue. The hypoglossal nerve lies on the hyoglossus just above its origin from the hyoid bone (**Fig. 21.7**).

4. Close to the attachment of the hyoglossus on the tongue, find the styloglossus muscle. It extends between the styloid process and lateral aspect of the tongue (refer to **Fig. 21.6**).

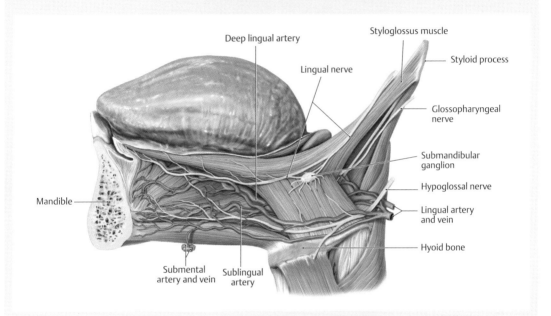

Fig. 21.6 Nerves and vessels of the tongue (left lateral view). (From: Schuenke M, Schulte E, Schumacher U. THIEME Atlas of Anatomy. Head, Neck, and Neuroanatomy. Illustrations by Voll M and Wesker K. © Thieme 2020.)

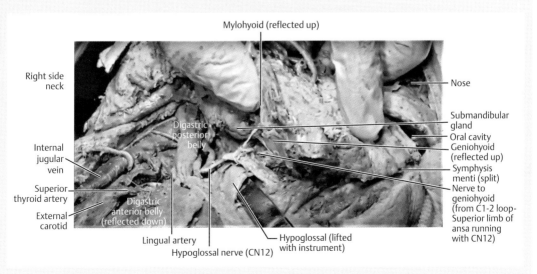

Fig. 21.7 Floor of the mouth: tongue.

5. Find the lingual artery lying deep to the hyoglossus muscle (refer to **Figs. 21.5** and **21.6**). It gives deep and dorsal lingual arteries. Similarly, see the formation of the lingual vein at the posterior margin of the hyoglossus muscle. It is formed by joining the branches of the deep and dorsal lingual veins.

6. It is difficult to visualize all the intrinsic muscles of the tongue in dissection; therefore, see bundles of these muscles in coronal section in **Fig. 21.8**.

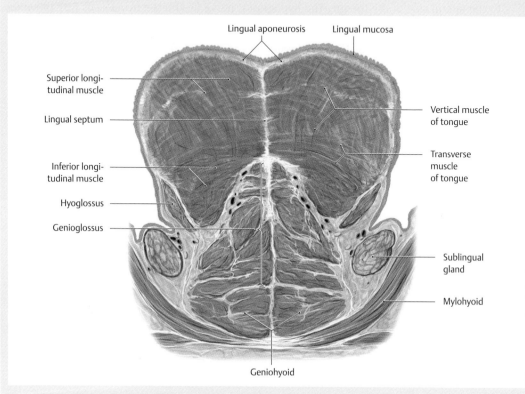

Fig. 21.8 Intrinsic muscles of the tongue (anterior view of a coronal section). (From: Schuenke M, Schulte E, Schumacher U. THIEME Atlas of Anatomy. Head, Neck, and Neuroanatomy. Illustrations by Voll M and Wesker K. © Thieme 2020.)

Muscles of the Tongue

A median fibrous septum is present in the midline of the tongue, which divides it into right and left equal halves. These are classified as extrinsic and intrinsic. The extrinsic muscles take their origin from outside the tongue (refer to **Fig. 21.6**), while the intrinsic muscles are confined within the tongue (**Fig. 21.8**).

Extrinsic Muscles of the Tongue

Extrinsic muscles of the tongue are described in **Table 21.1**.

Table 21.1   Extrinsic muscles of the tongue

Muscle	Origin	Insertion	Nerve supply	Action
Genioglossus	From the upper genial tubercle	On the dorsum of the tongue from the tip to the hyoid bone	Hypoglossal nerve	Protrusion of the tongue by the posterior fibers, while the anterior fibers retract the tip of the tongue. When both the muscles contract together the dorsum of the tongue is depressed
Hyoglossus	From the body and greater cornu of the hyoid bone	Posterior half of the lateral side of the tongue	Hypoglossal nerve	Depresses the side of the tongue
Styloglossus	Styloid process and stylohyoid ligament	Dorsolateral aspect of the tongue blends with the inferior longitudinal muscle of the tongue	Hypoglossal nerve	Pulls the tongue posterosuperiorly during swallowing
Palatoglossus	Palatine aponeurosis of the soft palate (inferior surface)	Posterolateral part of the tongue	Pharyngeal branch of the vagus which forms the pharyngeal plexus (through vagus-accessory complex)	Elevate the posterior part of the tongue or pull the soft palate inferiorly

Intrinsic Muscles of the Tongue

The intrinsic muscles of the tongue are described in **Table 21.2**.

Table 21.2   Intrinsic muscles of the tongue

Muscle	Location and extent	Nerve supply	Actions
Superior longitudinal	Present just beneath the mucous membrane of the dorsum and extends from close to the epiglottis to the anterior end of the tongue. It extends from the median septum to the lateral margin of the tongue	Hypoglossal nerve	Turns the tip of the tongue upward
Inferior longitudinal	Present on the inferior aspect of the tongue between the genioglossus and hyoglossus	Hypoglossal nerve	Turns the tip of the tongue downward
Transverse lingual	Fibers run from each side of the median septum to the lateral margin of the tongue	Hypoglossal nerve	Produces narrowing and lengthening of the tongue
Vertical lingual	Fibers run from the dorsal to the ventral lingual surface	Hypoglossal nerve	It flattens and broadens the tongue

Artery

The lingual artery is the main artery supplying the tongue (refer to **Fig. 11.4**; **Figs. 21.5** and **21.6**). Its four branches are as follows:

1. *Tonsillar branch*: It supplies the pharyngeal part of the tongue.

2. *Dorsal branches*: These branches supply the posterior portion of the tongue.

3. *Deep lingual branch*: It supplies the deep part of the tongue.

4. *Sublingual branch*: It supplies the anterior portion of the tongue.

Vein

The tongue is drained by the deep lingual and dorsal lingual veins. The deep lingual vein joins the sublingual vein and forms the vena comitans, which runs along the hypoglossal nerve (refer to **Fig. 21.6**). *All these veins drain directly or indirectly in the facial or internal jugular vein.*

Nerves

1. *Motor supply*: All the muscles of the tongue are innervated by the hypoglossal nerve except the palatoglossus, which is supplied by the pharyngeal plexus.

2. *General sensory supply*: The anterior two-thirds of the tongue is supplied by the lingual nerve (branch of the mandibular division of the trigeminal). The posterior one-third of the tongue is supplied by the glossopharyngeal nerve.

3. *Special (taste) sensation*: The chorda tympani (a branch of the facial nerve) carries the taste sensation from the anterior two-thirds of the tongue. The posterior one-third and circumvallate papillae are innervated by the glossopharyngeal nerve.

Lymphatic Drainage

There are two sets of lymphatic plexus, that is, the intramuscular plexus and submucosal plexus. The intramuscular plexus drains to the submucosal plexus. The following four areas of the tongue drain to different groups of the lymph nodes (**Fig. 21.9**):

1. *The posterior one-third of the tongue and circumvallate papillae*: This area on either side of the midline drains to the upper deep cervical (jugulodigastric) group of lymph nodes. Some area near the median plane may drain to both sides.

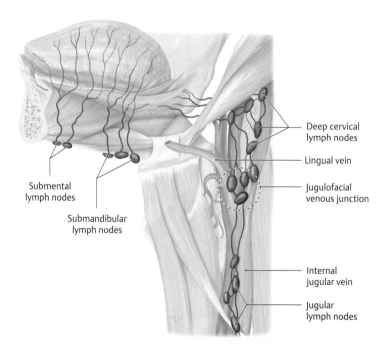

Fig. 21.9 Lymphatic drainage of the tongue (left lateral view). (From: Schuenke M, Schulte E, Schumacher U. THIEME Atlas of Anatomy. Head, Neck, and Neuroanatomy. Illustrations by Voll M and Wesker K. © Thieme 2020.)

2. *The central part of the anterior two-thirds*: This area on either side of the median septum drains to the inferior deep cervical (jugulo-omohyoid) group of lymph nodes. Some area near the median plane may drain to both sides.

3. *The lateral part (margin) of the anterior two-thirds*: This area drains to the submandibular group of lymph nodes. This then drains to the jugulo-omohyoid group of the deep cervical lymph nodes.

4. *The tip of the tongue*: This area drains to the submental group of lymph nodes, which in turn drains to the submandibular and jugulo-omohyoid groups of the deep cervical lymph nodes. The tip drains bilaterally (**Fig. 21.9**).

▌Clinical Notes

1. The hypoglossal nerve injury produces paralysis and wasting of the muscles of the tongue on the side of the injury. The protruded tongue deviates toward the side of the nerve lesion because of unopposed action of the tongue muscles on the normal side.

2. Many groups of lymph nodes drain the tongue from both the ipsilateral and contralateral sides; hence, cancer may spread in a wider area (on both the sides) (**Fig. 21.9**).

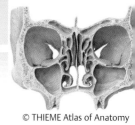
Learning Objectives

At the end of the dissection of the nasal cavity, you should be able to identify the following:

- Median *nasal septum.*
- Boundaries of the nasal cavity.
- Features of the lateral wall of the nasal cavity, that is, three *conchae* and three *meatuses* (meati), openings of various *paranasal air sinuses*, and *nasolacrimal duct.*
- Nasal branches of the pterygopalatine ganglion and sphenopalatine branch of the maxillary artery.
- Relationship of the paranasal sinuses to the orbit, anterior cranial fossa, and nasal cavity.

Introduction

The nasal cavity is divided into two narrow cavities, right and left, by the septum of the nose. The anterior openings of the nasal cavity are nostrils. Posteriorly, each nasal cavity opens into the nasopharynx through the *choanae*. The walls of the nasal cavities are formed by bones and cartilages. Each nasal cavity has a roof, floor, and medial and lateral walls, which are lined by the mucous membrane. The lateral wall of the nasal cavity is very uneven because of the three *conchae*. Lateral to the lateral wall of the nose are air sinuses which communicate with the nose through the *meatuses*.

The mucous membrane of the nose is mainly innervated by the *maxillary nerve*, which reaches the nasal mucosa through branches of the *pterygopalatine ganglion*, *anterior superior alveolar nerve*, and the *greater palatine nerve*. The main supply of blood to the nasal cavity is through the *sphenopalatine branch of the maxillary artery*.

The paranasal air sinuses are related to the nasal cavity and they all open in the lateral wall of the nose. The *maxillary air sinus* lies laterally to the lateral wall of the nasal cavity. The roof of the maxillary sinus is the floor of the orbit.

Surface Landmarks

Bones and Cartilages Forming the Nasal Cavity

In the sagittal section of the skull, passing through the nose, mouth, and pharynx, identify the bones forming the nasal cavity (**Fig. 22.1**).

On a dry skull, look for the bones forming the anterior nasal aperture. Note the presence of the median nasal septum, anterior nasal spine, and nasal notch of the right and left maxilla (refer to **Fig. 1.3**).

The walls of the nasal cavity are formed as follows:

1. *Medially* (median nasal septum) by the perpendicular plate of the ethmoid, vomer, and septal cartilage (refer to **Fig. 1.9a**).

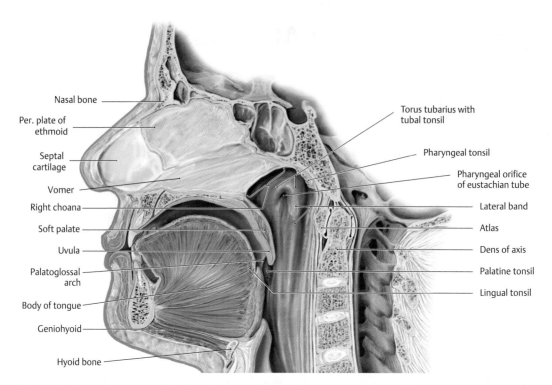

Fig. 22.1 Sagittal section of the head passing through the nose, mouth, and pharynx. (From: Schuenke M, Schulte E, Schumacher U. THIEME Atlas of Anatomy. Head, Neck, and Neuroanatomy. Illustrations by Voll M and Wesker K. © Thieme 2020.)

2. *Laterally* by the maxilla, lacrimal bone, ethmoid, inferior nasal concha, and perpendicular plate of the palatine bone (refer to **Fig. 1.9b** and **c**). The cartilages forming the lateral wall are nasal cartilages and alar cartilage.

3. *The roof* is formed by the nasal bone, cribriform plate of the ethmoid, and body of the sphenoid.

4. *The floor* is formed by the palatine process of the maxilla and horizontal process of the palatine bone (refer to **Fig. 1.9d**).

5. Identify the bony features on the lateral wall of the nose, that is, the sphenoethmoidal recess, superior, inferior, and middle conchae, the bulla ethmoidal, uncinate process, and maxillary hiatus (refer to **Fig. 1.9b** and **c**).

Dissection and Identification

You shall first dissect the median nasal septum on the specimen of the midsagittal section of the head that contains the nasal septum. This dissection should be followed by the dissection of the lateral wall of the nasal cavity.

A. Dissection of nasal septum (medial nasal wall).

1. By blunt dissection, strip the mucosa of the nasal septum to expose the *perpendicular plate of the ethmoid bone, vomer,* and *septal cartilage* (refer to **Fig. 22.1**).

2. To expose the nerve and vessel of the septum, carefully cut the septal cartilage and bones in piecemeal from the mucous membrane on the opposite side (that lines the other side of the nasal septum).

3. In the mucosa, find the *nasopalatine nerve* and *sphenopalatine artery*, which run from the sphenopalatine foramen to the *incisive canal* (**Figs. 22.2** and **22.3**). Also, observe anterior and posterior ethmoidal arteries.

4. Near the roof, observe the branches of the *anterior ethmoidal nerve* and olfactory nerve (**Fig. 22.2**).

B. Dissection of lateral wall of nose.

1. Now start dissecting the lateral wall of the nose (refer to **Fig. 1.9b** and **c**). First, identify an area superior to the nostril, the *vestibule*. The *atrium* is an area superior to the vestibule and anterior to the middle meatus (**Fig. 22.4**).

2. Cut the inferior concha to expose the inferior meatus. Remove the mucosa from the lateral wall of the inferior meatus and observe the opening of the *nasolacrimal duct* (**Fig. 22.5**).

3. Similarly, cut through the middle concha and observe the features in the middle meatus. Observe the *hiatus semilunaris* and *ethmoidal bulla*. On the surface of the ethmoidal bulla, identify the opening of the middle ethmoidal air sinus. In the *semilunar hiatus*, identify the opening of the *frontal air sinus, anterior ethmoidal sinus,* and *maxillary sinus* (**Fig. 22.5**).

4. Cut the superior nasal concha and identify the opening of the *posterior ethmoidal air sinus* in the superior meatus.

5. Identify the opening of the sphenoidal sinus in the *sphenoethmoidal recess* (**Fig. 22.4**).

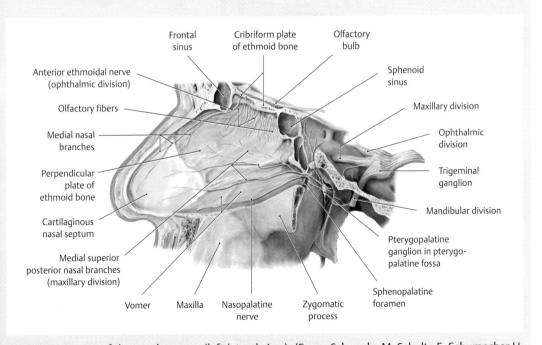

Fig. 22.2 Nerves of the nasal septum (left lateral view). (From: Schuenke M, Schulte E, Schumacher U. THIEME Atlas of Anatomy. Head, Neck, and Neuroanatomy. Illustrations by Voll M and Wesker K. © Thieme 2020.)

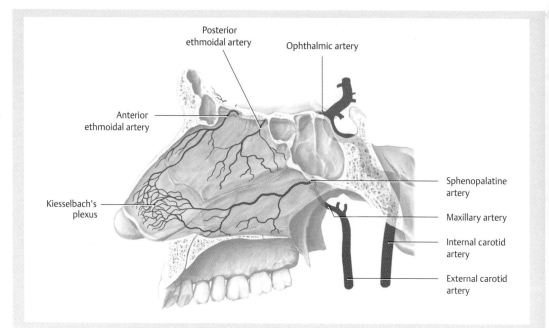

Fig. 22.3 Vascular supply of the nasal septum (left lateral view). (From: Schuenke M, Schulte E, Schumacher U. THIEME Atlas of Anatomy. Head, Neck, and Neuroanatomy. Illustrations by Voll M and Wesker K. © Thieme 2020.)

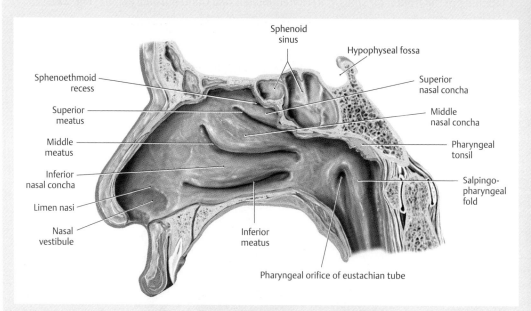

Fig. 22.4 Mucosa of the nasal cavity. (From: Schuenke M, Schulte E, Schumacher U. THIEME Atlas of Anatomy. Head, Neck, and Neuroanatomy. Illustrations by Voll M and Wesker K. © Thieme 2020.)

C. Exposure of pterygopalatine ganglion.

1. This is the time to dissect the pterygopalatine ganglion and the greater palatine nerve. Strip the mucosa from the medial pterygoid plate and perpendicular plate of the palatine bone. Break through the perpendicular plate of the palatine bone and expose the greater palatine nerve. Extend the exposure of the greater palatine canal above to the pterygopalatine ganglion and below up to the greater palatine foramen in the hard palate (**Fig. 22.6**).

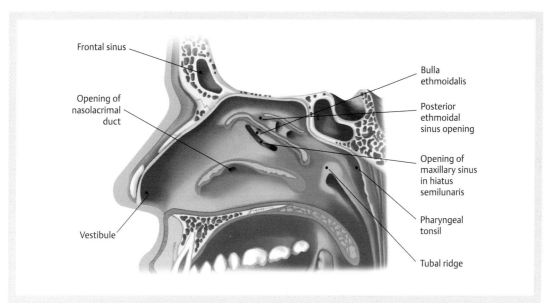

Fig. 22.5 Sagittal section through the nose and palate. The conchae have been cut away to expose the meatuses and the openings into them. The opening of the infundibulum is unusual.

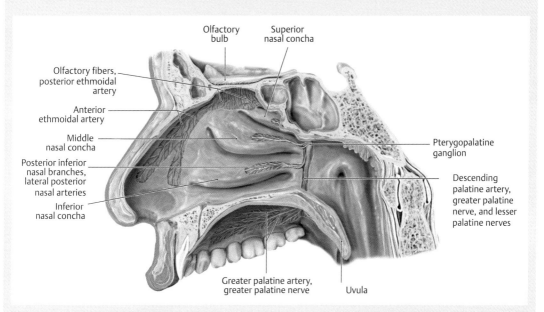

Fig. 22.6 Vessels and nerves of the right lateral nasal wall (left lateral view). (From: Schuenke M, Schulte E, Schumacher U. THIEME Atlas of Anatomy. Head, Neck, and Neuroanatomy. Illustrations by Voll M and Wesker K. © Thieme 2020.)

2. The pterygopalatine ganglion is present at the level of the sphenopalatine foramen. Identify the branches of the pterygopalatine ganglion. Trace the greater palatine nerve to the hard palate and follow the lesser palatine nerve terminating in the soft palate. Identify the descending palatine branch of the maxillary artery (refer to **Fig. 22.6**).

3. Strip away the thin medial walls of the ethmoidal air cells. Remove the mucous membrane lining these ethmoidal air cells till you reach the orbital lamina of the ethmoid. Remove this lamina which forms the medial wall of the orbit. You can now expose the medial surface of the medial rectus muscle.

4. Similarly, break away the medial wall of the maxillary sinus between the nasolacrimal duct (anteriorly) and greater palatine canal (posteriorly). This will expose the maxillary air sinus from the medial side. Observe the interior of the maxillary sinus.

5. Note the cavity of the sphenoidal sinus. It lies directly inferior to the hypophyseal fossa (refer to **Fig. 22.4**).

Nasal Septum

The nasal septum divides the nasal cavity into right and left cavities. It is partly bony and partly cartilaginous. The septum is formed by the perpendicular plate of the ethmoid and vomer, while cartilage is called the septal cartilage. It occupies the space between the perpendicular plate of the ethmoid and vomer, anteriorly (refer to **Fig. 1.9a** and **Fig. 22.1**). Bones and cartilage of the nasal septum are covered by fibrofatty tissue and mucous membrane. The mucosa of the upper part of the nasal septum is olfactory in nature and the remaining mucosa is respiratory in nature.

Lateral Wall of the Nasal Cavity

The skeletal framework of the lateral wall of the nose is formed by many bones (i.e., the maxilla, lacrimal bone, ethmoid, inferior nasal concha, and perpendicular plate of the palatine bone). The cartilages forming the lateral wall are nasal cartilages and alar cartilage. The lateral bony and cartilaginous wall is covered anteroinferiorly by the skin and a large part by the mucous membrane. It is divided into three regions, that is, the *vestibule, atrium,* and *the area of conchae and meatus* (refer to **Fig. 22.4**).

1. The vestibule is the lowest part of the lateral wall and is lined by the hairy skin of the nose.

2. The atrium is located above the vestibule and anterior to the middle meatus.

3. The region of conchae and meatuses presents three shelf-like projections known as superior, middle, and inferior conchae. Just below each concha is a shallow space, which is known as the meatus. Thus, there are three meatuses, that is, superior, middle, and inferior meatus.

4. The superior concha is a small projection from the ethmoid bone. It encloses a small space called the superior meatus.

5. The middle concha is also a projection from the ethmoid bone, below it encloses the middle meatus.

6. The inferior concha is the longest and is formed by an independent bone. It encloses below the inferior meatus.

7. The following openings of the paranasal air sinuses are seen in various meatuses on the lateral wall of the nose (refer to **Fig. 22.5**):

   a. *Superior meatus*: posterior ethmoidal air sinus.

   b. *Middle meatus*:

      i. On the ethmoidal bulla: middle ethmoidal air sinus.

      ii. In the hiatus semilunaris: frontal air sinus, anterior ethmoidal sinus, and maxillary sinus.

   c. *Inferior meatus*: nasolacrimal duct.

Nerves and Vessels of the Nasal Septum

1. The anterosuperior part of the septum is innervated by the anterior ethmoidal nerve, while the posteroinferior part by the nasopalatine nerve. Olfactory nerves carry a special sense of smell from the upper part of the septal mucosa (refer to **Fig. 22.2**).

2. The septum is richly supplied by blood, that is, by the anterior ethmoidal artery, sphenopalatine artery, and septal branch of the superior labial artery (refer to **Fig. 22.3**).

3. Venous blood drains ultimately to the ophthalmic vein, pterygoid venous plexus, inferior cerebral vein, and facial vein.

4. Lymph from the anterior half of the septum drains to the submandibular glands and from the posterior half to the deep cervical nodes.

The Little area (Kiesselbach area) is a small anteroinferior area of the nasal septum where it is rich in blood supply (**Fig. 22.3**). The rich supply of blood is due to anastomosis between various arteries supplying the septum. Nose bleeding is common because of tear in the area leading to a rupture of the artery or vein of plexus of Little's area.

Nerves and Vessels of the Lateral Wall

Sensory Nerve Supply

General sensations from the lateral wall are divided into four quadrants (**Fig. 22.7**):

1. Anterosuperior: *Anterior ethmoidal nerve* (from the ophthalmic nerve).

2. Anteroinferior: *Anterosuperior alveolar nerves* (from the maxillary nerve).

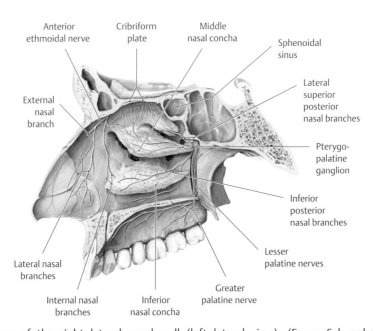

Fig. 22.7 Nerves of the right lateral nasal wall (left lateral view). (From: Schuenke M, Schulte E, Schumacher U. THIEME Atlas of Anatomy. Head, Neck, and Neuroanatomy. Illustrations by Voll M and Wesker K. © Thieme 2020.)

3. Posterosuperior: *Posterosuperior nasal branches* (from the pterygopalatine ganglion).

4. Posteroinferior: *Posteroinferior nasal branches* (from the greater palatine nerve).

Special sense of smell is carried through the olfactory nerve (first cranial nerve) from the mucosa of the superior nasal concha.

Autonomic Supply

Parasympathetic: It comes from the facial nerve forming a relay in the pterygopalatine ganglion and reaches the mucosa through the sphenopalatine nerve. These are secretomotor and vasodilator to the nasal mucosa.

Sympathetic: The postganglionic fibers come through the internal carotid artery to the pterygopalatine ganglion. Without relay in this ganglion, they pass to the nasal mucosa through the branches of the ganglion.

Arteries

1. The anterior part of the lateral wall is supplied by the *anterior ethmoidal artery* and *alar branch of the facial artery*.

2. The posterior part is supplied by the *sphenopalatine* and *greater palatine arteries* (**Fig. 22.8**).

Veins

Veins correspond to the arteries and drain in various venous plexuses: veins in the anterior part form a plexus and drain to the facial vein. Veins of the posterior part of the lateral wall drain to the pharyngeal plexus of veins, while veins of the middle part drain in the pterygoid plexus of veins.

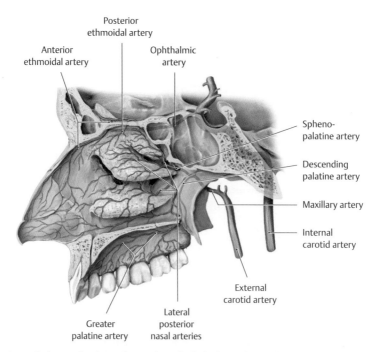

Fig. 22.8   Arteries of the right lateral nasal wall (left lateral view). (From: Schuenke M, Schulte E, Schumacher U. THIEME Atlas of Anatomy. Head, Neck, and Neuroanatomy. Illustrations by Voll M and Wesker K. © Thieme 2020.)

Pterygopalatine Ganglion

It is a parasympathetic ganglion which receives preganglionic fibers from the facial nerve. The pterygopalatine ganglion hangs from the maxillary nerve in the pterygopalatine fossa lateral to the sphenopalatine foramen (refer to **Figs. 22.6** and **22.7**).

It has *parasympathetic, sympathetic,* and *sensory roots*:

1. The *preganglionic parasympathetic fibers* come to the ganglion through the nerve of the pterygoid canal. The fibers arise from the superior salivatory and lacrimatory nucleus and relay in this ganglion. The postganglionic fibers innervate the lacrimal, nasal, and palatine glands.

2. *Postganglionic sympathetic fibers* come along with the internal carotid plexus. The deep petrosal nerve arises from the plexus and joins the greater petrosal nerve to form the nerve of the pterygoid canal. This nerve joins the pterygopalatine ganglion, but fibers do not relay in this ganglion. They are distributed along with the branches of the ganglion. The sympathetic fibers are vasoconstrictor.

3. *Sensory roots* of the pterygopalatine ganglion are derived from the maxillary nerve. They do not relay in the ganglion and are distributed along the branches of the ganglion.

Branches

The branches of the pterygopalatine ganglion are mostly derived from the maxillary nerve, though it carries the sensory, parasympathetic, and sympathetic fibers.

1. *Orbital branches*: These enter the orbit through the inferior orbital fissure and innervate the orbitalis muscle, and mucous membrane of the sphenoidal and posterior ethmoidal air sinuses.

2. *Greater and lesser palatine branches*: Greater and lesser palatine nerves innervate the mucous membrane of the lateral wall of the nose, hard palate, palatine tonsil, and soft palate.

3. *Nasal branches*: These enter the nasal cavity through the sphenopalatine foramen and are grouped in the *posterior superior lateral* and *posterosuperior medial nasal* branches.

4. *Pharyngeal branches*: These pass through the palatinovaginal canal to supply the mucous membrane of the pharynx and tympanic tube.

Irritation of the pterygopalatine ganglion in allergic states, as in the case of hay fever or cold, leads to running nose and eyes. Therefore, sometimes it is called the ganglion of hay fever.

Maxillary Sinus

The maxillary sinus is the largest air sinus of the body (**Fig. 22.9**). It is located inside the body of the maxilla. This sinus is pyramidal in shape whose apex is directed laterally and base medially. Height of the sinus is about 3 cm, length is 3 cm, and width is about 2.5 cm. It has five walls, that is, *anterior, posterior, roof, floor,* and *medial*.

Walls and Relations

1. The anterior wall is formed by the anterior (facial) surface of the maxilla. It contains the canals in which branches of the anterior and middle superior alveolar nerves run.

2. The posterior wall is formed by the posterior surface of the maxilla which is related to the pterygopalatine fossa and infratemporal fossa and their contents. The branches of the posterior superior alveolar nerve run in this wall.

3. The roof is the floor of the orbit. It is related to the infraorbital nerve and vessels.

4. The floor of the sinus is formed by the alveolar process of the maxilla. The roots of the premolar and first two molar teeth may project in it.

5. The medial wall forms a large part of the lateral wall of the nose. It has a large opening.

The maxillary sinus opens laterally in the middle meatus in an opening called hiatus semilunaris. The level of this opening is just below the roof. Hence, drainage of secretion/discharge from this sinus is difficult (**Fig. 22.9a** and **b**).

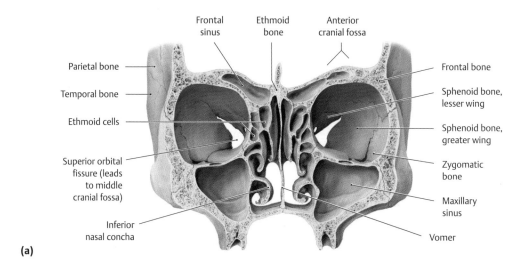

(a)

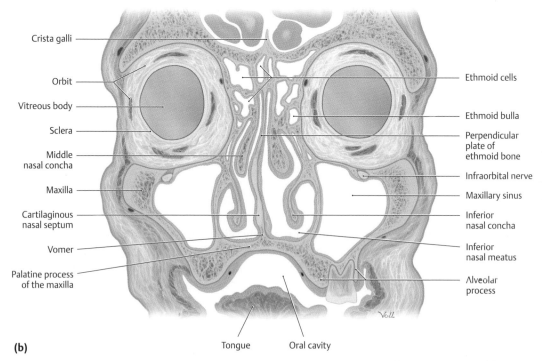

(b)

Fig. 22.9 **(a)** Coronal section of the skull through the nasal cavity, paranasal sinuses, and orbit. **(b)** Coronal section of the head passing through the nose, paranasal sinuses, and orbit. (From: Schuenke M, Schulte E, Schumacher U. THIEME Atlas of Anatomy. Head, Neck, and Neuroanatomy. Illustrations by Voll M and Wesker K. © Thieme 2020.)

Arteries and Veins

It is supplied by the *infraorbital artery*, *greater palatine artery*, and *posterior superior alveoloartery*. The veins drain to the infraorbital vein and greater palatine vein.

Nerves

It is supplied by the *infraorbital nerve* and branches from the *greater palatine nerve*.

Lymphatic Drainage

Lymph goes to the *submandibular group* of lymph nodes.

Ethmoidal Air Sinuses

The ethmoidal air sinuses are divided into three groups, that is, anterior, middle, and posterior. They consist of 10 to 15 air cells and lie in the labyrinth of the ethmoid bone (refer to **Fig. 22.9**).

The relations of the ethmoidal air sinuses are important as superiorly they are related to the anterior cranial fossa, medially to the nasal cavity, and laterally to the orbital cavity.

The anterior and middle ethmoidal sinuses open in the middle meatus while the posterior sinuses open in the superior meatus.

The ethmoidal air sinuses are supplied by the ophthalmic nerve (anterior and posterior ethmoidal branches). Arterial supply is through the ethmoidal arteries.

Sphenoidal Air Sinuses

The right and left sphenoidal air sinuses are separated by a thin septum in the body of the sphenoid. The important relations of sinus are hypophysis cerebri, optic chiasma, and cavernous sinus. Each sinus opens in the sphenoethmoidal recess (refer to **Fig. 22.4**).

Frontal Air Sinuses

The frontal air sinuses are paired air sinuses situated deep to the superciliary arches on either side of the medial line. They are related inferolaterally to the orbit, inferiorly to the nasal cavity, and laterally to the meninges and frontal lobe. They open in the middle meatus (refer to **Figs. 22.2** and **22.5**).

■ Clinical Notes

Little Area and Epistaxis

The Little area (Kiesselbach area) is a small anteroinferior area of the nasal septum where it is rich in blood supply. The rich supply of blood is due to anastomosis between various arteries supplying the septum. Nose bleeding is common because of tear in the area leading to rupture of the artery or vein of plexus of the Little area (refer to **Fig. 22.3**).

Sinusitis

1. The infection of the paranasal air sinus is known as sinusitis. It is usually secondary to the infection in the nose. It is characterized by prolonged, thick, purulent discharge from the nose and headache. In the X-ray, the infected sinus looks opaque.

2. As the opening of the maxillary sinus is just below the roof, the discharge of the sinus is difficult to drain to the nasal cavity. Therefore, the maxillary sinusitis is very common. The sinus can be drained and irrigated by a needle inserted through the inferior nasal concha.

3. Brain abscess may result due to the frontal or ethmoidal sinusitis as they are closely related to the frontal lobe of the brain.

Deviated Nasal Septum

Most of the time, the nasal septum is not in the midline but deviated to one side. Excessive deviation produces the unilateral nasal obstruction and is treated by the submucosal resection of the nasal septum.

Pterygopalatine Ganglion

Irritation of the pterygopalatine ganglion in allergic states, as in case of hay fever or cold, leads to running nose and eyes. Therefore, sometimes it is called the ganglion of hay fever.

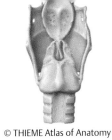

Introduction

The larynx is the organ of voice. It also plays an important role in respiration, phonation, and swallowing. It is the upper expanded part of the windpipe and lies in the neck opposite to the fourth to sixth cervical vertebrae (**Fig. 23.1**). The thyroid gland lies anterior to it and the pharynx posterior to it. Below, it is continuous with the trachea at the level of the sixth cervical vertebra.

The skeleton of the larynx is made up of many cartilages (thyroid, cricoid, epiglottic, arytenoids, corniculate, and cuneiform), membranes and ligaments (thyrohyoid membrane, median thyrohyoid ligament, cricothyroid membrane, cricotracheal membrane, and quadrangular membrane). There is a presence of intrinsic and extrinsic muscles of the larynx.

The larynx contains a valve called glottis that serves the double function of controlling the passage of air and production of sound. The intrinsic muscles of the larynx control the glottis, while the extrinsic muscles (suprahyoid and infrahyoid) control the position of the larynx in the neck.

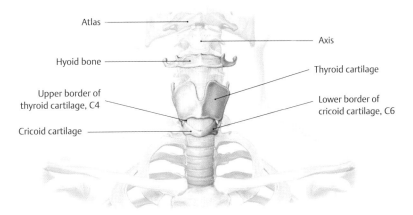

Fig. 23.1 Location of the larynx and anterior view of the laryngeal cartilages. (From: Schuenke M, Schulte E, Schumacher U. THIEME Atlas of Anatomy. Head, Neck, and Neuroanatomy. Illustrations by Voll M and Wesker K. © Thieme 2020.)

Surface Landmarks

Cartilages, Membranes, and Ligaments Forming the Laryngeal Skeleton (Video 23.1)

A large number of cartilages of the larynx are united with each other by ligaments and membranes, which form the rigid framework to keep the lumen of the larynx patent (**Figs. 23.2** and **23.3**). There are three paired (arytenoid, corniculate, and cuneiform) and three single (epiglottic, thyroid, and cricoid) cartilages.

Students should learn the details of these cartilages, membranes, ligaments, and joints of the larynx from a textbook of gross anatomy before commencing the dissection of the larynx.

Thyroid cartilage: It consists of two quadrilateral laminae which are joined anteriorly in the midline to form the laryngeal prominence. It is present below the hyoid bone and consists of the superior and inferior cornua or horns (refer to **Fig. 23.2**). The inferior horn of the thyroid cartilage articulates with the cricoid cartilage at the cricothyroid joint.

Cricoid cartilage: It lies below the thyroid cartilage. It is shaped like a ring with broad lamina located posteriorly and a narrow arch located anteriorly (**Figs. 23.1, 23.2,** and **23.3**). It articulates with the inferior horn of the thyroid cartilage on either side.

Cricothyroid membrane: It has two parts, that is, the median cricothyroid ligament (**Figs. 23.2** and **23.4**) and conus elasticus (cricovocal ligament) (refer to **Fig. 23.6b**). The cricothyroid membrane is attached to the whole length of

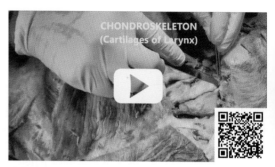

Video 23.1   Larynx–Part 1: external structure.

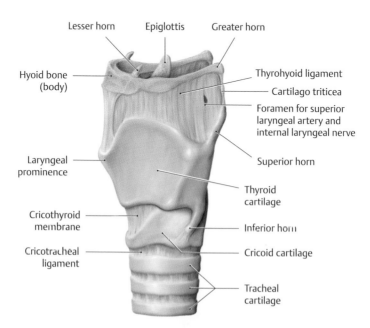

Fig. 23.2   Anterolateral view of the laryngeal cartilages and ligaments. (From: Schuenke M, Schulte E, Schumacher U. THIEME Atlas of Anatomy. Head, Neck, and Neuroanatomy. Illustrations by Voll M and Wesker K. © Thieme 2020.)

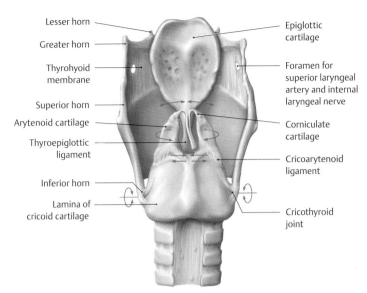

Fig. 23.3 Posterior view of the laryngeal cartilages. Arrows indicate the directions of movements at various inter cartilaginous joints. (From: Schuenke M, Schulte E, Schumacher U. THIEME Atlas of Anatomy. Head, Neck, and Neuroanatomy. Illustrations by Voll M and Wesker K. © Thieme 2020.)

the upper border of the arch of the cricoid cartilage. Anteriorly, the median part is known as the cricothyroid ligament, while the lateral part passes deep to the lamina of the thyroid cartilage and is known as the conus elasticus whose free margin forms the vocal ligament (**Fig. 23.6b**).

Cricotracheal membrane: This membrane extends between the lower border of the cricoid cartilage and the upper tracheal ring (refer to **Fig. 23.2**).

Epiglottic cartilage: It is a leaf-like cartilage which lies posterior to tongue and hyoid bone. It is broad above and narrows below (**Fig. 23.3**). Its lower end is attached anteriorly to thyroid cartilage just below notch by *thyroepiglottic ligament*. The *hyoepiglottic ligament* connects epiglottic cartilage to hyoid bone.

Thyrohyoid membrane (ligament): It is attached to the upper border of the hyoid bone above and to the lamina and superior cornu of the thyroid cartilage below (refer to Figs. **23.2** and **23.3**).

Arytenoid cartilages: These are paired cartilages situated on the superior border of the lamina of the cricoid cartilage. They form the synovial joint with the cricoid cartilage (**Fig. 23.3**). Each arytenoid cartilage is pyramidal in shape and has an apex and a base and two processes, that is, vocal and muscular processes (**Fig. 23.3**).

Quadrangular membrane: It extends between the lateral border of the epiglottic cartilage and the lateral border of the arytenoid cartilage. Its free upper border forms the aryepiglottic ligament, while lower free border forms the vestibular ligament (vestibular fold).

Corniculate cartilage: This is a very small cartilage situated above the arytenoid cartilage (**Fig. 23.3**).

Cuneiform cartilage: This is a rod-like small cartilage in the lower part of the aryepiglottic fold (**Figs. 23.5** and **23.6**).

Joints between the Laryngeal Cartilages

Two important joints of the larynx are described briefly as follows:

Cricothyroid joints: These joints are between the inferior horns of the thyroid cartilage and lateral surface of the cricoid cartilage. These are the synovial type of joints. The thyroid cartilage rotates forward and backward around a transverse axis passing through both the joints, when the cricoid cartilage is stationary. The forward rotation of the thyroid cartilage produces the tightening of the vocal cords while the backward rotation leads to slacking.

Cricoarytenoid joints: These joints are between the facets on the upper border of the lamina of the cricoid cartilage and bases of the arytenoid cartilages. The sliding and gliding movements bring two arytenoid cartilages close to each other (leading to adduction of the vocal cords) or away from each other (leading to abduction of the vocal cords). The pivotal rotation on a vertical axis leads to the rotation of the arytenoid cartilages. The vocal processes of the arytenoid cartilages are rotated laterally (leading to widening of the rima glottidis) or medially (leading to narrowing of the rima glottidis).

Dissection and Identification

A. Dissection to expose external laryngeal nerve, recurrent laryngeal nerve, and inferior thyroid artery.

1. On the external surface of the larynx, review the attachments of the cut ends of the sternothyroid and thyrohyoid muscles.

2. Identify the attachment of the inferior constrictor muscle to the thyroid and cricoid cartilages. Find the external laryngeal nerve on its surface as it is going to innervate the cricothyroid muscle (**Fig. 23.4**).

3. At the lower border of the inferior constrictor muscle, find the recurrent laryngeal nerve (and its inferior laryngeal branch) and inferior laryngeal artery (branch of the inferior thyroid artery). These nerves and vessels are present in the groove between the esophagus and trachea (refer to **Fig. 23.4a** and **b**).

B. Exposure of cricothyroid muscle and external laryngeal nerve.

1. Detach the inferior constrictor from its attachment to the cricoid and thyroid cartilages to expose the inferior horn of the thyroid cartilage to its articulation with the cricoid cartilage. This will expose the cricothyroid muscle completely. Trace the external laryngeal nerve to the cricothyroid muscle.

2. If the thyrohyoid muscle was not removed previously (**Fig. 23.4a**), cut through the thyrohyoid muscle and expose the thyrohyoid membrane. Clean the thyrohyoid membrane completely (**Fig. 23.2**).

3. On the surface of the thyrohyoid membrane, find the superior laryngeal vessels and internal laryngeal nerve (refer to **Fig. 23.4**). These vessels and the nerve penetrate the thyrohyoid membrane to supply the internal structures of the larynx.

4. Find a membrane extending between the upper border of the cricoid cartilage and lower border of the thyroid cartilage in the midline anteriorly; this is the cricothyroid ligament. More laterally, this membrane passes deep to the thyroid cartilage. It is known as the conus elasticus (**Fig. 23.6b**) and its upper free border will form the vocal ligament.

5. On the midsagittal section of the head and neck, see the sectioned surface of the larynx and identify the epiglottis and ligaments attaching the epiglottis to the hyoid bone (hyoepiglottic ligament) and to the thyroid cartilage (thyroepiglottic ligament). Dissect the glossoepiglottic fold.

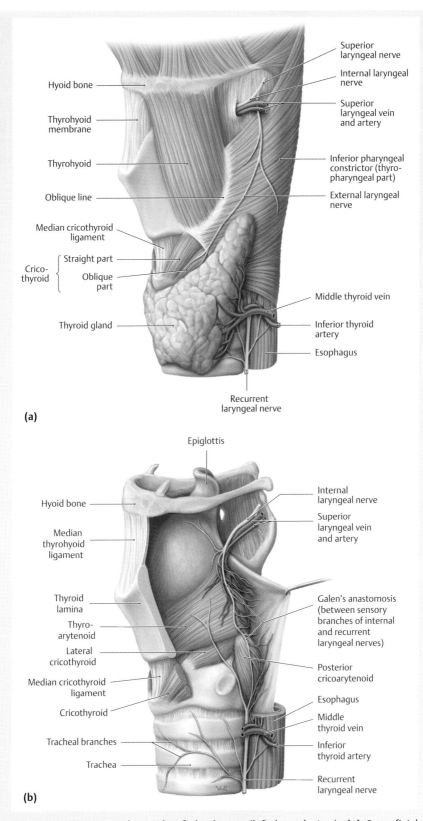

Fig. 23.4 Nerves and vessels of the larynx (left lateral view): **(a)** Superficial dissection and **(b)** deep dissection. (From: Schuenke M, Schulte E, Schumacher U. THIEME Atlas of Anatomy. Head, Neck, and Neuroanatomy. Illustrations by Voll M and Wesker K. © Thieme 2020.)

C. Dissection of vocal and vestibular folds (Video 23.2).

1. Study the interior of the mucous membrane covering the larynx and identify the vestibule of the larynx, vestibular fold, ventricle of the larynx, and vocal fold (**Fig. 23.5a** and **b**).

2. Identify the rima vestibuli, saccule of the larynx, and rima glottidis.

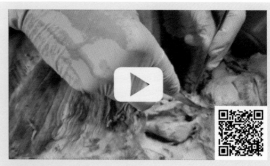

Video 23.2   Larynx–Part 2: internal structure.

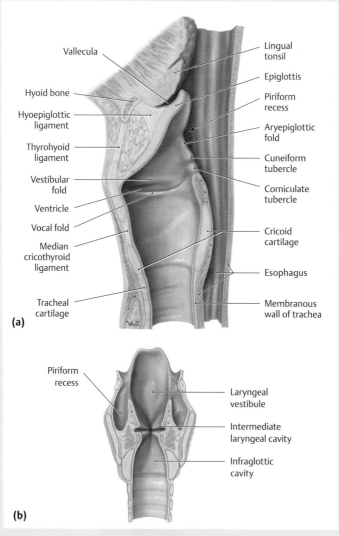

(a)

(b)

Fig. 23.5 Laryngeal mucosa covering the laryngeal cartilages, ligaments, membranes, and muscles: **(a)** Left lateral view of midsagittal section of larynx with the pharynx and esophagus cut along the midline and spread open. **(b)** Posterior view as seen in coronal section. (From: Schuenke M, Schulte E, Schumacher U. THIEME Atlas of Anatomy. Head, Neck, and Neuroanatomy. Illustrations by Voll M and Wesker K. © Thieme 2020.)

3. Cut the vestibular fold from the upper part of the arytenoid cartilage and strip it forward carefully to expose the thyroepiglotticus muscle (**Fig. 23.6d**).

4. Similarly, strip the mucous membrane from the inferior surface of the vocal fold and expose the conus elasticus and vocal ligament. Now strip the mucous membrane from the superior surface of the vocal fold and expose the thyroarytenoid muscle. See its continuity with the thyroepiglotticus.

D. Exposure of posterior cricoarytenoid muscle, transverse and oblique arytenoid muscles.

1. Now remove the mucosa from the posterior aspect of the cricoid cartilage to expose the posterior cricoarytenoid muscle. Superior to this, identify the transverse and oblique arytenoid muscles (**Fig. 23.6c**).

2. On the lateral side, detach the cricothyroid muscle and disarticulate the cricothyroid joint. Give a vertical incision to the thyroid lamina close to the midline. Reflect the thyroid lamina to expose the deeper part of the cricoid cartilage (**Fig. 23.6d**). Reflect the mucosa posteriorly. Immediately deep to the mucosa lie the internal laryngeal nerve (branch of the superior laryngeal, branch of the vagus) and inferior laryngeal nerve (continuation of the recurrent laryngeal nerve). These nerves are accompanied by the superior and inferior laryngeal vessels (**Fig. 23.4a** and **b**).

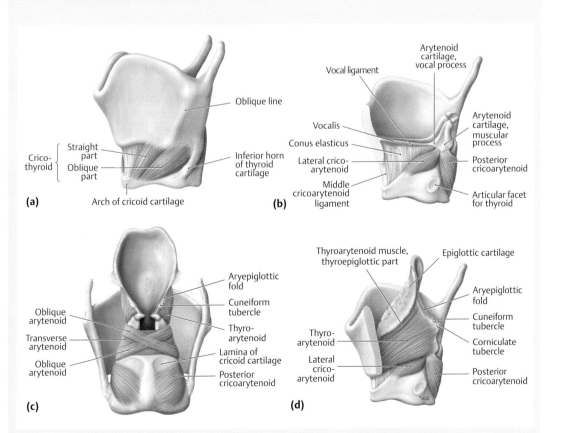

Fig. 23.6 **(a–d)** Intrinsic muscles of the larynx. (From: Schuenke M, Schulte E, Schumacher U. THIEME Atlas of Anatomy. Head, Neck, and Neuroanatomy. Illustrations by Voll M and Wesker K. © Thieme 2020.)

3. Identify the lateral cricoarytenoid muscle and above this find the thyroarytenoid muscle (refer to **Fig. 23.6**). The vocalis muscle is difficult to dissect as it is formed by the medial fibers of the thyroarytenoid muscle.

4. Now remove the thyroarytenoid and thyroepiglottic muscles along with the epiglottis to expose the conus elasticus, vocalis, and vocal ligament (**Fig. 23.6b**).

5. Dissect and identify the vocal and muscular processes of the arytenoid cartilage. Identify the corniculate cartilage above, at the apex of the arytenoid cartilage (**Fig. 23.3**).

Cavity of the Larynx (Video 23.3)

The cavity of the larynx is lined by the mucous membrane. In the median section of the larynx two folds are seen, upper vestibular and lower vocal fold (refer to **Fig. 23.5**). (*In the coronal section passing through the complete larynx, two pairs of folds are seen, that is, upper pair of vestibular and lower pair of vocal folds.*) Because of these folds, the cavity is divided into three parts, that is:

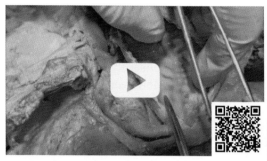

Video 23.3 Interior of larynx, trachea, laryngopharynx, and piriform fossa.

1. *Vestibule of the larynx*: It extends between the pharyngeal opening of the larynx and the vestibular folds. It has a long anterior wall formed by the mucous membrane covering the epiglottic cartilage. The short posterior wall is formed by the mucous membrane covering the arytenoid and corniculate cartilages. Laterally, the upper boundary is formed by the *aryepiglottic fold* containing the corniculate cartilage. The lower limit of the vestibule is formed by the *vestibular folds*. The space between the right and left vestibular folds is called the *rima vestibuli*.

2. *Ventricle and saccule*: The ventricle of the larynx is a narrow groove between the vestibular fold and vocal fold on each side (right and left sides). Laterally, it presents as a mucous membrane lined, deep, blind recess which extends posterosuperiorly. This is known as the saccule of the larynx.

3. The lower boundary of the ventricle is formed by the vocal fold. Each vocal fold consists of the conus elasticus, vocal ligament, and muscle covered by the mucous membrane. The vocal ligament is a free, thickened edge of the conus elasticus. It is attached anteriorly to the thyroid cartilage, close to the midline, and posteriorly to the vocal process of the arytenoid cartilage. The space between the right and left vocal folds is known as *rima glottidis*.

4. *Infraglottic part of the larynx*: This part is present below the vocal folds and is circular where it is bounded by the conus elasticus and internal aspect of the cricoid cartilage. Below the cricoid cartilage it is continuous with the trachea.

Muscles of the Larynx

The muscles of the larynx are grouped into extrinsic and intrinsic muscles. The *extrinsic muscles* are attached to the larynx and other structures, such as the hyoid bone and sternum. Extrinsic muscles include all the infrahyoid muscles and some suprahyoid muscles. The muscles such as stylopharyngeus and palatopharyngeus are also included in the extrinsic group. The extrinsic muscles keep the larynx in position. These muscles depress or elevate the larynx along with the hyoid bone, as during swallowing.

The *intrinsic muscles* are present on the lateral and posterior aspects of the larynx (**Table 23.1**). There are five lateral muscles (cricothyroid, lateral cricoarytenoid, thyroarytenoid, vocalis, and thyroepiglotticus) and three posterior muscles (posterior cricoarytenoid, transverse arytenoid, and oblique arytenoid) (refer to **Figs. 23.4** and **23.6**).

Table 23.1   Intrinsic muscles

Muscle	Origin	Insertion	Nerve supply	Action
Cricothyroid	From the anterior and lateral aspects of the cricoid cartilage	To the lower border of the lamina and anterior border of the inferior cornu of the thyroid cartilage	External laryngeal nerve (branch of the superior laryngeal)	It produces tension in the vocal folds
Thyroarytenoid	From the angle of the thyroid cartilage	To the anterolateral surface of the arytenoid	Recurrent laryngeal nerve	It produces relaxation of the vocal cord
Lateral cricoarytenoid	From the upper border of the arch of cricoid	To the muscular process of the arytenoid	Recurrent laryngeal nerve	Adductor of the vocal cord
Transverse arytenoid	From the muscular process and transverse border of the arytenoid of one side	To the muscular process and transverse border of the arytenoid of other side	Recurrent laryngeal nerve	Adductor of the vocal cord
Posterior cricoarytenoid	From the posterior surface of the lamina of the cricoid	To the posterior aspect of the muscular process of the arytenoid	Recurrent laryngeal nerve	Abductor of the vocal cord
Thyroepiglotticus	From the internal surface of the lamina of the thyroid cartilage	To the lateral margin of the epiglottis	Recurrent laryngeal nerve	It opens the inlet of the larynx
Vocalis	Fibers arise from various distances along the vocal ligament	To the anterolateral surface of the vocal process of the arytenoid	Recurrent laryngeal nerve	It helps in changing the pitch of the voice by increasing or decreasing the tension of the vocal ligament
Aryepiglotticus	From the apex of the arytenoid	To the lamina of the epiglottis	Recurrent laryngeal nerve	Brings the aryepiglottic folds together (closes the inlet of the larynx)
Oblique arytenoid	From the posterior aspect of the muscular process of one arytenoid	To the apex of the opposite arytenoid	Recurrent laryngeal nerve	They close the rima glottidis (sphincter of inlet of the larynx)

Nerves of the Larynx

Sensory Innervation

1. *Internal laryngeal nerve*: It is a branch from the superior laryngeal nerve (branch of the vagus nerve). It pierces the thyrohyoid membrane with the superior laryngeal artery. It supplies the

sensory fibers to the mucous membrane above the vocal folds. It also supplies the sensory fibers to the mucous membrane of the epiglottis and aryepiglottic folds (**Fig. 23.4**).

2. *Recurrent laryngeal nerve*: It is also a branch of the vagus nerve. It enters the larynx with the inferior laryngeal artery. It is sensory to the mucosa below the level of the vocal folds.

Motor Innervation

1. *External laryngeal nerve*: It is a branch from the superior laryngeal nerve and supplies the motor fibers to the cricothyroid muscle.

2. *Recurrent laryngeal nerve*: It is a branch of the vagus nerve and is motor to all the intrinsic muscles of the larynx (except the cricothyroid).

Vessels of the Larynx

1. The *superior laryngeal branch* of the superior thyroid artery runs with the internal laryngeal nerve. It pierces the thyrohyoid membrane and supplies the internal aspect of the larynx.

2. The *inferior laryngeal branch* of the inferior thyroid artery runs with the recurrent laryngeal nerve and supplies the mucosa of the lower part of the larynx.

3. The superior laryngeal vein drains into the superior thyroid vein, which in turn drains in the internal jugular vein. The inferior laryngeal vein drains into the inferior thyroid vein, which in turn drains to the left brachiocephalic vein.

▌Clinical Notes

1. *Laryngitis*: It is the inflammation of the larynx, which occurs usually during common cold. There occurs the swelling of the mucosa of the vestibule and aryepiglottic folds due to effusion of fluid. This can lead to obstruction in breathing.

2. *Injury to the internal laryngeal nerve*: This nerve is sensitive to the mucous membrane above the vocal folds. Any kind of irritation or entry of a foreign body leads to cough reflex. This is a protective phenomenon. Injury to this nerve may lead to the entry of a foreign body in the larynx.

3. *Injury to the recurrent laryngeal nerve*: If one side of the nerve is damaged, hoarseness of voice results. However, an injury to the nerves on both sides leads to a complete loss of voice due to paralysis of the intrinsic muscles of the larynx. The tracheostomy may become essential after bilateral paralysis. Injury to the recurrent laryngeal nerve may occur during thyroid gland surgery.

4. *Injury to the external laryngeal nerve*: This leads to paralysis of the cricothyroid muscle. It results in weakness of voice.

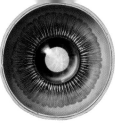
Introduction

The eyeball is an organ for sight, located in the anterior part of the orbit. It is almost a spherical
organ (diameter about 2.5 cm) enclosed in a fascial sheath (orbital fascia or Tenon capsule). This
sheath separates the eyeball from the orbital fat and extraocular muscles.

The eyeball has the following three coats (**Fig. 24.1**):

1. *Outer coat (fibrous coat)*: It consists of the *cornea* (anterior one-sixth part) and *sclera* (posterior
   five-sixth part).

2. *Middle coat (vascular coat)*: It consists of the *choroid, ciliary body*, and *iris*.

3. *Inner coat (nervous coat)*: It is formed by the *retina*.

The eyeball has two segments, that is, the anterior and posterior. The anterior segment includes
the cornea, iris, lens, and anterior and posterior chambers containing the aqueous humor. The
posterior segment is located posterior to the lens and contains the vitreous humor.

Surface Landmarks

1. On a dry skull, see the margins of the orbital opening (supraorbital, infraorbital, medial, and lateral) formed by the frontal, zygomatic, and maxillary bones (refer to **Fig. 1.3**).

2. In a living person, look for the cornea which is anterior one-fifth of the sphere, transparent and
   more convex than the posterior part. Note the limbus (sclerocorneal junction) and sclera. Sclera
   is a white opaque coat. Through the transparent cornea, you can observe the pupil surrounded
   by the iris.

3. The space between the iris and cornea is the anterior chamber and the space between the iris
   and lens is the posterior chamber. The aqueous humor fills the anterior and posterior chambers.

Dissection and Identification (Video 24.1)

The dissection on the fresh eyes of goat, ox, or buffalo, procured from the slaughter house, is recom-
mended. Fresh eyes should be stored in formaldehyde solution. One or two eyes should be kept in
the preservative solution for 2 or 3 days so that the vitreous body is hardened.

1. With the help of tooth forceps, pick up the conjunctiva and fascial sheath close to the limbus
   and cut these layers around the cornea.

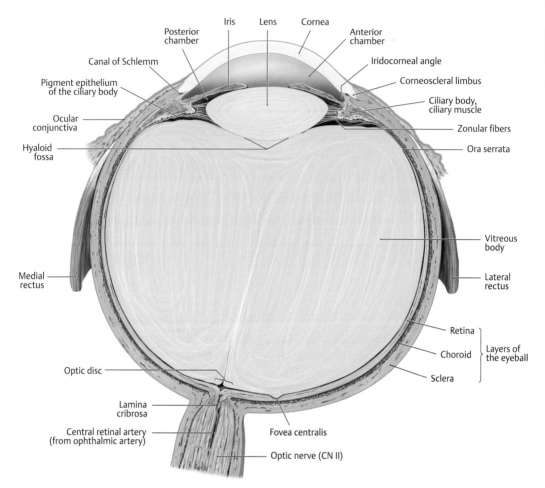

Fig. 24.1 Structure of the eyeball (superior view of the transverse section of the right eye). Posterior segment of eyeball consists of all structures lying posterior to lens, while anterior segment consists of lens and all structures anterior to it. (From: Schuenke M, Schulte E, Schumacher U. THIEME Atlas of Anatomy. Head, Neck, and Neuroanatomy. Illustrations by Voll M and Wesker K. © Thieme 2020.)

2. Reflect this bulbar fascia from the sclera toward the posterior side (toward the optic nerve). Note the vorticose veins posterior to the equator, and short and long ciliary vessels and nerves close to the entrance of the optic nerve (**Fig. 24.2**).

3. Make a coronal section through an eyeball just anterior to the equator and remove the vitreous body from the anterior segment of the section. This will expose the ciliary body, ciliary processes, and posterior aspect of the lens (**Figs. 24.3** and **24.4**).

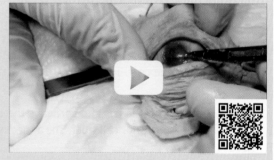

Video 24.1 Exenterated eyeball showing ocular muscles, lacrimal gland, and optic nerve.

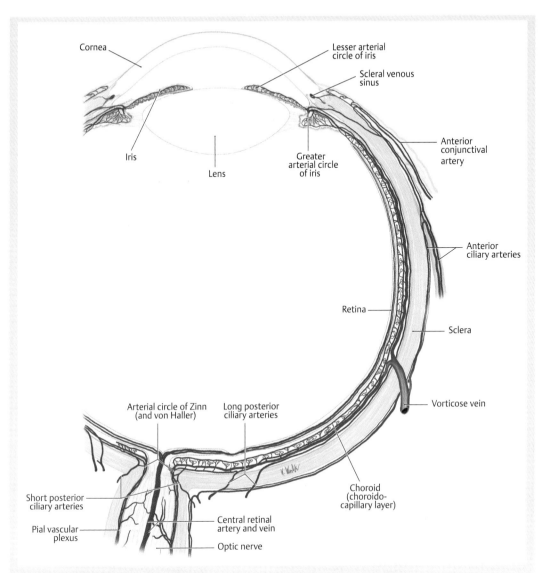

Fig. 24.2   Blood supply of the eyeball. (From: Schuenke M, Schulte E, Schumacher U. THIEME Atlas of Anatomy. Head, Neck, and Neuroanatomy. Illustrations by Voll M and Wesker K. © Thieme 2020.)

4. To expose the iris, remove the cornea by cutting around the sclerocorneal junction. This will expose the anterior surface of the iris.

5. In some hardened specimens, give a horizontal cut and note the hardened vitreous body (refer to **Fig. 24.1**).

6. Remove the lens by cutting through the suspensory ligaments. Incise the anterior surface of the lens (capsule of lens) and by applying pressure extrude the body of the lens from its capsule.

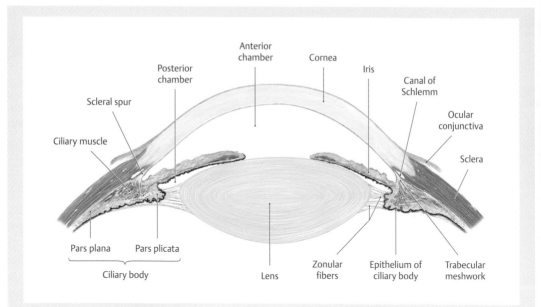

Fig. 24.3 Coronal section through the anterior segment of the eyeball. (From: Schuenke M, Schulte E, Schumacher U. THIEME Atlas of Anatomy. Head, Neck, and Neuroanatomy. Illustrations by Voll M and Wesker K. © Thieme 2020.)

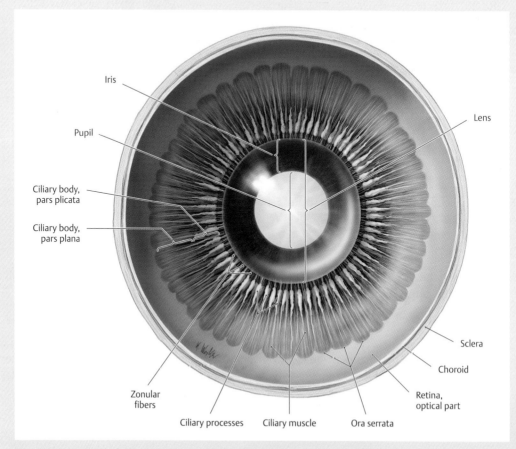

Fig. 24.4 Anterior half of the interior of the eyeball viewed from behind after the removal of the vitreous body. (From: Schuenke M, Schulte E, Schumacher U. THIEME Atlas of Anatomy. Head, Neck, and Neuroanatomy. Illustrations by Voll M and Wesker K. © Thieme 2020.)

Features of the Eyeball

The wall of the sphere of the eyeball is made up of three main layers from the outer to the inner side, that is, the *fibrous coat*, *vascular coat*, and *nervous coat*.

The *fibrous coat*: It is formed anteriorly by the cornea and posteriorly by the sclera (refer to **Fig. 24.1**).

1. The *cornea* is transparent. It is one-sixth of the fibrous coat of the eyeball. Cornea is not supplied by the blood vessels but is highly sensitive as it is richly supplied by the ophthalmic nerve.

2. The *sclera* is a thick opaque layer of posterior five-sixth of the fibrous coat. Anteriorly, the sclera is covered by the bulbar conjunctiva which is richly supplied by blood vessels and nerve. Few millimeters behind the limbus, the sclera gives attachment to the extraocular muscles. Near the equator in its posterior half, the sclera is penetrated by the *venae verticose*. Near the posterior pole of the eyeball, it is pierced by the optic nerve. Around the optic nerve, the sclera is pierced by the short and long ciliary nerves and vessels.

The *vascular coat*: This is a pigmented coat and consists of the choroid, ciliary body, and iris.

1. *The choroid*: It is a thin vascular layer. Its vessels are derived from the short ciliary arteries and it is drained by the varicose veins. It contains many pigmented cells which give it a dark brown color.

2. *Ciliary body*: It is an anterior continuation of the choroid and is situated between the limbus and choroid. It consists of the *ciliary ring*, *ciliary processes*, and *ciliary muscles*. The ciliary ring is a flattened circular band at the anterior end of the choroid. Ciliary processes are present between the ciliary ring and base of the iris. There are about 60 to 70 ciliary processes arranged radially, which are formed by infolding of the layer of the choroid. Ciliary processes give attachment to the suspensory ligaments of the lens. Ciliary muscles are smooth muscles arranged in two different strata, that is, the outer fibers run anteroposteriorly (meridional fibers) and the inner fibers run circularly. These fibers control the curvature of the lens for accommodation.

3. *Iris*: It is the anterior most part of the vascular coat and lies anterior to the lens. The iris has a central aperture, the pupil, and contains smooth muscles arranged in two layers, that is, circular and radial. These muscles on contraction cause constriction or dilation of the pupil, respectively. Thus, the iris acts as a diaphragm.

The *nervous coat*: The nervous coat is the innermost coat and is called the retina.

1. The optic part of the retina lines the internal surface of the choroid and is nervous in nature, that is, concerned with vision.

2. Anteriorly, the nonfunctional part of the retina is continuous forward on the ora serrata and lines the ciliary ring, ciliary processes, and posterior aspect of the iris. This part is non-nervous and, therefore, nonfunctional (**Fig. 24.4**, also refer to **Fig. 24.6**).

3. Histologically, there are many layers in the retina (**Fig. 24.5a**). It consists of the rods and cones, bipolar cells, and ganglion cells. Rods are used in dim light; cones are used in bright light. The axonal processes of the ganglion cells leave the retina as the optic nerve at a point known as the optic disc. It has no visual elements (rods and cones); therefore, is known as the blind spot (**Fig. 24.5b**).

4. About 3 mm lateral to the optic disc, there is a yellowish spot known as the *macula lutea*, with a depression in it (*fovea centralis*) (**Fig. 24.5b**). The vision is more acute in the macula due to the concentration of cones in this area.

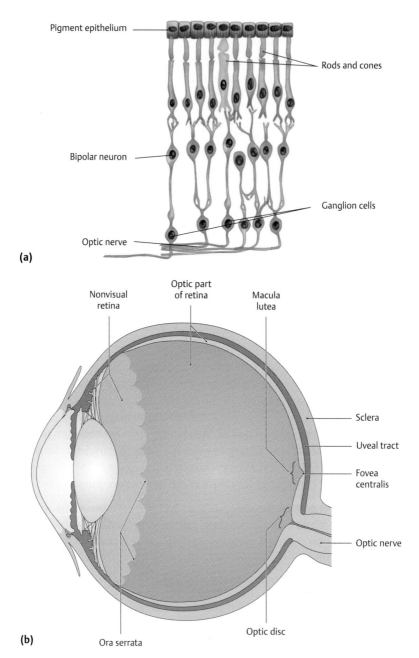

Fig. 24.5 **(a)** Layers of the retina (schematic diagram). **(b)** Retina as seen in transverse section of eyeball. (From: Schuenke M, Schulte E, Schumacher U. THIEME Atlas of Anatomy. Head, Neck, and Neuroanatomy. Illustrations by Voll M and Wesker K. © Thieme 2020.)

Segments of the eyeball: The eyeball has two segments, that is, the anterior and posterior segments (refer to **Fig. 24.1**).

1. *The anterior segment* consists of the lens and all the structures anterior to it, that is, the iris and cornea and anterior and posterior chambers.

2. The space between the iris and cornea is the *anterior chamber* and the space between the iris and lens is the *posterior chamber*. Anterior and posterior chambers communicate with each other through the pupil.

3. The aqueous humor fills the anterior and posterior chambers, which is produced by the ciliary processes. The aqueous humor is drained through the anterior chamber by the *canal of Schlemm* located in the sclera at the iridocorneal angle (**Fig. 24.6**).

4. The *posterior segment* is located posterior to the lens and consists of the vitreous humor, retina, and optic disc. The vitreous is a colorless, jelly-like substance containing water and mucoprotein.

Arterial Supply

All the arteries which supply the eyeball are branches of the ophthalmic artery (branch of the internal carotid artery). These are as follows (refer to **Fig. 24.2**):

1. *Central artery of the retina*: The retina is supplied by the central artery of retina which enters the optic nerve a few millimeters behind the eyeball. It is an end artery.

2. *Short posterior ciliary arteries*: About 10 to 20 branches of these arteries pierce the sclera around the entrance of the optic nerve to the sclera. They supply the choroid and sclera.

3. *Long posterior ciliary arteries*: These branches pass through the sclera to reach the ciliary body and iris, where they form the arterial circles of the iris.

4. *Anterior ciliary arteries*: These arteries are derived from the arteries of the four recti. They anastomose with the vessels of the posterior ciliary arteries.

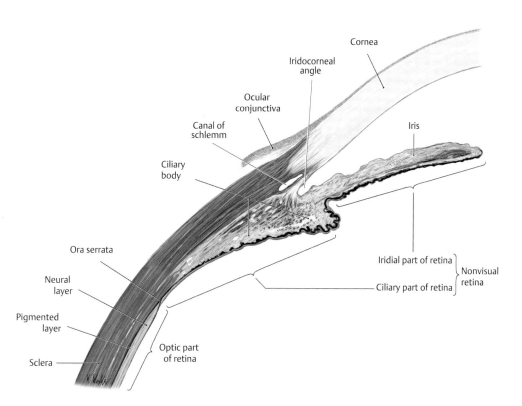

Fig. 24.6 A section through iridocorneal angle to show parts of nonvisual retina canal of Schlemm and ciliary body. (From: Schuenke M, Schulte E, Schumacher U. THIEME Atlas of Anatomy. Head, Neck, and Neuroanatomy. Illustrations by Voll M and Wesker K. © Thieme 2020.)

Venous Drainage

Blood is drained from the eyeball by four to six vorticose veins, which come out of the sclera behind the equator and open into the superior or inferior ophthalmic veins (refer to **Fig. 24.2**).

Nerves of the Eyeball

The nerves of the eyeball are as follows:

Long ciliary nerves: These are branches of the nasociliary nerve. They pass along the medial side of the optic nerve and pierce the sclera.

1. They contain the *sensory fibers* to innervate the eyeball.

2. They also contain the *sympathetic postganglionic fibers*, which enter the nasociliary nerve from the plexus around the internal carotid artery. It innervates the dilator of the pupil.

Short ciliary nerves: These nerves arise as 12 to 15 branches from the ciliary ganglion and pierce the sclera around the optic nerve. These branches run anteriorly and form a plexus to supply the cornea, ciliary body, and iris. Short ciliary nerves contain:

1. Sensory fibers to the cornea, iris, and ciliary body derived from the nasociliary nerve.

2. Postganglionic sympathetic fibers from the internal carotid plexus to the vessels of the eyeball.

3. Postganglionic parasympathetic fibers from the ciliary ganglion to the ciliary body and the sphincter of the pupil.

▌ Clinical Notes

1. Retinal detachment is the separation of the neural layer from the pigment layer of the retina.

2. Degenerative changes in the lens produce cataract.

3. Corneal grafts are successful as the cornea is avascular; hence, graft rejection is not there.

4. Occlusion of canal of Schlemm raises the intraocular tension leading to a disease called glaucoma.

5. Blockage in the central artery of the retina leads to sudden blindness as this artery is an end artery.

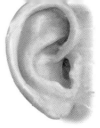

Learning Objectives

At the end of the dissection of the ear, you should be able to identify and understand the following:

- Parts of the external ear and parts of the external acoustic meatus (cartilaginous and bony parts).

- Walls of the middle ear cavity, auditory ossicles (malleus, incus, and stapes), tympanic membrane, and facial nerve.

- Stapedius tendon, tendon of tensor tympani, chorda tympani nerve, round window, oval window, and promontory.

- Facial nerve in the facial canal, genicular ganglion.

- Semicircular ducts, vestibule and cochlea, and branches of the vestibulocochlear nerve.

Introduction

The ear is an organ of hearing and balance. It is divided into three parts, that is, the *external ear, middle ear (tympanic cavity)*, and *internal ear (labyrinth)* (**Fig. 25.1**).

1. The external ear consists of the *auricle* and *external acoustic meatus*. It is separated from the middle ear by the *tympanic membrane* (**Fig. 25.1**).

2. The middle ear is located in the petrous temporal bone. It consists of a small cavity known as the tympanic cavity. It contains three small ossicles extending between the tympanic membrane and lateral wall of the internal ear (**Fig. 25.1**).

3. The internal ear consists of the bony labyrinth and membranous labyrinth (vestibulocochlear organ) on which the vestibulocochlear nerve ends.

For hearing, the sound waves have to pass through three subdivisions of the ear, that is, the external, middle, and internal ear.

Surface Landmarks

1. Examine the external ear (auricle and external acoustic meatus) of a living person and note the following: the helix, antihelix, concha, tragus of an auricle, and cartilaginous part of the external acoustic meatus (refer to **Fig. 25.2**).

2. On the external surface (base and lateral aspect) of a dry skull, identify the following bony features: the external acoustic meatus (bony part), mastoid process, stylomastoid foramen, jugular fossa, carotid canal, and pharyngotympanic tube groove/sulcus tubae (refer to **Fig. 1.5**).

3. On the internal aspect of the middle and posterior cranial fossae, review the following bony features: the internal acoustic meatus, tegmen tympani, and groove for greater petrosal nerve (refer to **Fig. 1.7**).

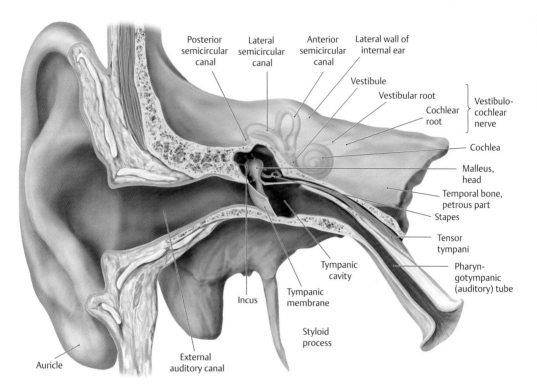

Fig. 25.1 Parts of the ear. (From: Schuenke M, Schulte E, Schumacher U. THIEME Atlas of Anatomy. Head, Neck, and Neuroanatomy. Illustrations by Voll M and Wesker K. © Thieme 2020.)

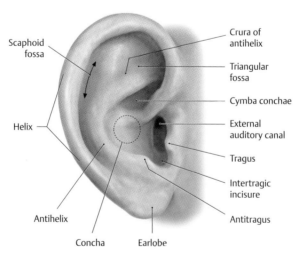

Fig. 25.2 Right auricle (lateral aspect). (From: Schuenke M, Schulte E, Schumacher U. THIEME Atlas of Anatomy. Head, Neck, and Neuroanatomy. Illustrations by Voll M and Wesker K. © Thieme 2020.)

Dissection and Identification

The dissection of the middle and internal ear is not always very satisfactory. One cannot expose the structures of the middle and internal ear completely due to their small size and their labyrinthine nature. The dissection of the ear is carried out either on the hard (calcified) petrous part of the temporal bone or the temporal bone is decalcified first by keeping it in a mild solution of acid for a few weeks. A decalcified petrous temporal bone becomes soft and allows its sectioning easily.

A. Dissection of the external acoustic meatus and tympanic membrane.

The auricle is completely cut to expose the cartilaginous part of the external acoustic meatus. The cartilaginous part of the meatus is cut through its anterior wall. Similarly, cut the tympanic plate, which forms the anterior wall of the bony part of the meatus. Try to expose the external surface of the tympanic membrane (**Fig. 25.3**).

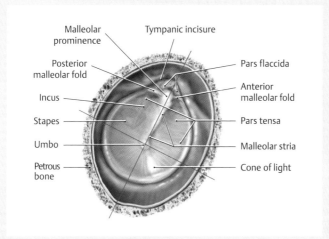

Fig. 25.3 Tympanic membrane (right tympanic membrane, lateral view). (From: Schuenke M, Schulte E, Schumacher U. THIEME Atlas of Anatomy. Head, Neck, and Neuroanatomy. Illustrations by Voll M and Wesker K. © Thieme 2020.)

B. Dissection of middle ear cavity.

1. To expose the middle ear cavity, gently break the tegmen tympani (forming the roof of the middle ear cavity) and remove the broken bony pieces. Observe the auditory ossicles within the tympanic cavity, as malleus and incus are easily seen from the superior view (refer to **Fig. 25.4**).

2. With the help of a fine forceps remove the incus. The malleus should remain attached to the tympanic membrane.

3. If you are dissecting on a decalcified specimen, it will be easier to give a cut to the temporal bone which extends parallel to the tympanic membrane and almost passes parallel to the superior border of the petrous temporal bone. This cut will pass through the middle ear cavity dividing its medial and lateral walls.

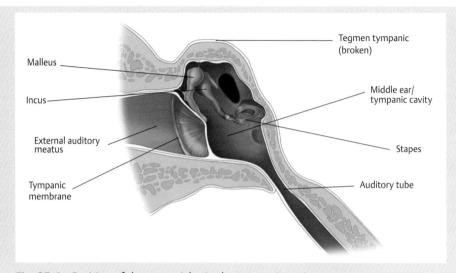

Fig. 25.4   Position of the ear ossicles in the tympanic cavity.

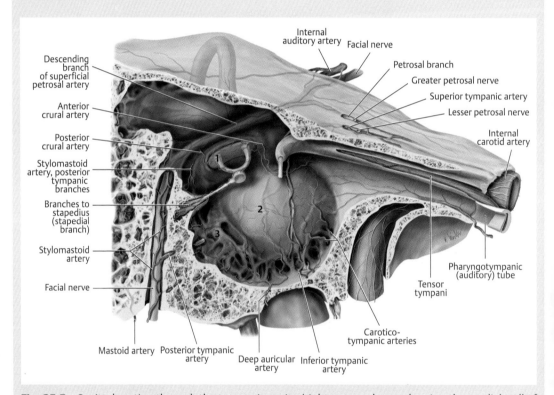

Fig. 25.5   Sagittal section through the tympanic cavity (right petrous bone, showing the medial wall of tympanic cavity). 1, Stapes on oval window; 2, promontory and 3, round window. (From: Schuenke M, Schulte E, Schumacher U. THIEME Atlas of Anatomy. Head, Neck, and Neuroanatomy. Illustrations by Voll M and Wesker K. © Thieme 2020.)

4. On the medial wall of the tympanic cavity, identify the stapes attached to the oval window. Also, identify the tendon of the stapedius muscle (**Fig. 25.5**).

5. Look for the promontory and round window.

6. On the lateral wall of the tympanic cavity, identify the internal aspect of the tympanic membrane and chorda tympani nerve (**Fig. 25.6**).

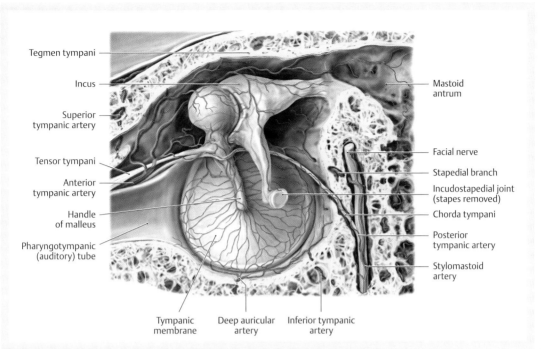

Fig. 25.6   Sagittal section through the tympanic cavity (right petrous bone, showing the **lateral** wall of tympanic cavity). Medial view of the right tympanic membrane. (From: Schuenke M, Schulte E, Schumacher U. THIEME Atlas of Anatomy. Head, Neck, and Neuroanatomy. Illustrations by Voll M and Wesker K. © Thieme 2020.)

C. Dissection of internal ear.

1. Now remove the roof of the internal acoustic meatus on a decalcified bone with the help of a scalpel. Follow the facial and vestibulocochlear nerves laterally. The facial nerve lies superficial to the vestibulocochlear nerve.

2. The facial nerve makes a sharp bend in the posterior direction and shows a swelling, the *geniculate ganglion*. The *greater petrosal nerve* arises from the ganglion and runs anteromedially (**Fig. 25.5**).

3. The cochlea of the internal ear lies in the area between the facial nerve, geniculate ganglion, and greater petrosal nerve.

4. The semicircular canals lie posterolateral to the facial nerve and in the dissected specimen will appear as a series of tiny holes in the bone.

5. You shall not be able to see more details of the internal ear as it is difficult to dissect the complete membranous labyrinth.

Description of the External Ear

The external ear consists of the auricle and external auditory meatus (**Fig. 25.1**). The auricle is made up of irregular elastic cartilage covered by a thin, tightly adhering skin. The thin skin contains hair follicles and sweat and sebaceous glands. The lateral concave surface of the ear shows various features, such as the helix, antihelix, scaphoid fossa, concha, tragus, antitragus, etc. The function of the auricle is to focus the sound waves toward the external auditory meatus.

The external auditory meatus is made up of a tubular canal about 25 cm in length. The wall of the lateral one-third of the canal is cartilaginous and the medial two-thirds is bony. It is an S-shaped passage extending between the concha and tympanic membrane. The canal is covered by a relatively thick skin in its lateral part and contains hair follicles, sebaceous gland, and ceruminous glands. The secretions of these glands form the ear wax. The medial two-thirds of the canal is lined by thin skin and contains very few hair follicles and glands.

Three vestigial muscles are attached to the auricle, that is, the *auricularis anterior, auricularis superior*, and *auricularis posterior*.

Description of the Middle Ear

The middle ear is sometimes called the tympanic cavity. It is a narrow slit-like cavity located in the petrous part of the temporal bone. It is present between the external ear (tympanic membrane laterally) and internal ear (lateral wall of the internal ear medially). The cavity communicates anteriorly with the auditory tube (*pharyngotympanic*) and posteriorly with the opening of the *mastoid antrum* (refer to **Fig. 25.6**). It contains three auditory ossicles (*malleus, incus*, and *stapes*), but these ossicles are covered by the mucous membrane of the tympanic cavity. Therefore, in the real sense the cavity contains only air. The *epitympanic recess* is a superior extension of the middle ear cavity above the level of the tympanic membrane. In this recess lies the upper end of the malleus and major part of the incus.

The cavity of the middle ear is a six-sided rectangular space in the petrous temporal bone. It consists of a roof, floor, and medial, lateral, anterior, and posterior walls.

1. *Roof*: It is formed by a thin plate of bone called tegmen tympani of the petrous temporal bone.

2. *Floor*: It is formed by a thin plate of bone separating the middle ear from the jugular fossa. The canaliculus for the tympanic branch of the glossopharyngeal nerve is located close to the medial wall.

3. *Anterior wall*: It is a narrow wall and has two openings, that is, the canal for the tensor tympani muscle and opening of the canal for the bony part of the auditory tube. Below it forms the posterior wall of the carotid canal.

4. *Posterior wall*: The upper portion of the posterior wall has a large irregular *aditus to the mastoid antrum*. Below this is the pyramidal eminence, which gives passage to the stapedius muscle. The opening of the posterior canaliculus of the chorda tympani nerve is located in this wall. The facial nerve canal lies below the pyramid.

5. *Medial wall*: It is the lateral wall of the internal ear. It presents a prominence of the facial canal in the posterosuperior part of the medial wall. Below this is a presence of the oval window (fenestra vestibuli) to which the foot plate of stapes is attached. Promontory is the round bulge in the middle of the medial wall. The tympanic plexus of nerve is present on its surface (**Fig. 25.7**). The round window is situated just posterior to the promontory.

6. *Lateral wall*: It is formed by the tympanic membrane (eardrum) and above by the lateral wall of the epitympanic recess (**Fig. 25.6**).

Tympanic Membrane

It is a thin and translucent oval membrane, which separates the middle ear from the external ear (refer to **Figs. 25.1** and **25.3**). It is about 1 cm in diameter and placed obliquely. It is made up of three layers, that is, the outer *cuticular*, intermediate *fibrous*, and inner *mucous layer*. Its periphery is attached to the bony rim at the medial end of the external auditory meatus. This sulcus is deficient in its upper part at the tympanic notch. The lateral process of the malleus is attached below this tympanic notch. The anterior and posterior malleolar folds converge to the lateral process of the malleus from the two ends of the tympanic notch. The part of the tympanic membrane between these two malleolar folds is lax; hence, it is known as pars flaccida. The rest of the tympanic membrane is known as pars tensa. The lower end of handle of the malleus is attached near the center of the tympanic membrane forming a bulge called the *umbo*. This bulge is toward the middle ear cavity. Therefore, the tympanic membrane looks concave when seen from the lateral (outer) surface.

Contents of the Middle Ear Cavity

As such the middle ear cavity only contains air and all the other structures lie outside the mucous membrane which is lining these structures.

Auditory ossicles: From the lateral to the medial side, these are the *malleus, the incus*, and *stapes* (refer to **Figs. 25.1** and **25.4**). They *transmit the sound vibrations from the external ear to the internal ear*.

1. *Malleus*: It is the largest ear ossicle and resembles a hammer. It consists of head, neck, and handle. It has two processes, the lateral and anterior processes. The handle is attached to the tympanic membrane, while the head articulates with the incus. The medial surface of the head also provides attachment to the tensor tympani tendon.

2. *Incus*: It has a body and a long and short process. The body articulates with the head of the malleus and the long process articulates with the head of stapes.

3. *Stapes*: It consists of head, neck, anterior and posterior limbs, and a base of footplate. The anterior and posterior limbs pass medially to join the oval base of the footplate. The footplate is attached to the oval window.

The ear ossicles are held together by the ligaments and articulations between them.

Muscles: There are two muscles in the middle ear, the tensor tympani and stapedius (refer to **Figs. 25.1, 25.5** and **Table 25.1**).

Table 25.1 Muscles in the middle ear

Muscle	Origin	Insertion	Nerve supply	Action
Tensor tympani	From the bony wall of its canal and from the cartilaginous part of the auditory tube	Medial aspect of the upper part of the handle of the malleus	Mandibular nerve trunk	It pulls the tympanic membrane inward to make it tense
Stapedius	From the inner wall of the pyramid	In the neck of the stapes	It is supplied by the facial nerve	It pushes the footplate of the stapes in the oval window; thus, it opposes the action of the tensor tympani

Chorda tympani nerve: It is a branch of the facial nerve and contains fibers of taste for the anterior two-thirds of the tongue and preganglionic parasympathetic fibers to submandibular and sublingual glands. It arises in the canal for the facial nerve just above the stylomastoid foramen. It then comes to the middle ear cavity through its posterior wall (through the posterior canaliculus). It lies in the substance of the tympanic membrane and crosses the neck of the malleus to enter the anterior canaliculus in the anterior wall of the middle ear cavity (refer to **Fig. 25.6**). It comes out at the base of the skull through the medial end of the squamotympanic fissure. At the base of the skull, it lies on the medial side of the spine of the sphenoid and then joins the lingual nerve.

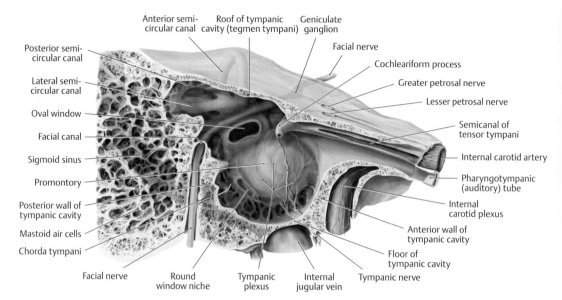

Fig. 25.7 Tympanic cavity clinically important anatomical relationships (oblique sagittal section showing the medial wall of the tympanic cavity). (From: Schuenke M, Schulte E, Schumacher U. THIEME Atlas of Anatomy. Head, Neck, and Neuroanatomy. Illustrations by Voll M and Wesker K. © Thieme 2020.)

Nerve Supply of the Middle Ear Cavity

The tympanic cavity is supplied by the tympanic plexus (refer to **Fig. 25.7**), which is formed by the tympanic branch of the glossopharyngeal nerve, and superior and inferior caroticotympanic nerves from the sympathetic plexus around the internal carotid artery. Plexus gives origin to the lesser petrosal nerve and a root to the greater petrosal nerve. Plexus supplies the mucosa of the middle ear cavity, auditory tube, and mastoid air cells.

Arterial Supply of the Middle Ear Cavity

1. Many branches from the *external carotid artery* supply the middle ear cavity: the tympanic branch of the maxillary, stylomastoid branch of the posterior auricular, and branch from the middle meningeal and from the ascending pharyngeal.

2. Tympanic branches from the *internal carotid artery* (**Fig. 25.5**).

Venous Drainage

Veins drain to the pterygoid venous plexus and superior petrosal sinus.

Lymphatic Drainage

Lymph from the mucosa of the cavity drains to the parotid group of lymph nodes and deep cervical groups.

Description of the Internal Ear

The internal ear is also located in the petrous part of the temporal bone. It consists of an outer bony labyrinth in which the membranous labyrinth is enclosed. Various parts of the membranous

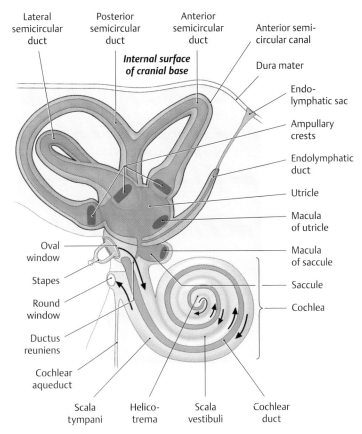

Fig. 25.8 Schematic diagram of the inner ear. (From: Schuenke M, Schulte E, Schumacher U. THIEME Atlas of Anatomy. Head, Neck, and Neuroanatomy. Illustrations by Voll M and Wesker K. © Thieme 2020.)

labyrinth are shown in **Fig. 25.8**. The internal ear is associated with two different kinds of sensations, that is, balance (equilibrium) and hearing. The portion associated with a balance is called the vestibular apparatus and that of hearing is known as the cochlear apparatus (refer to **Fig. 25.8**).

Vestibular Apparatus

Following are the parts of the vestibular apparatus: the utricle, saccule, and semicircular ducts.

Utricle and Saccule

The narrow sensory zones of the utricle and saccule are called *macula* (refer to **Fig. 25.8**). These zones bulge into the lumen and are bathed by the endolymph. Two types of cells are seen in the macula, that is, the *supporting cells* and *sensory epithelial hair cells*. The columnar supporting cells secrete the thick, gelatinous glycoprotein layer called the *otolithic membrane* that rests on the hair cells. The dense calcium carbonate crystals are present over the surface of this membrane. During the movement of the head in various planes, this membrane moves on the hair cells of the macula in the direction of the tilt and bends the hair bundles. The bending of hair triggers nerve impulses to the brain. Thus, the macula of the utricle and saccule are sites of hair cells for static and dynamic equilibrium.

Semicircular Ducts

The sensory zones of the semicircular ducts are situated in the ampulla (**Fig. 25.8**). In the floor of each ampulla, there is a transverse ridge called the *crista*. Each crista contains a group of *hair cells* and *supporting cells* covered by a mass of gelatinous material called the *cupula*. The hair cells have a tuft of stereocilia and a single cilium. When the head moves, the semicircular ducts also move with it. However, the endolymph, which is filled in the lumen of the canal, lags behind due to its inertia. When the stationary fluid comes in contact with the moving hair cells (through the cupula), the stereocilia bend. The bending of stereocilia leads to the generation of nerve impulse that passes along the eighth cranial nerve. Thus, the semicircular ducts are sites of hair cells for dynamic equilibrium.

Cochlear Apparatus

Anterior to the vestibule is the *cochlea*. It is a bony spiral canal that makes 2¾ turns around a central bony core called the *modiolus*. The lumen of the spiral canal is subdivided into three spiral chambers in the following way.

Scala Vestibuli

It is situated above the vestibular membrane.

Scala Tympani

It is situated below the basilar membrane.

The scala vestibuli and scala tympani are continuous with each other at the apex of the cochlea through an opening called the *helicotrema*. They contain the perilymph and are lined by the simple squamous epithelium.

Scala Media

It is also known as the cochlear duct. It is situated between the vestibular and basilar membranes. The cochlear duct is a small triangular-shaped membranous tube. It has three walls: the *floor* (the *basilar membrane*), *roof* (the *vestibular membrane*), and *outer wall* (*the stria vascularis*). The scala media contains the endolymph.

Organ of Corti

Resting on the basilar membrane is the *organ of Corti*. It is a complex epithelial structure, which contains the site of sound reception. The epithelium on the basilar membrane is columnar and highly specialized. The epithelium consists of supporting cells and about 16,000 hair cells. The supporting cells are of different types, that is, the phalangeal cells and the outer and inner pillar cells. The phalangeal cells are columnar in shape with a cup-shaped apex, which is occupied by the rounded base of a hair cell.

Hair cells are receptors for hearing and are present in two groups, that is, the inner hair cells and outer hair cells. The inner hair cells are arranged in a single row and extend the entire length of the cochlea, while the outer hair cells are arranged in three rows. There are about 30 to 100 stereocilia present on the apical end of each hair cell. Stereocilia are long, hair-like microvilli arranged in several rows of graded height. Both the outer and inner hair cells lack the single cilium as observed in the macula and crista. The peripheral processes of the bipolar neurons end in the hair cells of the spiral organ of Corti.

The spiral limbus bulges into the scala media from the inner angle, between the points of the modiolus origin of the vestibular membrane and the basilar membrane. The spiral limbus gives attachment to the *tectorial membrane*, which is a gelatinous sheet of glycoprotein. The tips of the stereocilia (hair) are embedded in the tectorial membrane.

Mechanism of Hearing

When sound waves strike the eardrum it starts vibrating. These vibrations are then transmitted to the ear ossicles. The stapes moves back and forth and pushes the membrane of the oval window. The vibration of the oval window generates waves in the perilymph of the scala vestibuli. From here, the waves are transmitted to the scala tympani and to the round window causing it to bulge in the middle ear. These waves of the scala vestibuli and scala tympani also push the vestibular membrane back and forth. This creates pressure waves in the endolymph inside the cochlear duct. This causes the basilar membrane to vibrate, which moves the hair cells against the tectorial membrane and bend the stereocilia. The hair cells thus produce receptor potentials, which in turn produce nerve impulse in the cochlear nerve of eighth cranial nerve. Through the auditory pathways, it reaches the hearing center in the brain which interprets the received impulse.

▌Clinical Notes

1. Pus may collect in the middle ear secondary to the infection of the throat or nose. This infection travels to the middle ear through the auditory tube.

2. The infection of the middle ear may spread to the neighboring area which contains important structures.

    a. It may rupture the tympanic membrane leading to the discharge of pus through the external acoustic meatus.

    b. Infection may spread to the mastoid air cells via aditus to the mastoid antrum. This condition is known as mastoiditis.

    c. It may cause meningitis and abscess of the temporal lobe of the brain when the infection goes to the middle cranial fossa through the tegmen tympani.

    d. Facial paralysis, if the facial nerve passing through the facial canal is affected.

    e. Thrombosis of the transverse and sigmoid sinus.

    f. The osteosclerosis of the edge of the oval window usually occurs at an old age leading to interference in the movements of the stapes. This is the most common cause of deafness during old age.

3. The excessive stimulation of the utricle and saccule causes motion sickness leading to headache, vertigo, nausea, and vomiting.

4. Exposure to excessive loud sound for a long time may lead to degenerative changes in the organ of Corti. This leads to deafness.

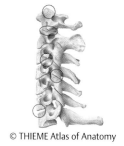

Learning Objectives

At the end of the dissection of the joints of the neck region, you should be able to identify and understand the following:

- Articular surfaces of the various joints.
- Structure of the intervertebral disc.
- Ligaments associated with various joints.
- Movements occurring at an individual joint.

Introduction

Three different types of joints are present in the neck region (**Fig. 26.1a and b**). These are:

1. Joints between the lower six cervical vertebrae, that is, the *intervertebral* joints.

2. Joint between the first cervical vertebra and occipital bone, that is, the *atlanto-occipital* joint.

3. Joint between the first and second cervical vertebrae (between the axis and atlas vertebrae), that is, the *atlanto-axial* joint.

The intervertebral joints of the cervical region are classified as the anterior and posterior intervertebral joints. The anterior intervertebral joints are between the two vertebral bodies and are of secondary cartilaginous variety (symphyseal joints). The posterior joints are between the articular processes of the adjacent vertebrae. These are of synovial variety and permit considerable range of movement.

The *atlanto-occipital joint*, on each side, is between the superior articular facets of the atlas and occipital condyles of the skull. These are of synovial variety. The *atlantoaxial joint* is between the atlas and axis vertebrae. The *atlanto-occipital* and *atlantoaxial joints* together are called *cranioverteberal joints*. The joints of neck region are strengthened by a number of ligaments (**Fig. 26.2a and b**).

Surface Landmarks

On a dry skull, review the bony features of the occipital condyles on the base of the skull (refer to **Fig. 1.5**). Also, learn the bony features of the axis (refer to **Fig. 1.15a and b**), atlas (refer to **Fig. 1.14a and b**), and typical cervical vertebrae (refer to **Fig. 1.13a and b**). On an articulated skeleton, observe the joints between the adjacent cervical vertebrae (refer to **Fig. 1.12**).

Dissection and Identification

The dissection of these joints is carried out on the hemisection of the neck, therefore procuring a hemisection of the neck.

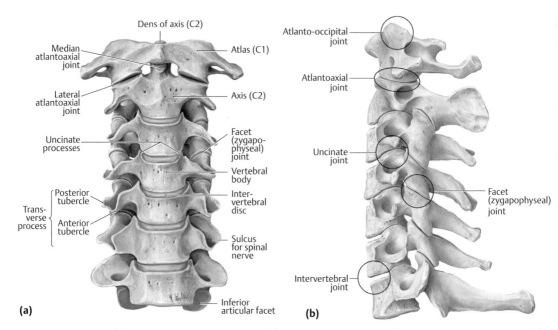

Fig. 26.1 Joints of the region (cervical region). **(a)** Various joints as seen from the anterior aspect of the cervical column. **(b)** Joints of the cervical column as seen in the lateral aspect. (From: Schuenke M, Schulte E, Schumacher U. THIEME Atlas of Anatomy. Head, Neck, and Neuroanatomy. Illustrations by Voll M and Wesker K. © Thieme 2020.)

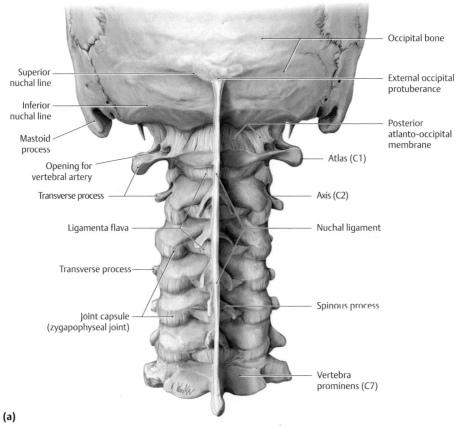

(a)

Fig. 26.2 **(a)** Ligaments of the joints of the neck region: Posterior view.

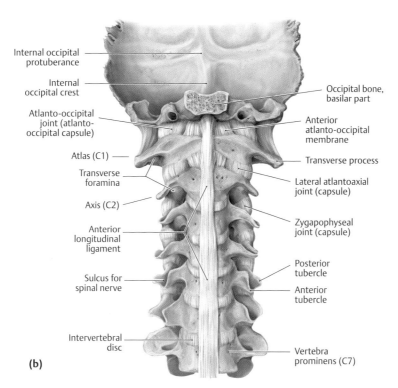

Internal occipital protuberance

Internal occipital crest

Atlanto-occipital joint (atlanto-occipital capsule)

Atlas (C1)

Transverse foramina

Axis (C2)

Anterior longitudinal ligament

Sulcus for spinal nerve

Intervertebral disc

Occipital bone, basilar part

Anterior atlanto-occipital membrane

Transverse process

Lateral atlantoaxial joint (capsule)

Zygapophyseal joint (capsule)

Posterior tubercle

Anterior tubercle

Vertebra prominens (C7)

(b)

Fig. 26.2   (b) Ligaments of the cervical region as seen from the anterior view after removal of the anterior skull base. (From: Schuenke M, Schulte E, Schumacher U. THIEME Atlas of Anatomy. Head, Neck, and Neuroanatomy. Illustrations by Voll M and Wesker K. © Thieme 2020.)

A. Dissection of atlanto-occipital, lateral atlantoaxial, and medial atlantoaxial joint.

1. On the anterior aspect of the specimen, cut through the anterior longitudinal ligament between the anterior arch of the atlas and anterior margin of the foramen magnum. Also, cut the anterior atlanto-occipital membrane (**Figs. 26.2** and **26.3**).

2. On the posterior aspect of the specimen, remove the remaining part of the posterior arch of the atlas and lamina of axis along with the posterior atlanto-occipital membrane and ligamentum flavum to expose the membrana tectoria (**Fig. 26.4a and b**).

3. Cut the divided membrana tectoria from the middle and reflect the cut ends upward and downward. This will expose the longitudinally divided cruciate ligament.

4. Cut through the divided longitudinal fibers of the cruciate ligament and alar ligament. Also, cut the apical ligament of dens (**Fig. 26.4c**).

5. Reflect the divided transverse ligament of the atlas. This will expose a synovial joint between the posterior surface of dens and transverse ligament of the atlas.

6. Now remove the fibrous capsule from the atlanto-occipital joint and expose the joint cavity and articulating surfaces (the occipital condyle and superior articular facet of the atlas) (refer to **Fig. 26.4d**).

7. Similarly, now cut through the articular capsule of the lateral atlantoaxial joint and expose the superior articulating surface of the axis (refer to **Fig. 26.4**). Similarly, expose the divided joint between the posterior surface of the anterior arch of the atlas and odontoid process.

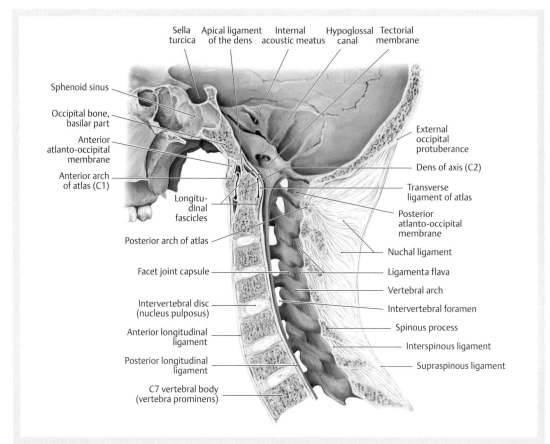

Fig. 26.3 Various ligaments in the midsagittal section of the neck region: left lateral view. (From: Schuenke M, Schulte E, Schumacher U. THIEME Atlas of Anatomy. Head, Neck, and Neuroanatomy. Illustrations by Voll M and Wesker K. © Thieme 2020.)

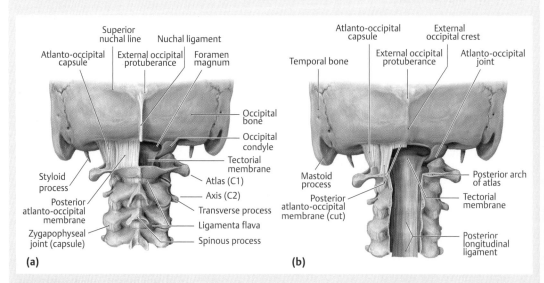

Fig. 26.4 Dissection from behind to show the main ligaments that connect the craniovertebral joints. **(a)** The right-half of posterior atlanto-occipital membrane is removed to expose the tectorial membrane. Note the presence of ligamentum flavum. **(b)** Membrana tectoria and posterior longitudinal ligament are exposed.

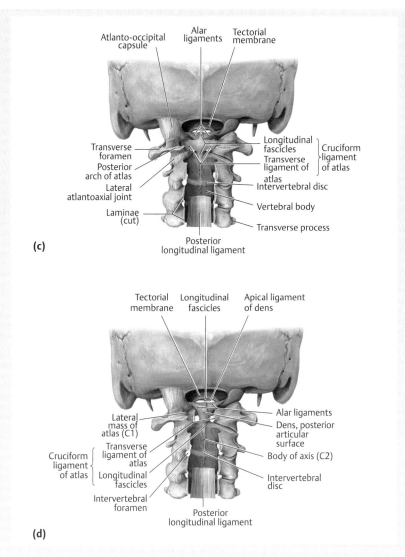

Fig. 26.4   Dissection from behind to show the main ligaments that connect the craniovertebral joints. **(b)** Membrana tectoria and posterior longitudinal ligament are exposed. **(c)** Note the cruciform and alar ligaments. **(d)** Apical ligament of dens, exposed atlanto-occipital and atlantoaxial joints. (From: Schuenke M, Schulte E, Schumacher U. THIEME Atlas of Anatomy. Head, Neck, and Neuroanatomy. Illustrations by Voll M and Wesker K. © Thieme 2020.)

B. Dissection of intervertebral joints (intervertebral disc joint and facet joint).

1. For the dissection of a typical cervical vertebral joint, remove the anterior and posterior longitudinal ligaments from the anterior and posterior surfaces of the cervical vertebral column.

2. On the longitudinal cut surface, observe the anulus fibrosus and nucleus pulposus of the intervertebral disc between the two adjacent bodies of the cervical vertebrae (**Fig. 26.3**).

3. Expose the articular facet joints by removing the remnants of the muscle and ligaments from the cervical articular processes and the laminae and spines.

4. Remove the articular capsule of the facet joints to expose the articular surfaces of the superior and inferior articular facets, respectively.

Description of the Typical Cervical Vertebral Joints

The typical cervical joints are present from the inferior surface of C2 downward to the upper surface of the seventh cervical vertebrae. There are series of *symphysis joints* between the vertebral bodies and *synovial joints* between the articular processes of the neural arches.

Joints between bodies: The bodies of these vertebrae are firmly bound with each other by the intervertebral disc. Each disc is composed of the outer *annulus fibrosus*, which surrounds the inner gelatinous mass called the *nucleus pulposus* (**Fig. 26.3**). Laterally, the intervertebral discs are replaced by the small *synovial joints* situated where the margins of the inferior vertebra overlap the vertebral body above.

The joints between bodies are supported by the anterior and posterior *longitudinal ligaments*. These ligaments are attached to the intervertebral discs and adjacent parts of the bodies. The movements produced at the joints between bodies are flexion extension and lateral bending.

Joints between the vertebral arches: The articular processes are united with each other by the synovial joints. The capsules of these joints are lax; therefore, a considerable range of movements can be produced. Besides these synovial joints, there are many ligaments which bind the adjacent neural arches, that is, the ligamentum flavum, supraspinous ligament, ligamentum nuchae, and intertransverse ligaments (refer to **Fig. 26.5c**). The movements between the arches are flexion, extension, and slight lateral bending.

Description of the Craniovertebral Joints

Atlantoaxial Joint

The joints between the atlas and axis vertebrae are three in number, that is, two lateral joints (one on each side) between the inferior articular facet of the atlas and superior articular facet of the axis, and one median joint between the anterior arch of the atlas and odontoid process of the axis. All three joints are synovial in variety. The median atlantoaxial joint is of *pivot* category while the lateral atlantoaxial joints are of *plane* category.

There are three ligaments extending between the dens and occipital bone. These are apical ligament of the dens, two alar ligaments, and membrane tectoria (**Fig. 26.5**). The other ligament of the joint is the transverse ligament. The movement of the atlantoaxial joint is rotation; the head along with the atlas rotates on the axis vertebra from side to side.

Atlanto-Occipital Joint

The joints are between the occipital condyles of the occipital bone and superior articular facets of the atlas vertebra. These are synovial joints of condyloid variety. Articular surfaces are covered by the hyaline cartilage and bones are united with each other by the articular capsule and lined by the synovial membrane.

The occipital bone and atlas vertebra are interconnected with the anterior and posterior *atlanto-occipital membranes*. The ligaments of craniovertebral joints are shown in **Fig. 26.5**. The movements of the atlanto-occipital joints are flexion, extension, and lateral bending.

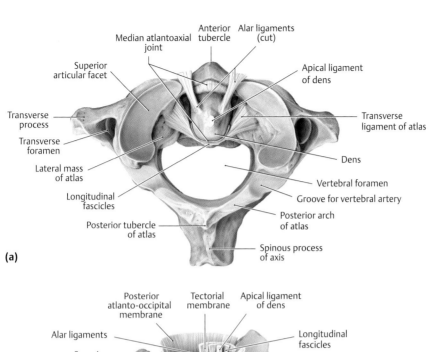

(a)

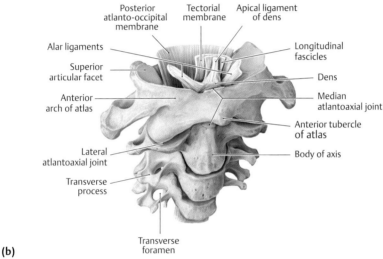

(b)

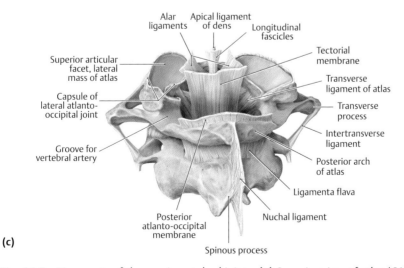

(c)

Fig. 26.5 Ligaments of the craniovertebral joints. **(a)** Superior view of atlas (C1) and axis (C2). **(b)** Anterosuperior view of C1–C4. **(c)** Posterosuperior view of atlas (C1) and axis (C2). (From: Schuenke M, Schulte E, Schumacher U. THIEME Atlas of Anatomy. Head, Neck, and Neuroanatomy. Illustrations by Voll M and Wesker K. © Thieme 2020.)

▮ Clinical Notes

1. Bilateral or unilateral dislocations of the facet joints are common at the lower cervical vertebral levels.

2. At the time of hanging, there occurs the fracture of the odontoid process and rupture of the transverse ligament followed by displacement of the atlas on the axis. This leads to the injury of the upper spinal cord resulting in death.

3. The osteoarthritis of the facet joints and formation of osteophytes are common in cervical vertebrae leading to compression of the spinal nerve at the intervertebral foramen.

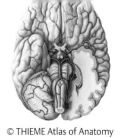

© THIEME Atlas of Anatomy

Learning Objectives

At the end of the dissection of the blood vessels of the brain, you should be able to identify and understand the following:

- Major subarachnoid cisterns.
- Superficial veins of the cerebral hemisphere, that is, the superior, middle, and inferior cerebral veins.
- Vertebral artery and its branches.
- Internal carotid, anterior cerebral artery, and middle cerebral artery.
- Formation of the circle of Willis and its central branches.

Students should note that we had already removed the brain from the cranial cavity (refer to Chapter 12). At that time, we had kept this brain in the preservative solution for future dissection. You should take out this brain and keep it in a tray. This brain is covered by two meninges, that is, the arachnoid and pia mater. The dura mater was left attached to the cranial cavity. The veins and arteries of the brain are present in the subarachnoid space. Refer to Chapter 12 for a quick review of the dura mater, dural folds, dural venous sinuses, arachnoid mater, arachnoid granulation, etc. You should also learn about the subarachnoid cisterns from a textbook of neuroanatomy.

Introduction of Brain

Before we proceed with the dissection of the brain, students should procure a full brain from the storage jar of the dissection hall/museum from which the meninges and blood vessels have been removed. On this specimen of the brain, learn the preliminary things about the gross structure of the brain with the help of your teacher and **Fig. 27.1**:

1. *Parts of the brain (forebrain, midbrain, and hindbrain) and cranial fossae in which they are lodged.*

2. *Preliminary observation of the sulci and gyri on the cerebral hemisphere.*

3. *Surfaces of the cerebral hemisphere and their lobes (superolateral, medial, and inferior surfaces; frontal, parietal, occipital, and temporal lobes).*

4. *Location and boundaries of the interpeduncular fossa.*

5. *Attachments of the cranial nerves at the base of the brain.*

Now procure a midsagittal section of the brain and with the help of your teacher learn about the medial surface of the cerebral hemisphere.

Parts of brain: The brain is a part of the central nervous system. It is located within the skull and consists of three major parts, i.e., forebrain, midbrain, and hindbrain (refer to **Fig. 27.1**).

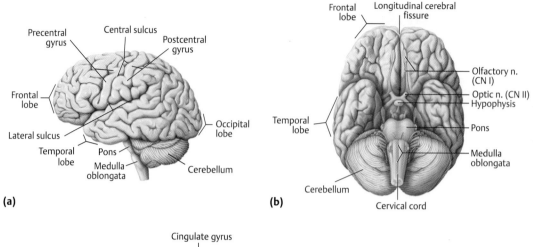

(a)

(b)

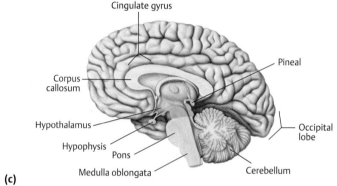

(c)

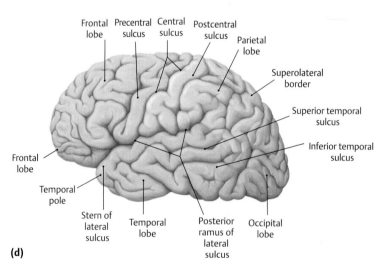

(d)

Fig. 27.1   Adult brain. **(a)** Left lateral view showing superolateral surface of cerebral hemisphere. **(b)** Basal view showing inferior (ventral) surface of brain. **(c)** Midsagittal section showing medial surface in the right half of brain. **(d)** Sulci, gyri, and lobes on superolateral surface of the left cerebral hemisphere.

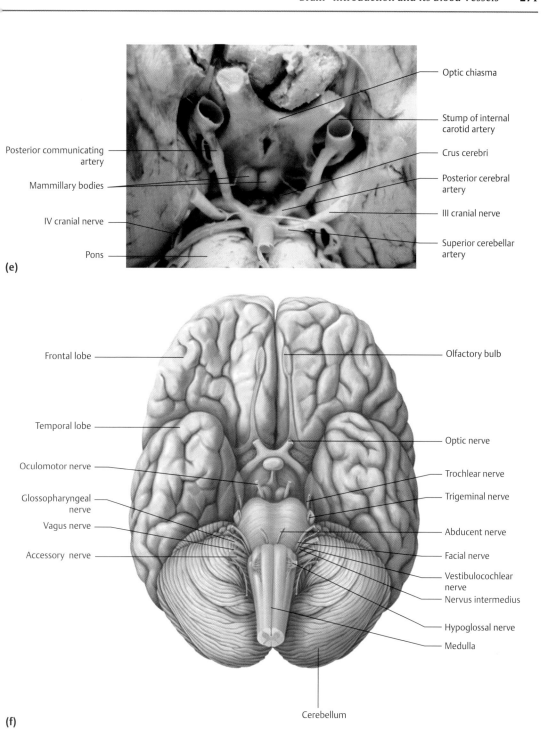

Fig. 27.1 Adult brain. **(e)** Photograph showing the interpeduncular fossa. **(f)** Attachment of various cranial nerves on the base (ventral surface) of brain. (Figure a-d, f: From: Schuenke M, Schulte E, Schumacher U. THIEME Atlas of Anatomy. Head, Neck, and Neuroanatomy. Illustrations by Voll M and Wesker K. © Thieme 2020; Figure e: Reproduced with permission from GP Pal, Illustrated Textbook of Neuroanatomy, Wolters Kluwer, 2013. (Courtesy Prof. SD Joshi, Director Prof., SAIMS, Indore.)

Forebrain: This is the largest part of the brain and consists of cerebrum and diencephalon (thalamus and hypothalamus). The cerebrum consists of two cerebral hemispheres separated from each other in midline by longitudinal fissure. The surface of each cerebral hemisphere is covered by gray matter which shows excessive folding. This folding consists of *sulci* (grooves) and *gyri* (ridges).

Each cerebral hemisphere presents three surfaces, i.e., superolateral surface, medial surface, and inferior surface. Each cerebral hemisphere is subdivided into four lobes, i.e., frontal, parietal, occipital, and temporal.

The diencephalon is situated deep inside the cerebral hemisphere and therefore except a small part of hypothalamus, diencephalon is not visible on surface. Each cerebral hemisphere encloses a large cavity (ventricle) known as *lateral ventricle.* Similarly, a narrow cavity is present between right and left diencephalon known as *third ventricle.*

Midbrain: It is a small part of the brain which joins forebrain with hindbrain. On the dorsal aspect midbrain shows two pairs of swellings: superior and inferior *colliculi.* The ventral surface of the midbrain presents right and left *crus cerebri.* Midbrain is traversed by cerebral aqueduct, which connects the third ventricle to fourth ventricle.

Hindbrain: It consists of pons, medulla, and cerebellum.

Pons is a white bulging mass located just below the midbrain on the ventral aspect of brain. It consists of mass of transverse fibers running between the two halves of cerebellum. This bundle of white fibers connecting pons to cerebellum is known as *middle cerebellar peduncle.*

Medulla is the caudal part of the hindbrain. It is conical in shape. Medulla continues above with the pons and below with the spinal cord. An anteromedian fissure divides the medulla into right and left halves. Two swellings are seen on each side of this anteromedian fissure: pyramid and olive.

Cerebellum: It is also called "small brain" because it is the second largest part of brain after cerebrum. Cerebellum is located posterior to pons and medulla. It consists of two lateral lobes (cerebellar hemispheres), which are connected with each other by a median structure, *vermis.* The fourth ventricle is present in hindbrain. Cavity of 4th ventricle is located posterior to pons and medulla and ventral to cerebellum.

Preliminary observation of the sulci and gyri on the cerebral hemisphere/Surfaces of the cerebral hemisphere and their lobes: Important sulci and gyri, on various surfaces of cerebral hemisphere that are located on different lobes are shown in **Figs. 27.1a–d**. You should learn preliminary aspects of cerebral hemisphere and brainstem with the help of your teacher and these figures. We shall learn all these in great details later in Chapter 31.

Location and boundaries of the interpeduncular fossa: This fossa is present on the ventral aspect of brain between right and left cerebral peduncles. It is bounded anteriorly by optic chiasma and optic tract, on sides by crus cerebri of cerebral peduncles and posteriorly by pons **(Fig. 27.1e)**. From anterior to posterior it contains tuber cinereum, infundibular stalk, mammillary bodies, and posterior perforated substance. Oculomotor nerve emerges from this fossa.

Attachments of the cranial nerves at the base of the brain: With the help of your teacher and **Fig. 27.1f** learn the attachments of all cranial nerves. Cranial nerves from 3rd to 12th are attached to brainstem. Cranial nerves 3rd and 4th take origin from midbrain, 5th from pons, 6th to 8th from the junction of pons and medulla, and 9th to 12th from medulla. All these nerves take origin from the ventral aspect of brainstem except 4th which arises from the dorsal aspect of midbrain.

Blood Vessels of the Brain

Only after studying the introductory aspects of brain, we shall dissect the arachnoid mater and study the subarachnoid cisterns, veins, and arteries lying in the subarachnoid space.

Introduction

The brain has a rich blood supply as it is metabolically highly active. It is supplied by a pair of vertebral arteries and a pair of internal carotid arteries. The vertebral arteries join each other to form the median basilar artery at the lower border of the pons. The basilar artery terminates in two posterior cerebral arteries. The internal carotid artery branches into two large arteries, that is, the middle cerebral and anterior cerebral. The circle of Willis is formed by the anastomosis of branches of the vertebral and internal carotid arteries.

The veins of the brain lie on the surface of the brain in the subarachnoid space. These veins drain their blood into the dural venous sinus.

Surface Landmarks

On a full brain, from which the meninges and blood vessels have been removed, review the following features:

1. Boundaries of the interpeduncular fossa.

2. Stem and posterior ramus of the lateral sulcus.

3. Longitudinal fissure.

4. Tentorial surface of the cerebral hemisphere.

Dissection and Identification

Observe the full brain which was removed from the cranial cavity. It is covered completely by the arachnoid membrane. However, sometimes it may so happen that the arachnoid membrane may get torn at certain places while removing the brain from the cranial cavity. Observe that the arachnoid membrane is very thin and almost transparent (**Fig. 27.2**). Veins are usually visible through the arachnoid membrane. As the cerebrospinal fluid (CSF) is not present in the subarachnoid space, the subarachnoid cisterns are difficult to visualize.

A. Dissection to expose the cisterns and veins on the surface of cerebral hemisphere (Videos 27.1 and 27.2).

1. With the help of scissors give an incision in the arachnoid membrane over the stem of the lateral sulcus. Extend this incision over the posterior ramus of the lateral sulcus. Over the stem of the lateral sulcus, a subarachnoid cistern is found (*cistern of the lateral sulcus*).

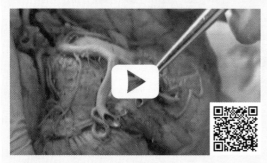

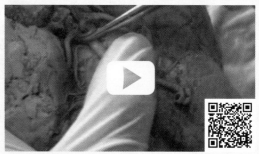

Video 27.1 Human brain: vertebrobasilar circulation of brain.

Video 27.2 Human brain: carotid middle cerebral, and anterior cerebral arteries.

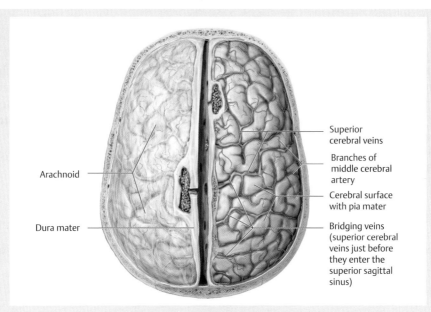

Fig. 27.2 Brain and meninges in situ (superior view). (From: Schuenke M, Schulte E, Schumacher U. THIEME Atlas of Anatomy. Head, Neck, and Neuroanatomy. Illustrations by Voll M and Wesker K. © Thieme 2020.)

2. Strip the arachnoid mater superiorly toward the superomedial border and inferiorly toward the inferolateral border of the cerebral hemisphere.

3. Observe the superficial middle cerebral vein lying in the lateral sulcus (**Fig. 27.3**). Trace the superior cerebral veins running upward and inferior cerebral veins on the surface of the temporal lobe.

4. Learn about the veins present on the inferior (**Fig. 27.4**) and medial surfaces (**Fig. 27.5**) of the cerebral hemisphere.

5. Once you have seen these veins, remove them from the surface of the cerebral hemisphere by stripping them carefully.

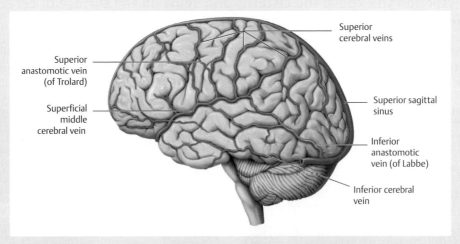

Fig. 27.3 Superficial veins of the brain (superficial cerebral veins: left lateral view). (From: Schuenke M, Schulte E, Schumacher U. THIEME Atlas of Anatomy. Head, Neck, and Neuroanatomy. Illustrations by Voll M and Wesker K. © Thieme 2020.)

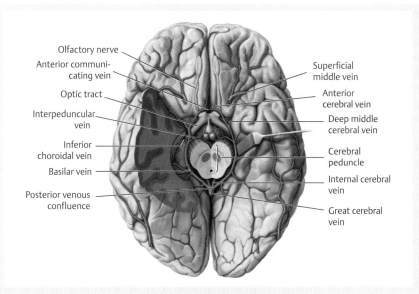

Fig. 27.4 Basal cerebral venous system. (From: Schuenke M, Schulte E, Schumacher U. THIEME Atlas of Anatomy. Head, Neck, and Neuroanatomy. Illustrations by Voll M and Wesker K. © Thieme 2020.)

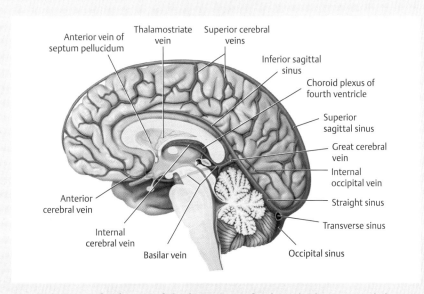

Fig. 27.5 Superficial veins of the brain (superficial cerebral veins: medial view). (From: Schuenke M, Schulte E, Schumacher U. THIEME Atlas of Anatomy. Head, Neck, and Neuroanatomy. Illustrations by Voll M and Wesker K. © Thieme 2020.)

B. Dissection of cerebral and cerebellar arteries and circle of Willis.

1. Observe the branches of the middle cerebral artery lying on the superolateral surface of the cerebral hemisphere (**Fig. 27.6**).

2. Divide the arachnoid membrane over the anterior aspect of the medulla oblongata and pons. This is the site of the cisterna pontis. This incision in the arachnoid membrane will expose the vertebral and basilar arteries (**Fig. 27.7**).

3. Divide the arachnoid membrane over the cerebellomedullary cistern. This will expose the posterior inferior cerebellar artery (**Fig. 27.7**).

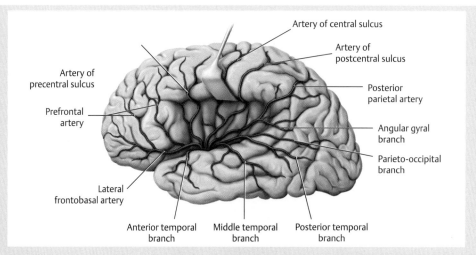

Fig. 27.6 Course and branches of the middle cerebral artery in the interior of the lateral sulcus (left lateral view). (From: Schuenke M, Schulte E, Schumacher U. THIEME Atlas of Anatomy. Head, Neck, and Neuroanatomy. Illustrations by Voll M and Wesker K. © Thieme 2020.)

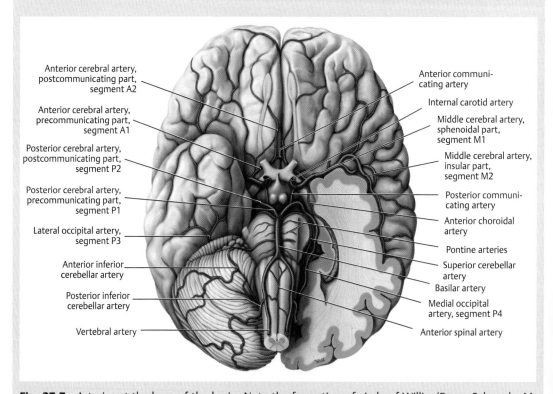

Fig. 27.7 Arteries at the base of the brain. Note the formation of circle of Willis. (From: Schuenke M, Schulte E, Schumacher U. THIEME Atlas of Anatomy. Head, Neck, and Neuroanatomy. Illustrations by Voll M and Wesker K. © Thieme 2020.)

4. Now extend the midline incision in the arachnoid membrane over the pons toward the interpeduncular fossa. This is the site of the interpeduncular cistern and contains the circle of Willis (refer to **Fig. 27.7**).

5. Find the stump of the internal carotid artery and trace the origin of the anterior and middle cerebral arteries. Follow the middle cerebral artery in the stem of the lateral sulcus (**Fig. 27.6**). Follow the anterior cerebral artery toward the longitudinal fissure.

6. Find the posterior cerebral artery and posterior communicating arteries in the interpeduncular fossa.

7. Now trace the central branches of the circle of Willis and cerebral arteries as they enter the anterior and posterior perforated substance.

Subarachnoid Cisterns

The arachnoid mater is a thin, delicate, transparent membrane. The pia mater closely adheres to the brain; therefore, it cannot be stripped off from the brain. The space between the pia (surface of the brain) and arachnoid is known as the subarachnoid space, which is filled with CSF. As the surface of the brain is irregular at certain places, the pia and arachnoid mater are widely separated from each other to form cisterns which are filled with pool of CSF (**Fig. 27.8**). Large cisterns are found around the brainstem and cerebellum, while small cisterns are seen in association with a few sulci and blood vessels.

Cerebellomedullary cistern or cisterna magna: It lies between the lower surface of the cerebellum and posterior surface of the medulla oblongata. It is the largest subarachnoid cistern.

Cisterna pontis: It lies on the anterior surface of the medulla and pons. It contains the vertebral and basilar arteries.

Interpeduncular cistern: It is present in front of the interpeduncular fossa. It contains the arterial circle of Willis.

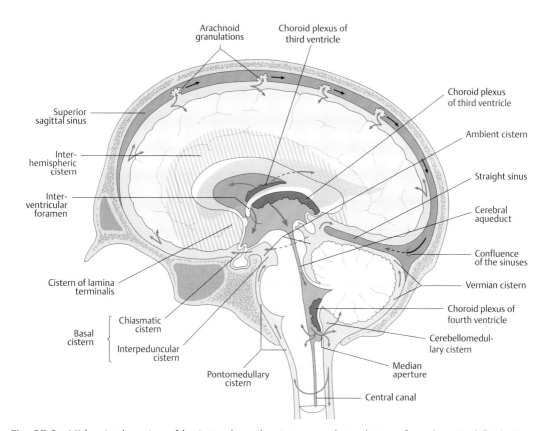

Fig. 27.8 Midsagittal section of brain to show the cisterns and circulation of cerebrospinal fluid. (From: Schuenke M, Schulte E, Schumacher U. THIEME Atlas of Anatomy. Head, Neck, and Neuroanatomy. Illustrations by Voll M and Wesker K. © Thieme 2020.)

Cistern of the lateral sulcus: It is present in the stem of the lateral sulcus, which contains the middle cerebral artery.

Cistern of the great cerebral vein: This cistern lies between the upper surface of the corpus callosum and splenium and contains the great cerebral vein.

Superficial Veins of the Cerebral Hemisphere

Superficial veins of the cerebral hemisphere are present on the external surface of the cerebral hemisphere in the subarachnoid space. These veins have a thin wall as they do not contain the muscle coat; therefore, the empty veins are difficult to visualize. Cerebral veins are also devoid of valves as they have to drain the blood toward gravity. The following major veins are present on the various surfaces of the cerebral hemisphere (refer to **Figs. 27.3–27.5**):

Veins on the superolateral surface of the cerebrum: These are the superior, middle, and inferior cerebral veins.

1. The superior cerebral veins are about 10 to 14 in number and drain the blood in the superior sagittal sinus.

2. The superficial middle cerebral vein is located in the lateral sulcus and drains to the cavernous sinus.

3. The inferior cerebral veins are present on the superolateral surface of the temporal lobe. Some of these drain to the superficial middle cerebral veins while the others drain to the transverse dural venous sinus.

Veins on the inferior surface of the cerebrum: This surface drains to the anterior cerebral vein, deep middle cerebral vein, and basal vein. On this surface, the basal vein is formed by the union of the anterior cerebral vein, deep middle cerebral vein, and striate veins.

Veins on the medial surface of the cerebrum: This surface shows the anterior cerebral vein, basal vein, and great cerebral vein. The great cerebral vein emerges beneath the splenium of the corpus callosum. The basilar vein joins the great cerebral vein. The great cerebral vein joins with the inferior sagittal sinus to form the straight sinus.

Arteries of the Brain

The brain derives its total blood supply from two internal carotid and two vertebral arteries.
Vertebral arteries: Each vertebral artery enters the subarachnoid space by piercing the dura and arachnoid mater just below the foramen magnum. It ascends through the foramen magnum by the side of the medulla and unites with its fellow at the lower border of the pons to form the basilar artery. The intracranial branches of the vertebral artery are as follows (refer to **Figs. 27.7** and **27.9**):

1. *Posterior spinal artery*: On either side, it passes inferiorly on the dorsal aspect of the medulla and spinal cord among the dorsal rootlets of the spinal nerve.

2. *Posterior inferior cerebellar artery*: On either side, it arises near the olive and runs downward and dorsally to supply the posterior part of the inferior surface of the cerebellum.

3. *Anterior spinal artery*: It is formed in the midline below the pons by the union of branches from the right and left vertebral arteries. It runs inferiorly in the anterior median fissure throughout the length of the spinal cord.

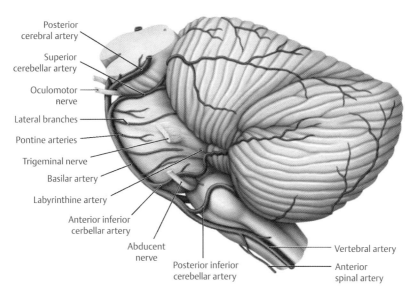

Fig. 27.9 Arteries of the brainstem and cerebellum (left lateral view). (From: Schuenke M, Schulte E, Schumacher U. THIEME Atlas of Anatomy. Head, Neck, and Neuroanatomy. Illustrations by Voll M and Wesker K. © Thieme 2020.)

Basilar artery: It runs in the median groove of the pons in the cisterna pontis. At the superior border of the pons, it divides into two posterior cerebral arteries. Following are the branches of the basilar arteries:

1. *Anterior inferior cerebellar arteries*: On each side, they supply the anterior part of the inferior surface of the cerebellum.

2. *Arteries of the labyrinth*: On each side, they accompany the vestibulocochlear nerve to enter the internal ear.

3. *Pontine arteries*: These are many branches which supply the pons.

4. *Superior cerebellar artery*: On each side, it winds around the lower aspect of the midbrain to reach the superior surface of the cerebellum. It supplies the parts of the pons, midbrain, and superior surface of the cerebellum.

5. *Posterior cerebral arteries*: The right and left posterior cerebral arteries lie at the superior border of the pons and run laterally to reach the tentorial surface of the cerebral hemisphere. Following are the branches of the posterior cerebral artery:

   a. *Central branches*: They enter the cerebrum through the posterior perforated substances to supply the thalamus and lentiform nucleus.

   b. *Posterior choroid artery*: It supplies the choroid plexus of the lateral and third ventricles of the brain.

   c. *Cortical branches*: These branches supply the cortex of the temporal and occipital lobes on the tentorial (inferior) surface.

Internal carotid arteries: On either side, the artery pierces the dura and arachnoid mater just medial to the anterior clinoid process. Here, it lies just below the anterior perforated substance and branches into the following (refer to **Fig. 27.7**):

1. *Ophthalmic*: This artery passes through the optic canal to go to the orbit.

2. *Anterior choroidal*: It supplies the choroid plexus in the inferior horn of the lateral ventricle.

3. *Posterior communicating*: It joins the proximal part of the posterior cerebral artery.

4. *Anterior cerebral artery*: It is the smaller terminal branch of the internal carotid artery. It passes forward and medially toward the longitudinal fissure. Here, the right and left cerebral arteries join each other through the anterior communicating artery. Now it runs on the corpus callosum. It gives central and cortical branches. The central branches pass through the anterior perforated substance to supply the deeper structures, such as the corpus striatum. The cortical branches supply the part of the orbital surface and medial surface of the cerebral hemisphere.

5. *Middle cerebral artery*: It is the larger terminal branch of the middle cerebral artery. First, it runs laterally in the stem of the lateral sulcus and then runs in the posterior ramus of the lateral sulcus. It gives central and cortical branches. The central branches pass through the anterior perforated substance to supply the caudate nucleus, internal capsule, and lentiform nucleus. The cortical branches supply the superolateral surface and adjacent part of the orbital surface and temporal pole.

The Circle of Willis

It is an arterial circle formed by the anastomosis of branches of the vertebral and internal carotid arteries. It is present in the interpeduncular fossa. This hexagonal circle is formed by the posterior cerebral, posterior communicating, internal carotid, and anterior cerebral and anterior communicating arteries (refer to **Figs. 27.7** and **27.10**). The circle of Willis gives origin to many *central* and *cortical branches*.

1. The *central branches* arise in four groups, that is, the anteromedial, anterolateral, posteromedial, and posterolateral. These branches supply the internal parts of the brain and pass through the anterior and posterior perforated substance.

2. The *cortical branches* ramify over the surface of the cortex.

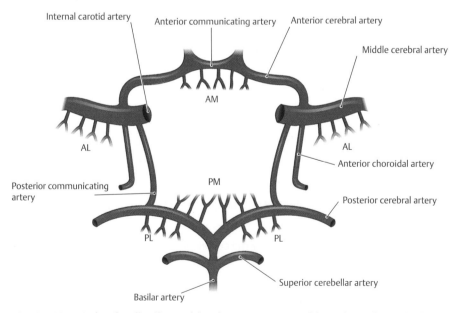

Fig. 27.10 Circle of Willis (formed by the anastomosis of branches of vertebral and internal carotid arteries). AL, anterolateral, AM, anteromedial, PL, posterolateral, PM, posteromedial groups of central arteries. (From: Schuenke M, Schulte E, Schumacher U. THIEME Atlas of Anatomy. Head, Neck, and Neuroanatomy. Illustrations by Voll M and Wesker K. © Thieme 2020.)

If one of the major branches forming the circle of Willis is blocked, then blood may bypass the blocked artery and supply the area of the blocked artery.

Imaging of Blood Vessels of Brain (Video 27.3)

The cerebral angiography is performed by injecting radio-opaque contrast media in common carotid or vertebral arteries. With the help of angiography (X-ray, CT or MRI) we may diagnose (find out) haemorrhage, blockage, stenosis, aneurysm and flow velocity of vessels of neck and brain.

Nowadays, X-ray angiography is being taken over by CT or MR angiography which can produce three-dimensional images of blood vessels through a test which is less invasive and stressful for the patients.

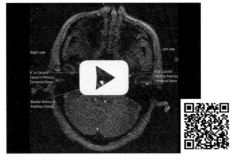

Video 27.3 Tracking brain circulation via 2D time of flight angiography (TOF) serial MRI axial slices with narration.

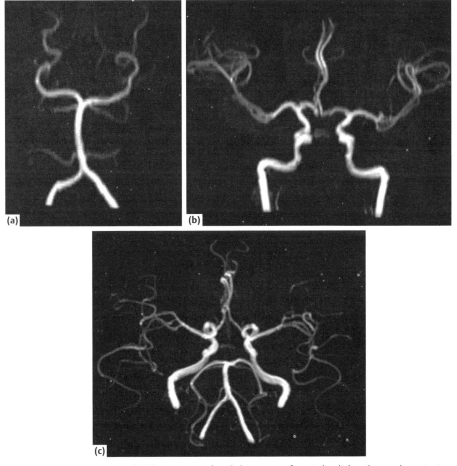

Fig. 27.11 Magnetic resonance (MR) angiography. **(a)** Image of vertebral, basilar and posterior cerebral arteries. **(b)** Internal carotid and its middle cerebral and anterior cerebral branches. **(c)** MR angiography showing circle of Willis which is formed by the branches of basilar and internal carotid arteries. (Reproduced with permission from Pal GP, Illustrated Textbook of Neuroanatomy, Wolters Kluwer, 2013) (Courtesy of Dr. Sangeet Choudhary, Chief radiologist, SRL Diagnostic, Indore).

■ Clinical Notes

1. The pressure on the internal jugular veins produces a marked rise in the intracranial venous pressure due to pooling of blood. This venous pressure can be measured by lumbar puncture with the help of a manometer. This confirms the continuity of the cranial and lumbar and subarachnoid spaces.

2. The blood–brain barrier is formed by the endothelial cells resting on the basal lamina and perivascular feet of the endocytes.

3. Occlusion, thrombosis, and aneurysm are very common in the cerebral vessels. Occlusion by thrombosis may result in infarction of the brain tissue. The rupturing of the artery may take place due to increase in blood pressure or aneurysm. This is known as cerebral hemorrhage.

4. Occlusion of central branches of the circle of Willis may lead to hemiplegia because of infarction of the motor fibers in the internal capsule.

5. Cerebral angiography is done in suspected cases of aneurysms, acute ischaemic stroke, vascular abnormalities etc. to look at the blood vessels of brain. Now a day MRI angiography is preferred over traditional angiography because it is less invasive and less painful (**Fig. 27.11**).

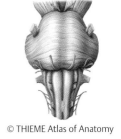

Medulla Oblongata

Learning Objectives

At the end of the dissection of the medulla, you should be able to identify and understand the following:

- Pyramid, pyramidal decussation, and its significance.
- Olive and olivocerebellar fibers passing through the inferior cerebellar peduncle.
- Tuber cinereum, nucleus of the spinal tract of the trigeminal.
- Gracile and cuneate tubercles and great sensory decussation.
- Inferior cerebellar peduncle.
- Nuclei of the ninth, tenth, eleventh, and twelfth cranial nerves and origin of these cranial nerves.

The *hindbrain* consists of the medulla, pons, and cerebellum (**Fig. 28.1**). It is continuous above with the midbrain and below with the spinal cord. Posteriorly, the upper parts of the medulla and pons are separated from the cerebellum by the cavity of the fourth ventricle. The medulla is connected posteriorly with the cerebellum through the inferior cerebellar peduncle. Similarly, the pons is connected with the cerebellum through the middle cerebellar peduncle.

The *brainstem,* the stem-like lower part of the brain, consists of three parts. From above downward these are midbrain, pons, and medulla oblongata (**Fig. 28.1**).

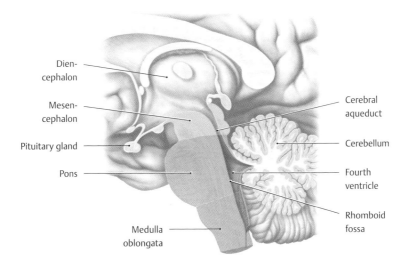

Fig. 28.1 Parts of hindbrain as seen in midsagittal section. (From: Schuenke M, Schulte E, Schumacher U. THIEME Atlas of Anatomy. Head, Neck, and Neuroanatomy. Illustrations by Voll M and Wesker K. © Thieme 2020.)

Introduction

The medulla oblongata is conical in shape and related anteriorly to the basilar part of the occipital bone in the posterior cranial fossa. It is about 3 cm long and 2 cm wide. The medulla is divided into an upper open part and lower closed part. The medulla gives attachment to the ninth through twelfth cranial nerves. The interior of the upper medulla consists of scattered masses of gray and white matters.

Surface Landmarks

1. Review the bony features of the posterior cranial fossa (refer to **Fig. 1.7**). The pons, medulla, and cerebellum lie in the posterior cranial fossa below the tentorium cerebelli.

2. The pons and medulla lie posterior to the basilar part of the occipital bone (clivus).

3. The lowermost part of the medulla passes through the foramen magnum. Inferiorly, it is continuous with the spinal cord at the level of origin of the first pair of the cervical spinal nerves.

Dissection and Identification

A. Dissection to expose brainstem.

1. Carefully remove the small blood vessels from the surface of the brainstem (refer to **Fig. 27.8**).

2. Look for the anteromedian fissure, pyramid, anterolateral sulcus, olives, posterolateral sulcus, and inferior cerebellar peduncle on the ventral surface of the medulla (**Fig. 28.2a**).

3. Locate the emergence of the glossopharyngeal, vagus, accessory, and hypoglossal nerves (**Fig. 28.2a,c**).

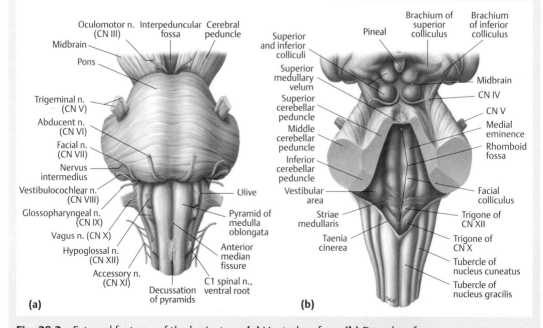

Fig. 28.2 External features of the brainstem. **(a)** Ventral surface, **(b)** Dorsal surface.

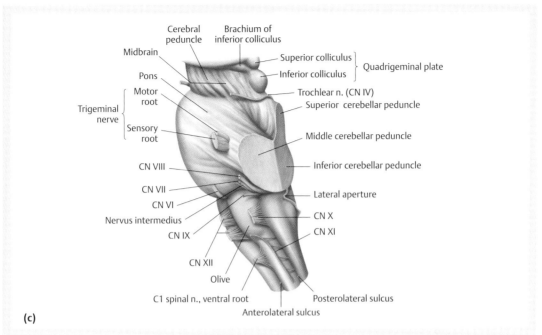

(c)

Fig. 28.2   (c) External features of the brainstem in lateral view. (From: Gilroy AM, MacPherson BR, Ross LM. Atlas of Anatomy. Second Edition. Illustrations by Markus Voll and Karl Wesker. © Thieme 2012.)

4. On the dorsal surface of the medulla, look for the posteromedian sulcus, fasciculus gracilis and fasciculus cuneatus, inferior cerebellar peduncle, and tuber cinereum (**Fig. 28.2b**).

5. At the upper end of the closed part, look for the gracile and cuneate tubercles.

6. The structures of the open part (floor of the fourth ventricle) will be seen later.

7. In a separate specimen of the medulla, study the cross-sections of the medulla at three different levels, that is, at the level of the pyramidal decussation, at the level of the gracile and cuneate tubercles, and at the level of the olives (**Fig. 28.3a–c**).

External Features of the Medulla

The medulla presents the ventral (anterior) and dorsal (posterior) surfaces (refer to **Fig. 28.2**). The ventral surface presents the anterior median fissure. The dorsal surface presents the posterior median sulcus in the lower closed part. The upper part of the dorsal surface forms the floor of the fourth ventricle.

Ventral surface of the medulla: On either side of the anterior median fissure the bulge is called the pyramid. The pyramid consists of the corticospinal (motor) fibers. At the lower medulla, most of the fibers of the pyramid cross to the opposite side (pyramidal decussation). Lateral to the pyramid, the *anterolateral sulcus* is present which gives attachment to the rootlets of the hypoglossal nerve. Lateral to the anterolateral sulcus, another bulge is present called the olive. Posterolateral to the olive, the *posterolateral sulcus* is present which gives attachment to the ninth, tenth, and eleventh cranial nerves. Posterior to the posterolateral sulcus, the *inferior cerebellar peduncle* is present on either side. The inferior cerebellar peduncles connect the medulla to the cerebellum.

The anteromedian fissure and posteromedian sulcus are continuous below, in the spinal cord, by the same names, respectively.

Dorsal surface of the medulla: It is divided into the lower *closed* and upper *open* parts:

1. *Closed part*: It shows the presence of the posteromedian sulcus, gracile tubercle, cuneate tubercle, and posterolateral sulcus. Lateral to the cuneate tubercle, an elevation is present which is called the *tuber cinereum*. It is produced by the spinal nucleus of the fifth cranial nerve and its tract.

2. *Open part*: The dorsal surface of the open part forms the lower part of the floor of the fourth ventricle. The central canal of the closed part of the medulla opens above in the floor of the sixth ventricle. This surface presents the *hypoglossal triangle (trigone of CN XII), vagal triangle (trigone of CN X)*, and *vestibular area* (**Fig. 28.2b**).

Internal Structure of the Medulla

The internal structure of the medulla is best studied by taking the transverse section of the medulla at three different levels:

1. At the level of the pyramidal decussation (refer to **Fig. 28.3a**).

2. At the level of the gracile and cuneate tubercles (refer to **Fig. 28.3b**).

3. At the level of the olives (refer to **Fig. 28.3c**).

   a. **At the level of pyramidal decussation (Fig. 28.3a).** This section resembles somewhat the spinal cord section. The most striking feature of this level is the pyramidal decussation and appearance of lateral corticospinal tract. The dorsal gray horn is replaced by the nucleus of the spinal tract of trigeminal nerve The gracile and cuneatus nuclei start appearing from the posterior gray column.

   b. **At the level of gracile** and **cuneate tubercles (at the level of great sensory decussation).** Three nuclei are seen in central gray mass, i.e., hypoglossal, vagus, and nucleus of solitary tract (**Fig. 8.3b**). Nucleus ambiguus is situated in the reticular formation. Fibers arising from the gracile and cuneatus nuclei (internal arcuate fibers) decussate in midline. This decussation is known as great sensory decussation. On the anterior aspect of the section pyramids are seen carrying corticospinal fibers. Ventral and dorsal spinocerebellar tracts are located on the lateral side of the section.

   c. **At the level of olives (at the level of open part of medulla, i.e., lower part of fourth ventricle).** No central canal is visible as it has opened in the floor of fourth ventricle. Note the changed position of hypoglossal, vagal, and nucleus of solitary tract (**Fig. 28.3c**). They all lie

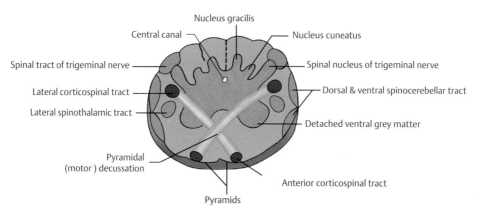

(a)

Fig. 28.3 Transverse section of the medulla oblongata at three different levels: **(a)** at the level of pyramidal decussation.

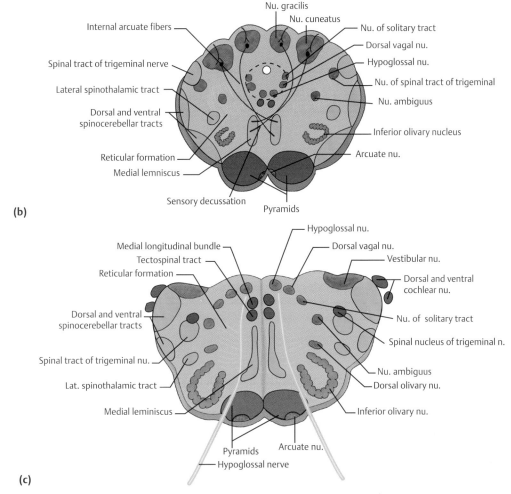

Fig. 28.3 Transverse section of the medulla oblongata at three different levels: **(b)** at the level of gracile and cuneate tubercle, and **(c)** at the level of olives.

now in the floor of fourth ventricle. The olivary nuclei are located in ventrolateral part of section, deep to olive. Note the appearance of inferior cerebellar peduncle.

Students should learn the detailed internal structure of the medulla from a textbook of neuroanatomy.

▌Clinical Notes

Lesions of the medulla may result due to various causes, that is, injury, congenital anomaly, and vascular lesions.

1. As the medulla contains respiratory and cardiovascular centers, an injury to the medulla may lead to sudden death. However, if the injury is nonfatal, it may affect the cranial nerves and the ascending or descending tracts. This may affect the function of the cranial nerve involved or cause paralysis of muscles on the opposite side (due to involvement of the corticospinal tract) and loss of sensations on the opposite side due to damage to the sensory tracts.

2. The vascular lesion may occur due to thrombosis or hemorrhage. Well-known vascular lesions of the medulla are the *medial medullary syndrome* (due to occlusion of the medullary branch of the anterior spinal artery) and *lateral medullary syndrome* (due to occlusion or thrombosis of the posterior inferior cerebellar artery) (Refer to **Fig. 27.9**).

Pons

Introduction

Pons is a part of the brainstem. It lies between the midbrain (above) and the medulla (below) in the posterior cranial fossa. The pons is situated above medulla oblongata, in front of the cerebellum. The ventral surface of the pons is convex, which on each lateral side is continuous with the middle cerebellar peduncle. The fifth cranial nerve is attached at the junction of the pons and middle cerebellar peduncle. The cranial nerves sixth to eighth are attached at the pontomedullary junction. The posterior surface of the pons is formed by the floor of the fourth ventricle.

Surface Landmarks

1. The ventral surface of the pons lies posterior to the basisphenoid bone (clivus) in the posterior cranial fossa.

2. The fifth cranial nerve is attached at the junction of the lateral part of the pons and middle cerebellar peduncle.

3. The ventral aspect lodges the basilar artery in the basilar groove.

Dissection and Identification

A. Dissection of pons.

1. There is nothing much to dissect in the pons. Carefully remove the small blood vessels and pia mater from the ventral surface of the pons.

2. Look for the basilar groove on the ventral aspect of the brain. Also, look for transversely running faint striations on the ventral aspect, which converges on the middle cerebellar peduncle.

3. Locate the emergence of the fifth, sixth, seventh, and eighth nerves (**Fig. 28.2a**).

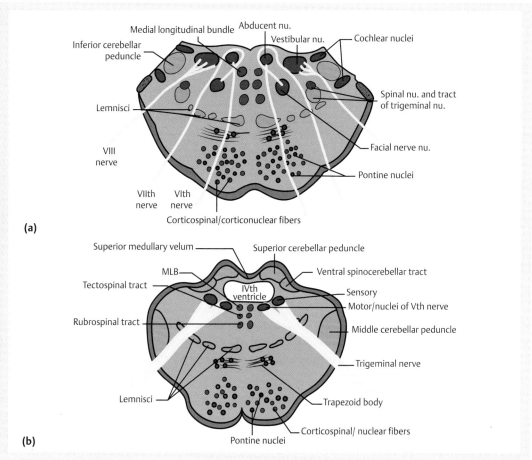

Fig. 28.4 Transverse section **(a)** at the lower level of pons. **(b)** the upper level of the pons. MLB, medial longitudinal bundle.

4. The structures of the posterior surface of the pons (forming the floor of the fourth ventricle) will be seen later.

5. In a separate specimen of the pons, study the cross-sections at two different levels, that is, at the level of the lower pons and upper pons (**Fig. 28.4**).

External Features of the Pons

The pons lies just above the medulla and below the midbrain. Thus, it acts as a bridge between the midbrain and medulla. It is about 2 to 3 cm long and presents the ventral and dorsal surfaces.

The ventral (anterior) surface of the pons is convex. It is bounded above by the superior border and below by the inferior border. In midline, it presents a sulcus known as the basilar groove which lodges the basilar artery. On the ventral aspect of the pons, transversely running faint striations are seen, which converge on the middle cerebellar peduncle. The middle cerebellar peduncle connects the pons to the cerebellum on each side.

At the inferior border (pontomedullary junction) of the pons, the sixth, seventh, and eighth cranial nerves are attached in order from medial to lateral. At the superior border of the pons, the cerebellar peduncles are attached (refer to **Fig. 28.1a**).

The dorsal (posterior) surface of the pons forms the upper part of the floor of the fourth ventricle (refer to **Fig. 28.1b**). This surface is covered by the cerebellum. We shall study the posterior surface of the pons after the removal of the cerebellum from its attachment to the brainstem.

Internal Structure of the Pons

The internal structure of the pons is best studied by taking the section of it at two different levels:

1. At the level of the lower pons, i.e., at the level of facial colliculi (refer to **Fig. 28.4a**).

2. At the level of the upper pons, i.e., at the level of trigeminal nuclei (refer to **Fig. 28.4b**).

The transverse section of the pons is divided into the ventral (basilar) and posterior (tegmentum) parts. The basilar part of the pons lies ventral to the trapezoid body while the tegmental part lies dorsal to it.

Structure of Basilar Part

The basilar part contains the transversely running fiber (pontocerebellar) and vertically running (corticopontine, corticonuclear, and corticospinal) white fibers. This part also contains scattered masses of gray matter called the pontine nuclei **(Fig. 28.4)**. The structure of the basilar part is the same throughout the pons (both in upper and lower levels).

Structure of Tegmental Part

The tegmentum of the pons is the direct upward continuation of the medulla. This part consists of many tracts and cranial nerve nuclei (V, VI, VII, and VIII). The structure of tegmentum is different in upper and lower parts of pons. Thus, we will study separately the structure of tegmentum in upper and lower parts of pons.

1. **Structure of tegmentum in the lower part of pons**—Various nuclei are seen at this level. These are abducent and vestibular nuclei at the floor of the fourth ventricle. The ventral and dorsal cochlear nuclei are present in relation to inferior cerebellar peduncle. The motor nucleus of facial nerve is located in reticular formation. Note the location of other nuclei with the help of **Fig. 28.4a**.

   Various lemnisci (medial, trigeminal, spinal, and lateral) are present posterior to trapezoid body. Inferior cerebellar peduncle is present in the lateralmost area of tegmentum **(Fig. 28.4a)**.

2. **Structure of tegmentum in the upper part of pons**—Note the presence of motor and sensory nuclei of trigeminal nerve. The nucleus of lateral lemniscus is present lateral to the lateral lemniscus.

   All the lemnisci are present in the same position as they were present at the lower level. The ventral spinocerebellar tract now forms superior cerebellar peduncle.

   For more on internal structure of the pons, students might refer to a textbook of neuroanatomy.

▋ Clinical Notes

The occlusion or hemorrhage of the pontine branches of the basilar arteries results in various syndromes, that is, the *Raymond syndrome, Millard–Gubler syndrome,* and *Foville syndrome.*

1. *Raymond syndrome*: It results in hemiplegia on the opposite side (due to involvement of the corticospinal tract) and medial squint on the same side (due to involvement of the abducens nerve).

2. *Millard–Gubler syndrome*: This results in hemiparesis on the opposite side (due to involvement of a few fibers of the corticospinal tract) and paralysis of the face on the same side (due to involvement of the facial nerve).

3. *Foville syndrome*: This results in paralysis of the facial muscles due to involvement of corticonuclear fibers and medial squint on the same side due to involvement of abducens nerve.

Midbrain

Learning Objectives

At the end of the dissection of the midbrain, you should be able to identify and understand the following:

On the external surface:

- Crura cerebri and interpeduncular fossa.
- Attachment of the oculomotor nerve.
- Superior and inferior colliculi, frenulum veli.
- Brachia of the superior colliculus and inferior colliculus.

In the internal structure:

- Tectum and cerebral peduncle parts, in the cross-section of the midbrain.
- Crus cerebri, substantia nigra, and tegmentum parts of cerebral peduncle in the cross-section of the midbrain.
- Red nucleus and tegmental decussation.
- Structure of the superior and inferior colliculi.

Introduction

The midbrain is the uppermost part of the brainstem. It connects the hindbrain with the cerebrum. It measures about 2.5 cm in length and traverses the tentorial notch. However, most of it lies in the posterior cranial fossa. The midbrain is traversed by the cerebral aqueduct that connects the third ventricle superiorly to the fourth ventricle inferiorly.

The midbrain shows the ventral, dorsal, and right and left lateral surfaces. The third cranial nerve originates from its ventral surface while the fourth nerve originates from its dorsal surface. The dorsal surface shows the presence of the colliculi.

Surface Landmarks

1. In the posterior cranial fossa of a dry skull, identify the clivus, posterior aspect of the dorsum sellae, and site of presence of the tentorial notch.

2. Identify the crus cerebri at the base of the brain where they form the lateral boundaries of the interpeduncular fossa.

3. Identify the pineal gland, splenium of the corpus callosum, and anterior lobe of the cerebellum which overlap the dorsal aspect of the midbrain.

Dissection and Identification

Dissection of Midbrain

1. Carefully remove the small blood vessels and pia mater from the surfaces of the midbrain.

2. Look for the interpeduncular fossa on the ventral aspect of the midbrain. Also, look for the attachment of the oculomotor nerve on the medial aspect of the crus cerebri.

3. The structures on the posterior surface of the midbrain are hidden by the pineal gland, splenium of the corpus callosum, and anterior lobe of the cerebellum. Gently push the anterior lobe of the cerebellum downward and splenium upward to observe the dorsal aspect of the midbrain.

4. In a separate specimen of the midbrain, study the cross-sections at two different levels, that is, at the level of the inferior colliculi and at the level of the superior colliculi.

External Features of the Midbrain

The midbrain presents the ventral, dorsal, and right and left lateral surfaces (refer to **Fig. 28.2a–c**).

Ventral Surface of the Midbrain

The ventral aspect presents two crura cerebri. Each crus cerebri emerges from the cerebral hemisphere and runs toward the pons. The lateral boundaries of the interpeduncular fossa are formed by the right and left crus cerebri. The interpeduncular fossa contains the posterior perforated substance and mammillary bodies and tuber cinereum. The oculomotor nerve emerges from the medial aspect of the crus cerebri.

Dorsal Surface of the Midbrain

This surface presents four rounded bodies called the colliculi. They are arranged in two pairs, that is, two superior (superior colliculi) and two inferior (inferior colliculi). These four colliculi are separated from each other by a cruciform sulcus. The lower end of vertical limb of cruciform sulcus ends in a frenulum veli. The trochlear nerve emerges from the either side of the frenulum veli. After taking origin from the dorsal aspect, the nerve winds around the lateral aspect of the midbrain to appear on its ventral aspect of the midbrain.

Lateral Surface of the Midbrain

On the right and left lateral surfaces of the midbrain, two bands of white fibers are seen. These bands are known as the superior and inferior brachium. The superior brachium connects the superior colliculus with the lateral geniculate body, while the inferior brachium connects the inferior colliculus with the medial geniculate body.

Internal Structure of the Midbrain

To understand the internal structure of midbrain we shall first study its transverse section (**Fig. 28.5**). In this section, the cerebral aqueduct is surrounded by gray matter. A transverse line drawn through the cerebral aqueduct divides the midbrain into two parts, that is, *tectum* and *cerebral peduncles*. The part lying behind the transverse line is called the tectum and the part lying ventral to the line is called the cerebral peduncles (**Fig. 28.5**).

Cerebral Peduncles

Each cerebral peduncle is made up of three parts, that is, the *crus cerebri, substantia nigra*, and *tegmentum*. The crus cerebri and substantia nigra remain the same throughout the midbrain. The structure of the tegmentum varies at the upper and lower levels of the midbrain.

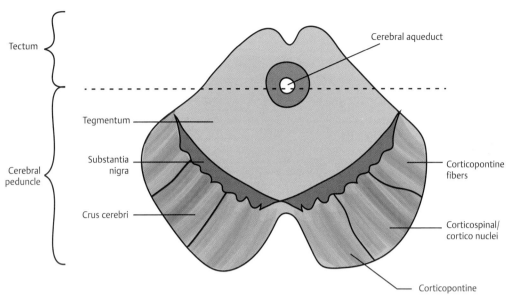

Fig. 28.5   Parts of midbrain (schematic diagram).

The crus cerebri consists of the descending fibers (motor fibers), which begin in the cerebral cortex and terminate at various levels of the brain and spinal cord. The substantia nigra is a mass of gray matter but it looks black because it contains melanin pigment and iron. The dopamine is synthesized in the substantia nigra.

The tegmentum contains gray and white matter, whose structure varies at the level of the superior and inferior colliculi.

Tectum

At the upper level, the tectum consists of a pair of superior colliculi and at the inferior level it consists of a pair of inferior colliculi. These colliculi are a collection of gray matter (nuclei). The inferior colliculus is a nucleus in the pathway of hearing. The superior colliculus is a nucleus in the pathway of vision.

Internal Structure of Midbrain at Various Levels

The internal structure of the midbrain is best studied by taking the section of it at two different levels:

1. At the level of the inferior colliculi (**Fig. 28.6a**).

2. At the level of the superior colliculi (**Fig. 28.6b**).

Transverse Section of Midbrain at the Level of Inferior Colliculus

1. *Structure of tegmentum*—The central gray matter contains trochlear and mesencephalic nuclei. Trochlear nucleus gives origin to nerve which comes out from the dorsal aspect of midbrain (**Fig. 28.6a**). Decussation of superior cerebellar peduncles is located ventral to central gray matter. Various lemnisci (medial, trigeminal spinal, and lateral) are located dorsomedial to substantia nigra.

2. *Structure of tectum*—It contains gray matter of inferior colliculus.

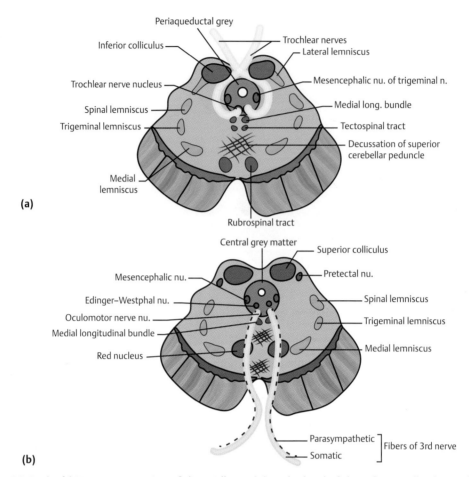

Fig. 28.6   (a, b) Transverse section of the midbrain **(a)** at the level of the inferior colliculus and **(b)** at the superior colliculus.

Transverse Section of Midbrain at the Level of Superior Colliculus

1. *Structure of tegmentum*—The oculomotor, mesencephalic, and Edinger-Westphal nuclei are present in periaqueductal gray. The red nucleus is prominent collection of gray matter posterior to substantia nigra. Note the location of dorsal and ventral tegmental decussation close to midline.

2. *Structure of tectum*—It contains superior colliculus and pretectal nucleus **(Fig. 28.6b)**.

▌Clinical Notes

Midbrain lesions may occur due to trauma, pressure (due to surrounding tumor), tumor of the midbrain itself, and vascular lesions. Well-known vascular lesions are the Weber and Benedikt syndromes.

1. *Weber syndrome*: This results due to the occlusion of the posterior cerebral artery supplying the crus cerebri of the upper midbrain. The clinical features of the syndrome are hemiparesis of the opposite side and paralysis (lateral squint) on the same side of the extraocular muscles innervated by the oculomotor nerve.

2. *Benedikt syndrome*: This lesion extends more posteriorly than the Weber syndrome and involves red nucleus and contralateral fibers of the cerebellum. In addition to the clinical features of the Weber syndrome, the patient also suffers from the cerebellar syndrome.

CHAPTER
29   Cerebellum

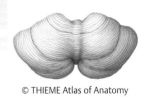

© THIEME Atlas of Anatomy

Learning Objectives

At the end of the dissection of the cerebellum, you should be able to identify and understand the following:

- Surfaces, fissures, and lobes.
- Vermis on the superior and inferior surface.
- Superior, middle, and inferior cerebellar peduncles.
- Arbor vitae cerebelli.
- Cerebellar nuclei (fastigial, globose, emboliform, and dentate).

Introduction

Cerebellum is the largest part of the hindbrain. It is located in the posterior cranial fossa behind the pons and medulla, below the tentorium cerebelli. There is a presence of the cavity of the fourth ventricle between the pons and the upper part of the medulla anteriorly, and cerebellum posteriorly. The cerebellum is connected to the midbrain, pons, and medulla through the superior, middle, and inferior cerebellar peduncles, respectively.

Functionally, the cerebellum is concerned with the movements of the skeletal muscles of the body, that is, it coordinates the voluntary movements and maintains the muscle tone. It is also involved in the maintenance of posture and equilibrium.

Surface Landmarks

1. Review the bony features of the posterior cranial fossa (refer to **Fig. 1.7**). The pons, medulla, and cerebellum lie in the posterior cranial fossa below the tentorium cerebelli.

2. Observe the internal occipital crest which gives attachment to the falx cerebelli. The falx cerebelli lies between the right and left cerebellar hemispheres on its inferior aspect.

3. Review the foramen magnum through which the tonsils of the cerebellum may herniate.

4. Note the vermis, fissure prima, horizontal fissure, posterolateral fissure, and flocculonodular lobe in the cerebellum.

Dissection and Identification

A. Dissection of cerebellum—fissures and lobes (Videos 29.1 and 29.2).

1. Remove the meninges and small blood vessels from the surface of the cerebellum.

2. Identify the right and left lobes of the cerebellum and superior and inferior vermis connecting the lobes (**Fig. 29.1a** and **b**).

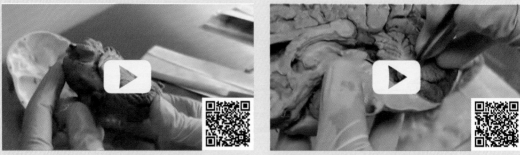

Video 29.1   Cerebellar dissection: Part I.   **Video 29.2**   Cerebellar dissection: Part II.

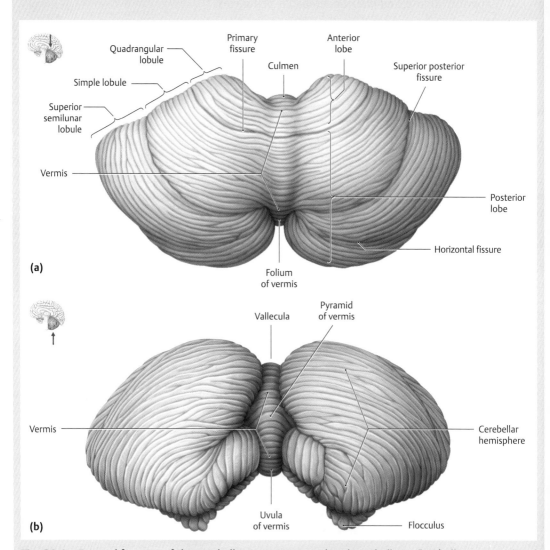

Fig. 29.1   External features of the cerebellum, as seen in isolated cerebellum. Cerebellum was isolated from brainstem by cutting its connection with all the cerebellar peduncles on both the sides: **(a)** superior view; **(b)** inferior view.

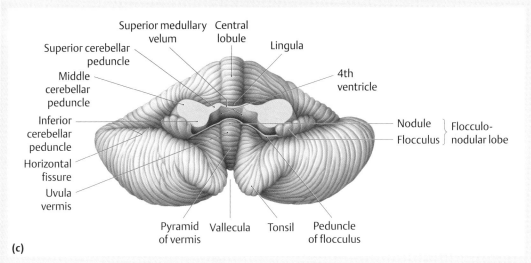

Fig. 29.1 External features of the cerebellum, as seen in isolated cerebellum. Cerebellum was isolated from brainstem by cutting its connection with all the cerebellar peduncles on both the sides: **(c)** anterior view. (From: Schuenke M, Schulte E, Schumacher U. THIEME Atlas of Anatomy. Head, Neck, and Neuroanatomy. Illustrations by Voll M and Wesker K. © Thieme 2020.)

3. Identify the superior and inferior surfaces of the cerebellum.

4. Locate the fissures, that is, the fissura prima, horizontal fissure, and posterolateral fissure. Identify the anterior, middle (posterior), and flocculonodular lobes.

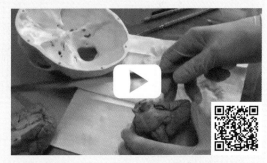

Video 29.3   Deep nuclei of cerebellum.

B. Dissection of cerebellar peduncles (Video 29.3).

1. Gently depress the superior surface of the cerebellum downward to expose the superior cerebellar peduncles and superior medullary velum. Note that the superior medullary velum lies between the right and left superior cerebellar peduncles and is covered by a thin layer of gray matter.

2. Now remove the upper portion of the cerebellum and lateral portions of the pons (**Fig. 29.2**). Identify the middle cerebellar peduncle extending from the lateral aspect of the pons to the cerebellum. Similarly, identify the inferior cerebellar peduncle connecting the medulla to the cerebellum.

3. With the help of blunt dissection, in one of the cerebellar hemispheres trace the fibers of the middle cerebellar peduncle going in the cerebellum. While tracing these fibers you will have to remove some gray and white matter from the surface of the cerebellum. Similarly, trace the fibers of the inferior peduncle from the medulla toward the cerebellum. Note that these fibers are going deep to the fibers of the middle peduncle. Lastly, follow the fibers of the superior cerebellar peduncle toward the cerebellum. These fibers lie deep (medial) to the middle and inferior peduncles (**Fig. 29.2**).

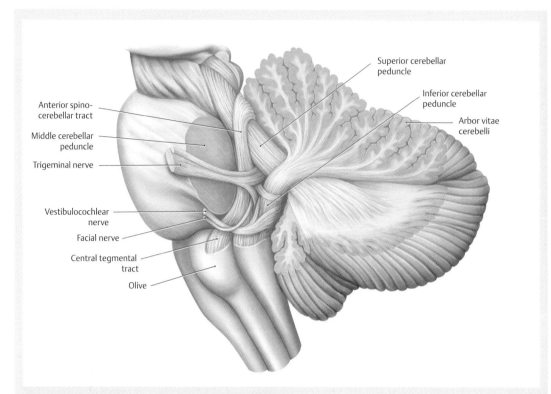

Superior cerebellar peduncle

Inferior cerebellar peduncle

Arbor vitae cerebelli

Anterior spino-cerebellar tract

Middle cerebellar peduncle

Trigeminal nerve

Vestibulocochlear nerve

Facial nerve

Central tegmental tract

Olive

Fig. 29.2 Dissection of cerebellar peduncles. (From: Schuenke M, Schulte E, Schumacher U. THIEME Atlas of Anatomy. Head, Neck, and Neuroanatomy. Illustrations by Voll M and Wesker K. © Thieme 2020.)

C. Dissection of intracerebellar nuclei.

To dissect the nuclei of the cerebellar hemisphere, with the help of a scalpel you should carefully scrape out the cerebellar tissue along the course of the superior cerebellar peduncle toward the cerebellum. You should gradually scrape off the cerebellar tissue deeper and deeper till the dentate nucleus is visualized. This nucleus is a crumpled bag of gray matter buried in the mass of white matter, close to the midline. The other cerebellar nuclei (fastigial, globose, and emboliform) are too small and difficult to visualize. These nuclei lie anteromedial to the dentate nucleus (**Fig. 29.3**).

D. Exposure of inferior medullary velum, median aperture of fourth ventricle and choroid plexus.

On the inferior surface of the cerebellum, on one side, gently detach the tonsil out of its bed. This will expose the thin inferior medullar velum, which forms the roof of the inferior part of the fourth ventricle. Near the midline, identify the median aperture of the fourth ventricle and note the presence of the choroid plexus on the ventricular surface of the inferior medullary velum. This plexus runs from the median aperture toward the lateral recess of the fourth ventricle.

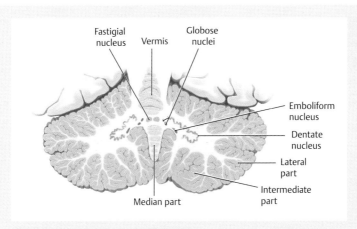

Fig. 29.3 Nuclei of the cerebellum. (From: Schuenke M, Schulte E, Schumacher U. THIEME Atlas of Anatomy. Head, Neck, and Neuroanatomy. Illustrations by Voll M and Wesker K. © Thieme 2020.)

External Features of the Cerebellum

The cerebellum consists of right and left cerebellar hemispheres connected with each other in the midline with the vermis (refer to **Fig. 29.1**). Each cerebellar hemisphere presents a superior and an inferior surface.

The superior surface of the right and left cerebellar hemispheres is flattened and presents a superior vermis in the midline. The inferior surface of the cerebellum is convex and presents a deep depression between the right and left cerebellar hemispheres. This depression is known as the vallecula. In the floor of this vallecula lies the inferior vermis.

The horizontal fissure is present at the junction of superior and inferior surfaces. The primary fissure is present on superior surface (**Fig. 29.1a**), while posterolateral fissure is present on inferior surface behind flocculonodular lobe (**Fig. 29.1c**). Cerebellum is divided into anterior, middle (posterior), and flocculonodular lobes with the help of the primary fissure and posterolateral fissure (**Fig. 29.4**). The posterior (middle) lobe extends on both the superior and inferior surfaces and, therefore, is the largest lobe of the hemisphere.

Location of Lobes of Cerebellum

Anterior lobe of cerebellum—It is located on superior surface anterior to primary fissure.

Middle or Posterior lobe of cerebellum—It is a large lobe which extends on both, superior and inferior, surfaces of cerebellar hemisphere. It is present between primary fissure and posterolateral fissure.

Flocculonodular lobe—It is located on the inferior surface in front of posterolateral fissure. It is the smallest lobe of cerebellum.

The surface of the cerebellum is covered by gray matter called the cerebellar cortex. The gray matter of the cerebellar cortex is arranged in a series of parallel ridges known as folia. Deep to the cerebellar cortex lies the white matter.

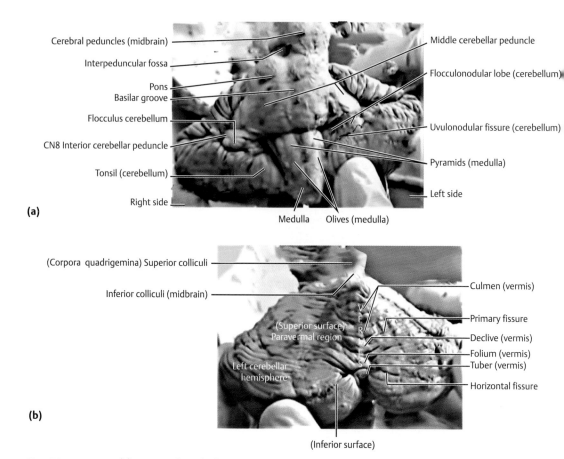

Fig. 29.4   External features of cerebellum: **(a)** anterior and **(b)** posterior views.

The cerebellum is connected to the midbrain, pons, and medulla through the superior, middle, and inferior cerebellar peduncles, respectively. Afferent and efferent fibers enter and leave the cerebellum through these peduncles.

The parts of the cerebellum can also be distinguished according to their phylogenetic development, i.e., archicerebellum, paleocerebellum, and neocerebellum. Flocculonodular lobe is considered to be the oldest in phylogenetic development and thus called "archicerebellum." The anterior lobe of cerebellum and parts of vermis are called paleocerebellum, while lateral portion of posterior lobe is called "neocerebellum."

Internal Structure of the Cerebellum

Cerebellar cortex and white matter of the cerebellum: A midsagittal section of the cerebellar hemisphere shows the central core of the white matter and superficially folded gray matter of the cortex. The white matter shows the tree-like complex branching on which the gray matter of the cortex is applied. This arrangement is called the *arbor vitae cerebelli* (refer to **Fig. 29.2**). The histological structure of the cortex is uniform throughout the cerebellum. The cortex consists of three layers, that is, the molecular layer, Purkinje layer, and granular layer (**Figs. 29.5** and **29.6a**). *Cerebellar nuclei*: These are present in the central mass of the white matter close to the midline, in each cerebellar hemisphere. Four cerebellar nuclei (*fastigial, globose, emboliform,* and *dentate*) are present in the central core of the white matter of each hemisphere (refer to **Figs. 29.3** and **29.6b**).

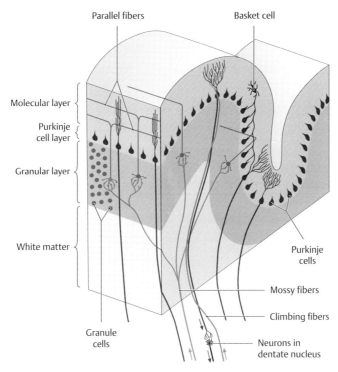

Fig. 29.5 Internal structure of the cerebellum. (From: Schuenke M, Schulte E, Schumacher U. THIEME Atlas of Anatomy. Head, Neck, and Neuroanatomy. Illustrations by Voll M and Wesker K. © Thieme 2020.)

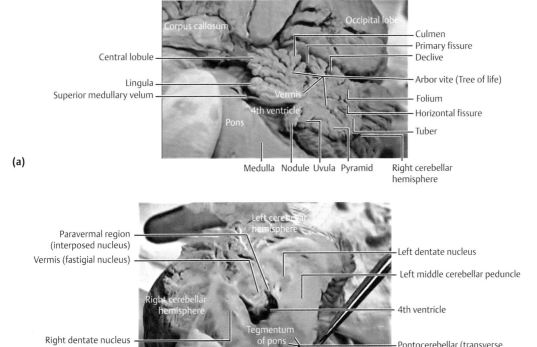

Fig. 29.6 Sections of cerebellum: **(a)** sagittal and **(b)** axial.

■ Clinical Notes

Lesion of the cerebellum may occur due to degeneration, trauma, tumor, and vascular causes.

1. *The lesion of the vermis (paleocerebellar syndrome)*: It may lead to ataxia, cerebellar nystagmus, and speech disorders.

2. *The lesion of the flocculonodular lobe (archicerebellar syndrome)*: It may lead to cerebral ataxia, vertigo, and vomiting.

3. *The lesion of the lateral part of cerebellar hemisphere (neocerebellar syndrome)*: This results due to lesion in the lateral part of the cerebellar hemisphere. The syndrome is characterized by ataxia, negative finger–nose test, intentional tremor, asynergy, nystagmus, and hypotonia.

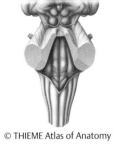
Introduction

The fourth ventricle is situated in the hindbrain. It is located between the lower pons and upper part of the medulla anteriorly and the cerebellum posteriorly. The fourth ventricle communicates above with the third ventricle through the cerebral aqueduct of the midbrain, below with the central canal of the lower medulla and spinal cord. The cavity communicates posteriorly with the cerebellomedullary cistern (subarachnoid space).

The floor of the fourth ventricle is formed by the dorsal aspect of the pons and the upper medulla. The roof of the ventricle is formed by the superior and inferior medullary vela. The cavity of the fourth ventricle is lined by the ependyma and contains the choroid plexuses. The cavity is filled with cerebrospinal fluid (CSF) (**Figs. 30.1** and **30.2**).

Surface Landmarks

1. Gently pull the superior surface of the cerebellum downward to see the superior medullary velum extending between the two superior cerebellar peduncles (**Fig. 30.1**).

2. Similarly, lift the inferior surface of the cerebellum along with the flocculus to see the median aperture and right and left lateral apertures. See the choroid plexus protruding through the opening of these apertures.

Dissection and Identification (Video 30.1)

A. Dissection to expose the floor of fourth ventricle.

1. We have already given a midline incision in the cerebellum to divide it into two separate hemispheres.

2. This cut passes through the roof of the fourth ventricle and extends below to the median aperture.

3. Remove the cerebellar hemisphere of one side by cutting through its cerebellar peduncles. This will expose half of the floor of the fourth ventricle (**Fig. 30.3**).

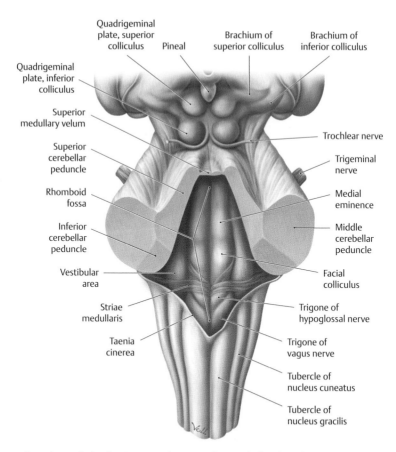

Fig. 30.1   Posterior view of the brainstem showing floor of the fourth ventricle. (From: Schuenke M, Schulte E, Schumacher U. THIEME Atlas of Anatomy. Head, Neck, and Neuroanatomy. Illustrations by Voll M and Wesker K. © Thieme 2020.)

B. Dissection to expose the roof of fourth ventricle and its choroid plexus.

1. On the attached hemisphere, in the midsagittal section, look for the roof (superior medullary velum, cerebellar recess, and inferior medullary velum) (**Fig. 30.2**). Note the extent of the lateral recess by passing the tip of a seeker along the lateral recess toward the lateral aperture.

2. Observe the choroid plexus on the ventricular surface of the inferior medullary velum. Trace the choroid plexus from the median aperture to the lateral recess. Gently reflect the inferior medullary velum downward to expose this choroid plexus.

3. Now remove the cerebellar hemisphere of the other side also by cutting through the cerebellar peduncles. This will expose the complete floor of the fourth ventricle.

4. Examine the floor of the fourth ventricle.

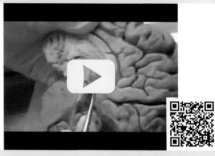

Video 30.1   Ventricles of brain.

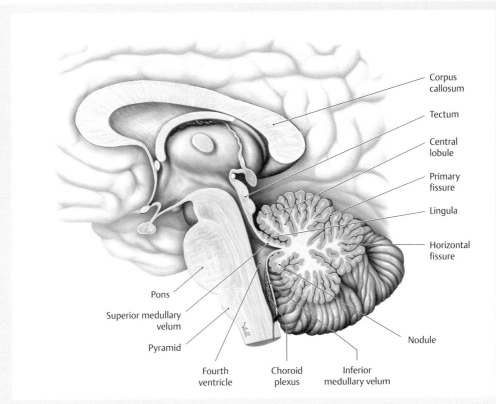

Fig. 30.2 Midsagittal section through diencephalon, brainstem, and cerebellum viewed from the left side, displaying the internal structure of the fourth ventricle and cerebellum. (From: Schuenke M, Schulte E, Schumacher U. THIEME Atlas of Anatomy. Head, Neck, and Neuroanatomy. Illustrations by Voll M and Wesker K. © Thieme 2020.)

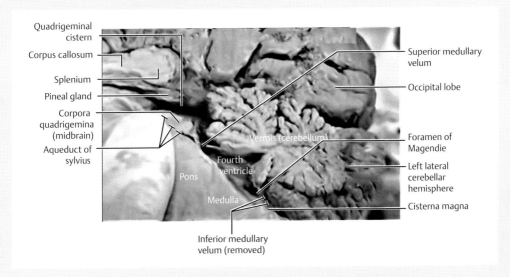

Fig. 30.3 Fourth ventricle as seen in midsagittal section of brain.

Features of the Fourth Ventricle

The cavity of the fourth ventricle is better appreciated in the midsagittal section of the brain (refer to **Fig. 30.2**). The cavity of the fourth ventricle is present in the hindbrain between the lower pons and upper medulla. The fourth ventricle consists of a floor, roof, and lateral boundaries. Fourth ventricle communicates with subarachnoid space through two openings in the roof, i.e., **foramen of Magendie** and **foramen of Luschka**.

Roof of the fourth ventricle: The roof is formed by the superior and inferior medullary vela. The roof is covered by the ependyma.

Above the cerebellar recess, it is formed by the thin superior medullary velum with the lingula of the cerebellum. The superior medullary velum extends between two superior cerebellar peduncles. Cerebellar recess is **median dorsal recess** which extends toward the cerebellum in midline. It is located between superior and inferior medullary vela.

Below the cerebellar recess, roof is formed by the inferior medullary velum, which extends in the midline up to the **median aperture** (foramen of Magendie). Laterally, the inferior medullary velum forms the bed of the tonsil and extends laterally till the posterior surface of the inferior cerebellar peduncle (where the **lateral recess** is located). The lateral recess of the fourth ventricle, on either side, is located between the inferior cerebellar peduncle and the flocculus of cerebellum. Through this recess fourth ventricle communicates with subarachnoid space (through foramen of Luschka).

The choroid plexuses of the fourth ventricle extend between the margins of the median aperture to the lateral aperture (through the lateral recess). Thus, CSF of fourth ventricle comes to subarachnoid space and cerebellomedullary cistern through median aperture and foramen of Luschka.

Floor of the fourth ventricle: The floor is diamond shaped and covered by the ependyma (refer to **Fig. 30.1**). It is formed by the posterior surface of the pons and upper half of the medulla oblongata. At the junction of the pons and medulla, the transversely running fibers, striae medullaris, are located. Thus, the upper part of the floor (above the striae medullaris) is the pontine part and the lower part is the medullary part. Superiorly, the floor extends up to the cerebral aqueduct and inferiorly up to the central canal.

The floor is divided into right and left halves by a median sulcus. On each side of the median sulcus, a longitudinal elevation is seen. This is known as the medial eminence. Near the lower end of the pons this shows a swelling called the facial colliculus, deep to which lies the abducens nerve nucleus. The sulcus limitans is a groove situated lateral to the medial eminence. The vestibular area is seen lateral to the sulcus limitans.

In the medullary part of the floor, two triangles, that is, the hypoglossal and vagal triangles are seen. The taenia is a white ridge along the inferolateral margin of the floor.

Lateral boundaries: On each side, the fourth ventricle is bounded by the superior cerebellar peduncles above and by the inferior cerebellar peduncles and cuneate and gracile tubercles below.

▮ Clinical Note

The circulation of CSF through the fourth ventricle may be blocked due to the presence of a tumor in the fourth ventricle. This may lead to the production of internal hydrocephalus resulting in dilation of the third and lateral ventricles.

Cerebrum: External Features

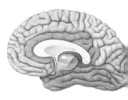

© THIEME Atlas of Anatomy

Introduction

The forebrain consists of the *cerebrum* and *diencephalon* (thalamus, hypothalamus). The cerebrum is the major part of the brain. It consists of the right and left *cerebral hemispheres*, which are partially separated from each other, in the midline, by the *longitudinal fissure* (**Fig. 31.1**). The longitudinal fissure contains the *falx cerebri* which is the fold of the dura mater and separates the right and left cerebral hemispheres. The surface of each cerebral hemisphere is covered by the gray matter (*cerebral cortex*), which is thrown into folds, that is, the *sulci* and *gyri*.

Deep to the cerebral cortex, the central core of each cerebral hemisphere is formed by the white matter. The white matter of the cerebral hemisphere contains collections of gray matter, that is, *caudate* and *lentiform* nuclei. Cerebrum encloses right and left *lateral ventricles* and *third ventricle*.

Surface Landmarks

1. With the help of a dry skull, review the relation between the brain and cranial cavities of the skull (refer to **Fig. 1.7**).

2. Also, review the relation of various parts of the brain with the falx cerebri and tentorium cerebelli.

3. See the relation of the frontal, temporal, and occipital poles of the cerebrum with the skull bones.

4. Review the position of the longitudinal fissure, central sulcus, stem of the lateral sulcus, and its posterior ramus in relation to the skull.

Dissection and Identification

A. Dissection of midsagittal section of brain to get right and left cerebral hemispheres.

1. We have already removed the meninges and blood vessels from the surface of the cerebrum. The surfaces of the cerebral hemispheres are now clearly seen. The cortex is covered with the pia mater.

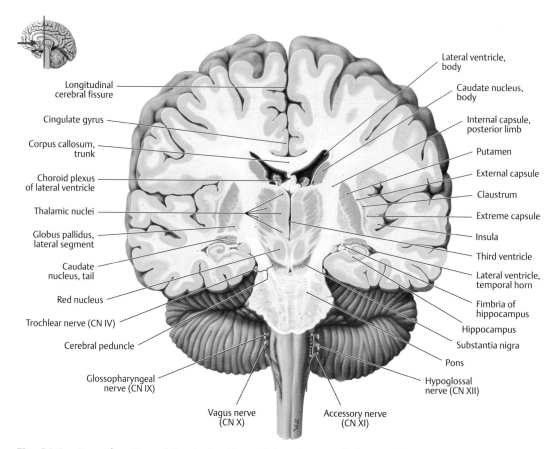

Fig. 31.1 Coronal section of the brain. (From: Schuenke M, Schulte E, Schumacher U. THIEME Atlas of Anatomy. Head, Neck, and Neuroanatomy. Illustrations by Voll M and Wesker K. © Thieme 2020.)

2. Give a transverse cut in the midbrain above the level of the superior colliculi. Thus, the midbrain and hindbrain are now separated from the forebrain (cerebrum and diencephalon).

3. Gently separate the two cerebral hemispheres at the longitudinal fissure so that at the bottom of this fissure, the upper surface of the corpus callosum becomes visible.

4. With the help of a brain knife, divide the corpus callosum exactly in the median plane. Continue the division of the corpus callosum till both the right and left hemispheres are completely separated (**Fig. 31.2a**).

B. Identification of structures seen on midsagittal section of brain.

1. Now the medial surface of each cerebral hemisphere is completely visible. Note the parts of the corpus callosum, fornix, and septum pellucidum (refer to **Fig. 31.2b**). Also, note the choroid plexuses.

2. On the medial surface, identify the thalamus and hypothalamus separated from each other by the subthalamic sulcus. This surface of the thalamus and hypothalamus forms the lateral wall of the third ventricle (**Fig. 31.2 a and b**).

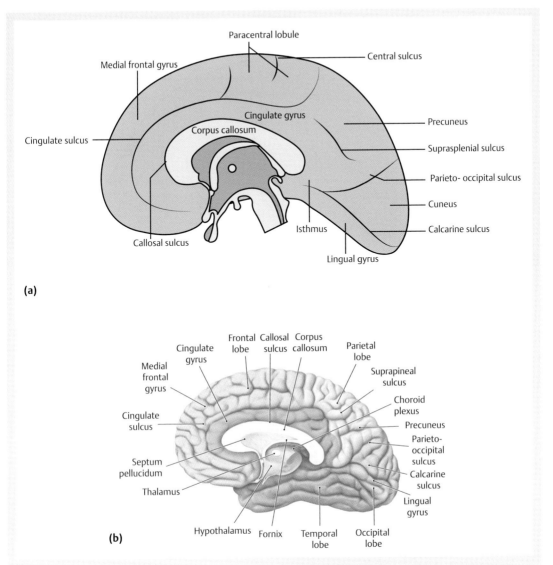

Fig. 31.2 **(a)** Schematic diagram showing sulci and gyri on medial surface of right cerebral hemisphere. **(b)** Sulci and gyri on the medial surface of the right cerebral hemisphere. (Figure b: From: Schuenke M, Schulte E, Schumacher U. THIEME Atlas of Anatomy. Head, Neck, and Neuroanatomy. Illustrations by Voll M and Wesker K. © Thieme 2020.)

C. Identification of structures seen on superolateral, medial, and inferior surfaces of cerebral hemisphere (Videos 31.1 and 31.2).

1. Now examine the sulci and gyri of the superolateral surface (**Fig. 31.3**), medial surface, and inferior surface of the cerebral hemisphere.

2. On the medial surface, gently pull the parahippocampal gyrus laterally to find the dentate gyrus, hippocampal gyrus, and the fimbria (**Figs. 31.4** and **31.5**).

3. To see the presence of stria in the visual cortex, cut a slice through the calcarine sulcus. The white stria of Gennari runs through the substance of the cortex parallel to its surface.

4. To examine the insula (the hidden cortex on the superolateral surface), pull the parietal and temporal operculum (**Fig. 31.6**).

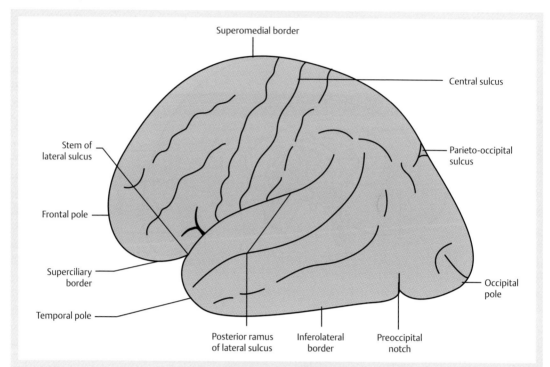

Fig. 31.3 Schematic diagram showing poles, border, and sulci and gyri on the superolateral surface of left cerebral hemisphere.

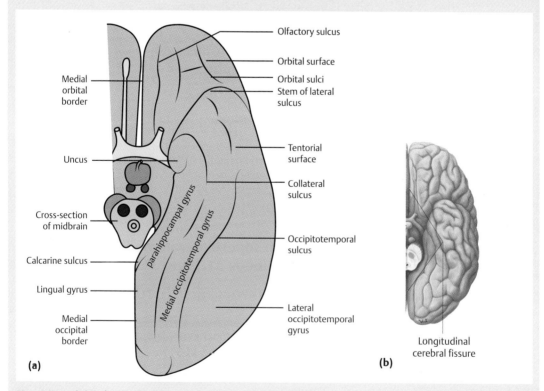

Fig. 31.4 **(a)** Schematic diagram showing borders and sulci and gyri on the inferior surface of left cerebral hemisphere. **(b)** Sulci and gyri on the inferior surface of left cerebral hemisphere. (Figure b: From: Schuenke M, Schulte E, Schumacher U. THIEME Atlas of Anatomy. Head, Neck, and Neuroanatomy. Illustrations by Voll M and Wesker K. © Thieme 2020.)

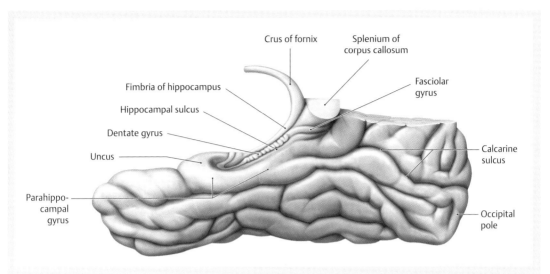

Fig. 31.5 Dissection to show hidden parts deep to uncus and parahippocampal gyrus. (From: Schuenke M, Schulte E, Schumacher U. THIEME Atlas of Anatomy. Head, Neck, and Neuroanatomy. Illustrations by Voll M and Wesker K. © Thieme 2020.)

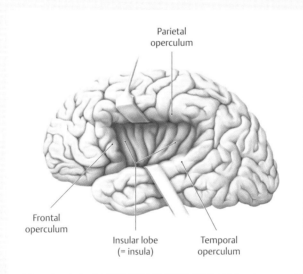

Fig. 31.6 Exposure of insula (lateral view of the left hemisphere). (From: Schuenke M, Schulte E, Schumacher U. THIEME Atlas of Anatomy. Head, Neck, and Neuroanatomy. Illustrations by Voll M and Wesker K. © Thieme 2020.)

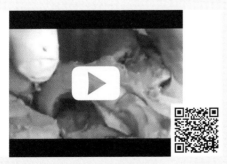

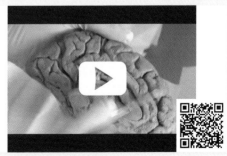

Video 31.1   Hippocampus and fornix.   **Video 31.2**   Papez circuit.

External Features of the Cerebrum

The cerebrum consists of two cerebral hemispheres, which are separated from each other by a longitudinal fissure (**Fig. 31.1**). The longitudinal fissure is situated in the median plane and contains the falx cerebri, arachnoid mater, arteries, and veins.

Poles, Surfaces, and Borders

Each cerebral hemisphere consists of three borders (superomedial, inferomedial, and inferolateral), three poles (frontal, temporal, and occipital), and three surfaces (superolateral, medial, and inferior; refer **Figs. 31.2–31.4**).

1. The location of the frontal, temporal, and occipital poles can be seen with the help of **Figs. 31.2** and **31.3**.

2. The superomedial border is the upper border which extends between the frontal and occipital poles.

3. The inferomedial border is divided into the *medial orbital* and *medial occipital* borders (**Fig. 31.4a**).

4. The inferolateral border extends between the temporal and occipital poles.

5. The superolateral surface is large and lies between the superomedial and inferolateral borders (refer to **Fig. 31.3**).

6. The medial surface lies between the superomedial and inferomedial borders and is only seen after the midsagittal section of the brain (refer to **Fig. 31.2**).

7. The inferior surface lies between the inferomedial and inferolateral borders and is divided into the orbital and tentorial surfaces by the stem of the lateral sulcus (**Fig. 31.4**).

Important Sulci on the Superolateral Surface and Lobes of the Cerebral Hemisphere

These sulci are used to divide the cerebral hemisphere into various lobes. These are the central sulcus, posterior ramus of the lateral sulcus, parietooccipital sulcus, and preoccipital notch. These sulci divide the cerebral hemisphere into frontal, parietal, temporal, and occipital lobes (**Figs. 31.2** and **31.3**). These lobes are named after the bones of the skull covering them, for example, the parietal bone covering the parietal lobe and the frontal bone covering the frontal lobe, etc.

Important Sulci and Gyri of the Cerebral Hemisphere

A brief account of a few important sulci and gyri, found on the surfaces of the cerebral hemisphere, is given here. Students should refer to a textbook for details of these sulci and gyri.

Superolateral surface: There is a presence of a precentral sulcus, which runs parallel to the central sulcus (refer to **Fig. 31.3**). The precentral gyrus is located between the central and precentral sulci. The precentral gyrus is a primary motor area. Note the presence of the superior and inferior frontal sulci and superior, middle, and inferior frontal gyri.

The parietal lobe shows the presence of the postcentral sulcus, which runs parallel to the central sulcus. Between these two sulci is the postcentral gyrus. It is a somatic sensory area of the cortex. The other sulcus is the interparietal sulcus, which is placed between the superior and inferior parietal lobules.

The temporal lobe consists of two sulci, that is, the *superior* and *inferior temporal sulci*, which separate the *superior, middle,* and *inferior temporal gyri*. The insular lobe is a hidden part of the cerebral cortex. The insula is a hidden cortex between the parietal and temporal lobes. This can be seen by pulling the parietal and temporal operculum away from each other (refer to **Fig. 31.6**).

The occipital lobe contains the terminal end of the *calcarine sulcus* and *lunate sulcus*.

Medial surface: The medial surface shows the following major sulci: *callosal, cingulate, parieto-occipital*, and *calcarine* (refer to **Fig. 31.2**). Following are the major gyri: *medial frontal, cingulated, precuneus*, and *cuneus*.

In the midsagittal section of the cerebrum, observe the parts of the corpus callosum (genu, trunk, and splenium) below the callosal sulcus. Also, note the presence of the fornix and septum pellucidum.

Inferior surface: The *orbital surface* shows the olfactory sulcus and orbital sulci. The gyri on this surface are gyrus rectus and four orbital gyri (**Fig. 31.4a**). The orbital surface shows the olfactory bulb and tract. The olfactory tract splits into the medial and lateral stria posteriorly, enclosing the anterior perforated substance. The *tentorial surface* presents the collateral and occipitotemporal sulci and medial occipitotemporal, lateral occipitotemporal, and parahippocampal gyri. The parahippocampal gyrus ends in the *uncus*.

Limbic Lobe and Hippocampus

The limbic system consists of the cortical and subcortical structures. The cortical structures include the limbic lobe and hippocampal formation. The limbic lobe consists of the subcallosal gyrus, cingulate gyrus, parahippocampus, and uncus. Hippocampus formation consists of the hippocampus, dentate gyrus, gyrus fasciolaris, indusium griseum, and longitudinal striae (refer to **Figs. 31.5** and **31.7**). Functionally, the limbic system is concerned with emotions and recent memory.

Functional Areas of the Cerebral Cortex

Functionally, the cerebral cortex consists of three different types of areas, that is, sensory, motor, and association. The sensory cortex receives and interprets the sensory impulses; the motor cortex is concerned with the initiation of movements, while the association cortex is concerned

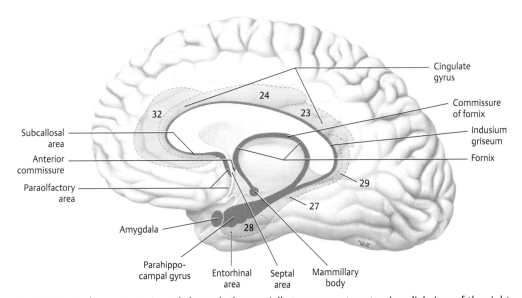

Fig. 31.7 Limbic system viewed through the partially transparent cortex (medial view of the right hemisphere). (From: Schuenke M, Schulte E, Schumacher U. THIEME Atlas of Anatomy. Head, Neck, and Neuroanatomy. Illustrations by Voll M and Wesker K. © Thieme 2020.)

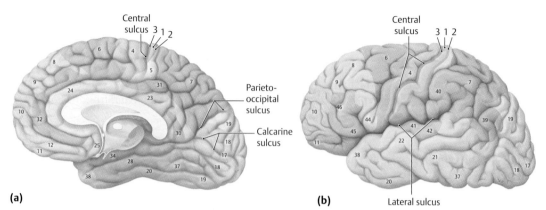

Fig. 31.8 Functional area of the cerebral cortex: **(a)** Midsagittal section of the right cerebral hemisphere (viewed from the left side). **(b)** Lateral view of the left cerebral hemisphere. (From: Schuenke M, Schulte E, Schumacher U. THIEME Atlas of Anatomy. Head, Neck, and Neuroanatomy. Illustrations by Voll M and Wesker K. © Thieme 2020.)

with functions such as intelligence, memory, emotions, personality, judgment, and reasoning. Brodmann in the early 20th century developed the brain map (by giving numbers 1–47 to the cortical areas) based on the cellular architecture of the cerebral cortex. This map reflects the functional organization of the cortex (**Fig. 31.8a** and **b**).

1. Primary motor area: Precentral gyrus (area 4) is concerned with the contraction of the skeletal muscles.

2. Primary somatic sensory area: Postcentral gyrus (areas 3, 1, 2) is concerned with the reception and interpretation of the sensory impulses.

3. Sensory speech area of Wernicke: The sensory speech area (area 22) is located in the posterior part of the superior temporal gyrus.

4. Motor speech area: It is located in the inferior frontal gyrus (areas 44, 45).

5. Primary visual area: It is situated on either side of the calcarine sulcus (area 17).

6. Primary auditory area: It is located on the superior surface of the superior temporal gyrus (areas 41 and 42).

Functional Imaging of Brain

Functional imaging includes EEG, PET scanning, functional MRI, and MR spectroscopy. Most of these kinds of imaging of brain are useful in identifying the increased or decreased metabolic activities of particular part of brain. Thus, we may assess the normal function of particular parts of brain including brain tumour or brain diseases.

Electroencephalography (EEG): The electrical activity of brain can be recorded by this procedure.

PET (Positron Emission Tomography) scanning: In this procedure radioactively labelled, metabolically active chemicals are injected into blood stream. Sensors in the PET scanner detects the radioactivity as the compound accumulates in various regions of brain (**Fig. 31.9**).

fMRI (functional MRI): This procedure measures signal changes in the brain which are due to changes in neuronal activities (**Fig. 31.10**).

Magnetic Resonance Spectroscopy (MRS): It is used to measure the levels of different metabolites in body tissues. This technique is used to diagnose brain tumour, stroke, seizure disorders, Alzheimer's disease, depression, Parkinson's disease etc.

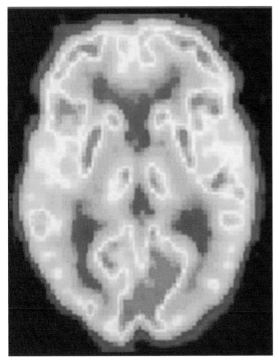

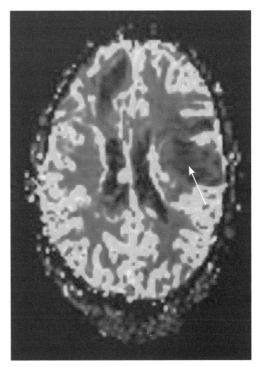

Fig. 31.9 Positron Emission Tomography (PET) scan of brain. Note that there is higher concentration of radioactive chemicals in cortex (red area is of gray matter) and low in white matter (green areas). The brain on color map shows metabolic activity in increasing order as black < dark blue < green < yellow < red < pink < white. (Reproduced with permission from Pal GP, Illustrated Textbook of Neuroanatomy, Wolters Kluwer, 2013) (Courtesy of Dr. Jay Kumar Rai, Head Nuclear Medicine, SAIMS, Indore).

Fig. 31.10 Functional Magnetic Resonance Imaging (fMRI) of brain. The arrow indicates the tissue in brain showing decreased neuronal activity due to presence of tumor. (Reproduced with permission from Pal GP, Illustrated Textbook of Neuroanatomy, Wolters Kluwer, 2013) (Courtesy of Dr. Sangeet Choudhary, Chief Radiologist, SRL Diagnostic, Indore).

▌Clinical Notes

1. In the precentral gyrus (primary motor area) and postcentral gyrus (primary sensory area), the body is represented upside down. Hence, the area of lesions of these gyri is diagnosed accordingly.

2. The motor speech area is always located in the dominant cerebral hemisphere, that is, in the left cerebral hemisphere in right-handed persons.

3. Similarly, the sensory speech area is also located in the dominant cerebral hemisphere.

Structures Seen on the Midsagittal Section of the Forebrain

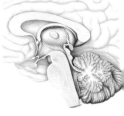

© THIEME Atlas of Anatomy

At the end of the observation of the midsagittal section of the forebrain, you should be able to identify and understand the following:

- Parts of the corpus callosum.
- Location of the fornix, anterior commissure, and interventricular foramen.
- Septum pellucidum.
- Posterior commissure, pineal gland, and pineal recess.
- Medial surface of the thalamus and hypothalamus separated from each other by the hypothalamic sulcus.
- Walls of the third ventricle.

Introduction

Most parts of the thalamus and hypothalamus are hidden deep inside the cerebral hemispheres. Similarly, the cavities of the ventricles are located deep in the brain. The bundles of white matter, such as the corpus callosum, fornix, and others, are also located within the cerebral hemispheres. All these structures may be visualized in the midsagittal section of the brain. Hence, the study of the midsagittal section of the brain is very useful to learn the gross anatomy of the brain.

Dissection and Identification

Identification of structures seen at midsagittal section of brain.

1. Observe the parts of the corpus callosum on the midsagittal section of the brain (**Fig. 32.1**).

2. Trace the bundle of the white fibers in the fornix between the anterior commissure and splenium.

3. Pass a bristle at the anterior end of the fornix in the interventricular foramen to appreciate the communication between the lateral and third ventricles.

4. Observe the septum pellucidum extending between the corpus callosum and fornix. You may cut and remove the septum to expose the central part of the lateral ventricle.

5. Observe the pineal recess and anterior and posterior commissures.

6. Locate the interthalamic adhesion. Identify the subthalamic sulcus, which extends between the interventricular foramen and cerebral aqueduct.

7. Identify the structures forming the walls, roof, and floor of the third ventricle.

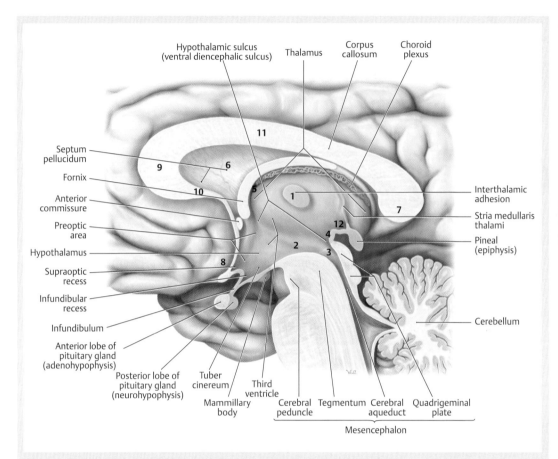

Fig. 32.1 Midsagittal section of the brain viewed from the left side. 1, Interthalamic adhesions; 2, subthalamic sulcus; 3, cerebral aqueduct; 4, posterior commissure; 5, interventricular foramen; 6, septum pellucidum; 7, splenium; 8, lamina terminalis; 9, Genu of corpus callosum; 10, Rostrum of corpus callosum; 11, trunk of corpus callosum and 12, Habenular commissure. (From: Schuenke M, Schulte E, Schumacher U. THIEME Atlas of Anatomy. Head, Neck, and Neuroanatomy. Illustrations by Voll M and Wesker K. © Thieme 2020.)

Structures Seen on the Midsagittal Section

We have already divided the forebrain at the midsagittal (median) plane. Now the medial surface of the right and left halves of the bisected brain is available for study. Note the following structures carefully.

Corpus Callosum

In the midsagittal section, the corpus callosum is seen as a C-shaped mass of white matter. It has four parts—rostrum, genu, trunk, and splenium **(Fig. 32.1)**. The fibers of the corpus callosum interconnect the cortical areas of one cerebral hemisphere with the corresponding cortical areas of the opposite cerebral hemisphere. Thus, the fibers of the corpus callosum are classified as the commissural fibers.

Fornix

Fornix is a bundle of white fibers which in the midsagittal section extends between the anterior commissure and the splenium **(Fig. 32.1)**. It is a paired structure, but the right and left fornix are fused beneath the trunk of the corpus callosum. The fused part of the fornix is called the body of the fornix. It lies above the medial margin of the superior surface of the thalamus from which it is separated by the tela choroidea and ependymal roof of the third ventricle. The body of the fornix is suspended from the corpus callosum by the septum pellucidum. Posterior to the anterior part of the fornix is the presence of the small interventricular foramen. Fornix consists of efferent fibers from the hippocampus.

Septum Pellucidum

The septum pellucidum is a thin vertical partition, which separates the right and left lateral ventricles from each other. Thus, it forms the medial wall of the lateral ventricle. It extends between the fornix and corpus callosum. It consists of two parallel laminae that may be separated from each other by the cavity of the septum pellucidum.

Anterior Commissure

Anterior commissure is a bundle of white fibers located anterior to the column of the fornix. The commissural fibers cross the midline to connect the anterior perforated substance and parts of the temporal lobes of the two cerebral hemispheres.

Posterior Commissure

Posterior commissure is present in the lower stalk of the pineal gland. It connects the nucleus of the posterior commissure, nucleus of the Cajal, and nucleus of the Darkschewitsch of right and left sides.

Habenular Commissure

The habenular commissure consists of white fibers, which connect the habenular nuclei of the two sides. It is located in the upper stalk of the pineal gland.

Pineal Gland

In the midsagittal section of the brain, the pineal gland is located inferior to the corpus callosum. The gland is attached to the brain by a pineal stalk. The third ventricle extends into the stalk as pineal recess. The pineal gland acts as an endocrine gland, which produces melatonin.

Thalamus

In the midsagittal section of the brain, only the medial surface of the thalamus is visible. The medial surface of the thalamus is lined by the ependyma and forms the upper part of the third ventricle, which lies above the hypothalamic sulcus. The hypothalamic sulcus extends from the interventricular foramen to the upper end of the cerebral aqueduct. The right and left thalami may be interconnected in midline by a band of gray matter known as the *interthalamic adhesion*. The thalamus is the principal relay station of the sensory impulses.

Hypothalamus

The hypothalamus is present in the lateral wall and floor of the third ventricle. It lies below the thalamus. The thalamus and hypothalamus, on the medial surface, are separated from each other by the hypothalamic sulcus. Some parts of the hypothalamus can be seen in the interpeduncular fossa, which also forms the floor of the third ventricle.

Third Ventricle

The third ventricle is a narrow space situated in the midline between two diencephalons (between two thalami and hypothalami). The cavity of the third ventricle has two lateral walls formed by the thalamus and hypothalamus (**Fig. 36.5**). It also consists of an anterior wall, a posterior wall, a roof, and a floor (**Fig. 32.1**). The anterior wall is formed by the anterior commissure and lamina terminalis. The floor is formed by the structures present in the interpeduncular fossa. Floor, from anterior to posterior, consists of supraoptic recess, infundibulum (infundibular recess), tuber cinereum, and area of mamillary body. The roof is formed by the ependyma stretching between two thalami. The posterior wall is formed by the suprapineal recess, habenular commissure, pineal recess, and posterior commissure.

The cavity of the third ventricle communicates with the right and left lateral ventricles through the interventricular foramen. Below, it also communicates with the fourth ventricle through the cerebral aqueduct.

Circumventricular Organs

There are certain areas located close to midline ventricles (in relation to third and fourth ventricles) and show the deficiency of blood brain barrier (BBB). These areas are known as circumventricular organs which serve very important functions. These areas are as under:

1. The median eminence

2. The organum vasculosum of lamina terminalis (OVLT)

3. The subfornical organ (below the fornix)

4. The pineal gland

5. The sub-commissural organ (below posterior commissure)

All the above circumventricular organs are related to third ventricle.

The area postrema. It is related to fourth ventricle.

All these circumventricular organs are demonstrated nicely on midsagittal section of brain (with the commentary on their functions) in **Video 32.1**.

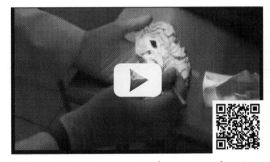

Video 32.1 Circumventricular organs, location, cytoarchitecture description.

▌Clinical Notes

1. Obstruction in the circulation of cerebrospinal fluid (CSF) at the level of the third ventricle leads to the accumulation of CSF in the lateral ventricles. This results in *hydrocephalus* in infants and *raised intracranial pressure* in adults.

2. The obstruction or dilatation of the ventricles can be visualized by the procedure called *ventriculography*.

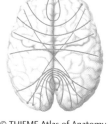
Learning Objectives

At the end of the dissection of the white matter of the cerebrum, you should be able to identify and understand the following:

- Fibers of the cingulum, longitudinal bundles, and uncinate fasciculus in a dissected cerebrum.
- In a midsagittal section of the cerebrum, identify the parts of the corpus callosum, and in the dissected lobe, identify and understand the significance of forceps minor, forceps major, and tapetum.
- In the dissected cerebrum, locate the corona radiata.
- In a horizontal section of the cerebrum, identify the parts of the internal capsule.
- See the continuity of the corona radiata with the crus cerebri after removal of the lentiform nucleus.

Introduction

The bundles of nerve fibers (axons) of the cerebrum are known as the white matter. Each cerebral hemisphere consists of an enormous mass of white matter which lies deep to the cerebral cortex. These fibers connect various parts of the brain with each other.

1. Fibers connecting the parts of the cortex of the same cerebral hemisphere with each other are called *association fibers*. These may be *short association fibers* (which pass from one part of the gyrus to another part of the same or neighboring gyrus) or *long association fibers* (which pass from one lobe to the other). Examples of long association fibers are *cingulum, superior longitudinal bundle, inferior longitudinal bundle, uncinate fasciculus,* etc. (**Fig. 33.1**).

2. The parts of the right and left cerebral hemispheres are connected by fibers which cross the midline. These fibers are known as *commissural fibers*. Examples of important commissural fibers are *corpus callosum* (**Fig. 33.2**), *anterior commissure, posterior commissure, fornix,* etc.

3. Fibers which connect the cerebral cortex with other parts of the central nervous system (brain and spinal cord) are called *projection fibers*. Examples of projection fibers are ascending and descending bundles of white fibers passing through the *corona radiata* and *internal capsule* (**Fig. 33.3**).

Dissection and Identification

A. Dissection of the cingulum association fibers.

We shall dissect the medial surface of the cerebral hemisphere to expose the cingulum association fibers:

1. The cingulum bundle lies deep to the gyrus cinguli. With the handle of a knife, scrape away the gray matter of the gyrus cinguli and parahippocampal gyrus. This will expose the cingulum bundle, which lies just above the corpus callosum.

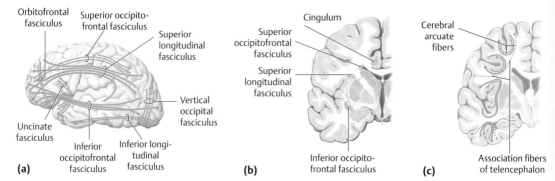

Fig. 33.1 Association fibers. **(a)** Lateral view of the left cerebral hemisphere. **(b)** Coronal section of the right cerebral hemisphere showing long association fibers. **(c)** Coronal section of the right cerebral hemisphere showing short association fibers. (Reproduced From: Schuenke M, Schulte E, Schumacher U. THIEME Atlas of Anatomy. Head, Neck, and Neuroanatomy. Illustrations by Voll M and Wesker K. © Thieme 2020.)

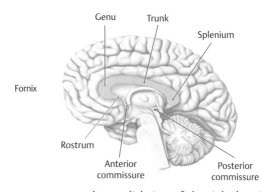

Fig. 33.2 Corpus callosum as seen on the medial view of the right hemisphere. Notice the parts of the corpus callosum, that is, rostrum, genu, trunk, and splenium. (From: Schuenke M, Schulte E, Schumacher U. THIEME Atlas of Anatomy. Head, Neck, and Neuroanatomy. Illustrations by Voll M and Wesker K. © Thieme 2020.)

2. Trace this bundle anteriorly up to the anterior perforated substance.

3. Trace the bundle posteriorly, where it goes around the splenium of the corpus callosum.

4. Trace this bundle further forward in the parahippocampal gyrus till the uncus.

B. Dissection of the superior longitudinal bundle.

To expose the superior longitudinal bundle and uncinate fasciculus, we have to remove the folds of the hemisphere (opercula) hiding the insular cortex:

1. With the help of a scalpel cut the orbital, frontoparietal, temporal opercula, and tip of the temporal pole. This will expose the insula.

2. With the help of the handle of a knife, remove the brain tissue at the upper border of the insula. This will expose the superior longitudinal bundle.

3. Remove the insular cortex. This will expose the claustrum, a thin layer of gray matter. Scrape away the thin layer of the claustrum. Deep to the claustrum, the white matter of the external capsule is exposed.

4. Superior to the rounded smooth zone of white matter, look for the radiating fan-shaped layer of white matter going toward the superior longitudinal bundle. These radiating fibers are a part of the corona radiata.

C. Dissection of the uncinate fasciculus.

In continuation with the above dissection, we shall dissect the uncinate fasciculus:

1. With the help of the handle of a knife, remove the brain tissue lying superficial to the stem of the lateral sulcus (frontotemporal area, limen insulae). This will expose the hook-shaped uncinate fasciculus.

2. Notice that its fibers are fanning out into the orbital surface of the frontal and temporal lobes.

D. Dissection of the corona radiata.

In continuation with the dissection of the superior longitudinal bundle and uncinate fasciculus, dissect the fibers of the corona radiata. The corona radiata is an example of projection fibers **(Fig. 33.3)**:

1. Remove the thin layer of the external capsule to expose the lateral surface of the lentiform nucleus.

2. Now remove the superior longitudinal bundle completely. Similarly, remove the uncinate fasciculus.

3. Now trace the white fibers which radiate in a fan-like fashion all around the margin of the lentiform nucleus. All these fibers are extending from the cerebral cortex of various lobes and lie deep to the lentiform nucleus.

E. Dissection of the internal capsule.

In a horizontal section of the cerebrum, observe the parts of the internal capsule, that is, the anterior limb, genu, posterior limb, and retrolentiform part **(Fig. 33.3; Video 33.1)**. The internal capsule lies deep to the lentiform nucleus and is continuous above with the corona radiata and below with the crus cerebri (cerebral peduncle).

In continuation with the dissection of the corona radiata, remove the lentiform nucleus, in piecemeal, from the lateral side of the internal capsule. See the continuity of the fibers of the internal capsule inferiorly with the fibers on the lateral surface of the crus cerebri (cerebral peduncle).

F. Dissection of the inferior longitudinal bundle.

Now turn the cerebral hemisphere to look at the inferior surface of the temporal lobe and tentorial surface of the occipital lobe.

1. With the blunt dissection, remove the superficial brain tissue between the temporal and occipital lobes.

2. This will expose the bundle of fibers that runs between the occipital and temporal lobes.

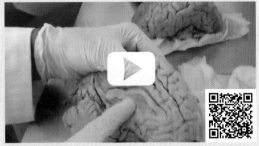

Video 33.1   Caudate nucleus, lentiform nucleus, thalamus, and internal capsule.

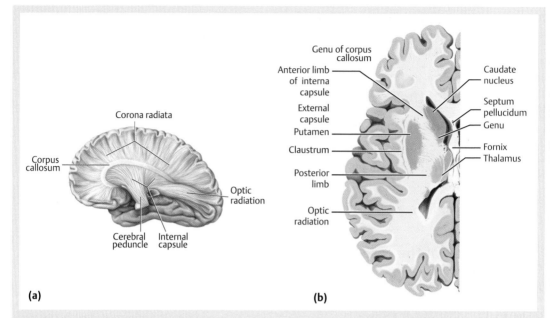

Fig. 33.3 (a,b)   Dissection of the corona radiata and internal capsule. (From: Schuenke M, Schulte E, Schumacher U. THIEME Atlas of Anatomy. Head, Neck, and Neuroanatomy. Illustrations by Voll M and Wesker K. © Thieme 2020.)

G. Dissection of the corpus callosum (Fig. 33.4).

After the dissection of the cingulum, we may dissect the corpus callosum in the cerebral hemisphere:

1. Remove the cingulum from the upper surface of the corpus callosum.

2. Start removing the brain tissue, in piecemeal, that lies above the superior surface of the corpus callosum.

3. Follow the fibers of the genu part of the corpus callosum forward and laterally, toward the medial surface of the frontal lobe. These fibers form the *forceps minor.*

4. Posterior to the fibers of the forceps minor, lift the fibers of the genu and from the body of the corpus callosum and tear them laterally. You will note that the horizontally running fibers of the corpus callosum are intersected by the vertically running fibers of the *corona radiata.*

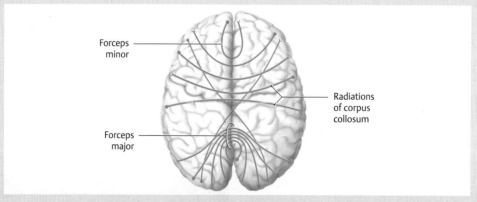

Fig. 33.4   Fibers of the corpus callosum. Fibers of genu, trunk, and splenium are also shown. (From: Schuenke M, Schulte E, Schumacher U. THIEME Atlas of Anatomy. Head, Neck, and Neuroanatomy. Illustrations by Voll M and Wesker K. © Thieme 2020.)

5. Follow the fibers of the splenium toward the cuneus, deep to the parieto-occipital sulcus. These fibers form the forceps major, which lies superior to the calcarine sulcus.

6. The calcarine sulcus and fibers of the forceps major indent the medial wall of the posterior horn of the lateral ventricle. Fibers of the forceps major form the *bulb of the posterior horn* and the calcarine sulcus produces a ridge known as the *calcar avis*. This can be confirmed by a coronal section passing through the occipital lobe.

7. Anterior to the fibers of the forceps major the fibers of the splenium run laterally; they form the roof of the posterior horn of the lateral ventricle. After forming the roof, these fibers turn downward to form the lateral wall of this ventricle. These fibers form the *tapetum* and terminate in the occipital and temporal lobes.

Description of the White Matter

Association Fibers

Association fibers are classified as short and long association fibers. The short association fibers pass from one part of the gyrus to another part of the same gyrus or to the adjacent gyrus. The long association fibers run for a long distance, that is, they connect to two different cerebral lobes of the same hemisphere (**Fig. 33.1**).

Cingulum: This bundle of long association fibers is present on the medial surface of the cerebral hemisphere. These fibers are present deep to the cingulated and parahippocampal gyri. Thus, they almost form a complete circle.

Superior longitudinal bundle: This bundle runs on the superolateral surface of the cerebral hemisphere above the level of the insula. Fibers of this bundle connect various parts of the frontal, parietal, occipital, and temporal lobes. Fibers run in both directions.

Inferior longitudinal bundle: This bundle connects the occipital and temporal lobes near their inferior surfaces.

Uncinate fasciculus: This bundle hooks around the stem of the lateral sulcus and connects the frontal and temporal lobes.

Commissural Fibers

These fibers connect the corresponding regions of the right and left cerebral hemispheres and, as a result, cross the midline.

Corpus callosum: The corpus callosum had the highest number of commissural fibers. In the sagittal section, it shows four parts, that is, the rostrum, genu, trunk, and splenium (**Fig. 33.2**). The fibers of the rostrum join the orbital surface of the two cerebral hemispheres. The fibers of the genu connect to the anterior part of the right and left frontal lobes. If seen in the transverse section, these fibers look like the limbs of forceps. Therefore, these fibers are called *forceps minor.* The trunk contains fibers to the remainder of frontal lobe and to the parietal lobe. The splenium contains fibers going to the parietal, occipital, and temporal lobes of the two sides. The fibers of the splenium form the *forceps major* and *tapetum.* The fibers of the tapetum are closely related to the posterior and inferior horns of the lateral ventricle.

Commissural fibers conduct nerve impulses from the gyri of one cerebral hemisphere to the corresponding gyri of the opposite cerebral hemisphere. Thus, both the cerebral hemispheres act as a single entity for bilateral responses and learning activity.

Anterior commissure: The anterior commissure is the bundle of white fibers that crosses the midline in the lamina terminalis. These fibers connect the temporal lobes of the right and left sides.

Posterior commissure: This bundle of white fibers is present in the inferior stalk of the pineal gland. This commissure connects the *interstitial nucleus of the Cajal* and *nucleus of the posterior commissure* of the two sides.

Habenular commissure: The habenular commissure is present in the superior stalk of the pineal gland and connects the habenular nuclei of the two sides.

Projection Fibers

Projection fibers are present in the form of *corona radiata* and *internal capsule* (**Fig. 33.3**).

Corona radiata: Fibers of the corona radiata pass between the cerebral cortex and other parts of the brain and spinal cord. It consists of both the afferent and efferent fibers. The efferent fibers begin in the cerebral cortex and pass inferiorly through the internal capsule. The afferent fibers mainly come through the thalamus and pass toward the cerebral cortex.

Above the internal capsule and lentiform nucleus, the fibers of the corona radiata spread out like a fan into the cerebral cortex. The fibers of the corona radiata are intersected by the fibers of the corpus callosum.

Internal capsule: The fibers of the internal capsule are a continuation of the fibers of the corona radiata and they connect the cerebral cortex to the centers in the thalamus, brainstem, and spinal cord, in both the directions. These fibers of the internal capsule, while passing through the cerebrum, lie between the large grey masses, that is, the caudate nucleus and thalamus medially and lentiform nucleus laterally. The fibers of the internal capsule are arranged compactly and are continuous below with the crus cerebri of the midbrain. In the horizontal section of the cerebrum, the internal capsule appears like a "V" with its concavity directed laterally. The internal capsule consists of the following parts: the anterior limb, genu, posterior limb, retrolentiform part, and sublentiform part (**Fig. 33.5**).

The anterior limb lies between the caudate nucleus and lentiform nucleus, while the posterior limb lies between the thalamus and lentiform nucleus. The anterior and posterior limbs meet each other at the genu, at an angle which opens laterally. The retrolentiform part of the internal capsule consists of fibers which lie behind the posterior end of the lentiform nucleus. Fibers passing below the lentiform nucleus constitute the sublentiform part of the internal capsule. The internal capsule consists of both the motor and sensory fibers (**Table 33.1**).

Table 33.1   Motor and sensory fibers in various parts of the internal capsule

Parts of the internal capsule	Sensory fibers	Motor fibers
Anterior limb	Thalamus to the prefrontal cortex	From the frontal lobe to the pontine nucleus
Genu	Thalamus to the frontal and parietal lobes	From the frontal lobe to the motor nuclei of the cranial nerve
Posterior limb	Thalamus to the frontal and parietal lobes	From the cortex to the substantia nigra, striate nucleus, red nucleus, and spinal cord
Retrolentiform part	Thalamus to the occipital lobe and optic radiation	From the parietal and occipital lobes to the pontine nuclei
Sublentiform part	Thalamus to the temporal cortex and auditory radiation	From the temporal and parietal lobes to the pontine nucleus

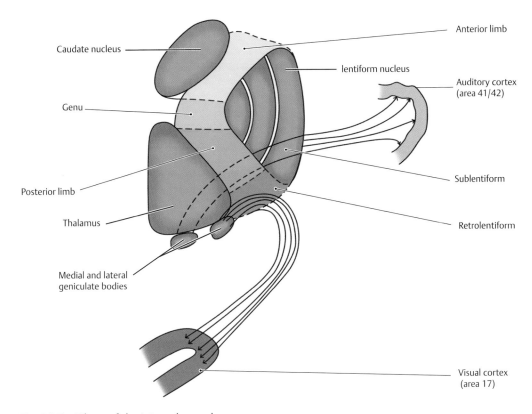

Fig. 33.5   Fibers of the internal capsule.

▌Clinical Notes

As the internal capsule consists of a compact bundle of motor and sensory fibers, occlusion of blood supply due to thrombosis or hemorrhage can result in paralysis and loss of sensation on the opposite half of the body, that is, hemiplegia. The most common vessel affected is the lateral striate branch of the middle cerebral artery (Charcot artery of the cerebral hemorrhage). This artery supplies the posterior limb of the internal capsule.

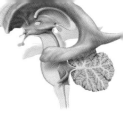

© THIEME Atlas of Anatomy

Learning Objectives

At the end of the dissection of the lateral ventricle, you should be able to identify and understand the following:

- C-shaped lateral ventricle with its subdivisions, that is, the anterior horn, body, posterior horn, and inferior horn.
- The floor, roof, medial, and anterior walls of the anterior horn which is located in the frontal lobe.
- The central part or the body of the lateral ventricle extends between the interventricular foramen and splenium. Identify the sloping floor which is formed by the thalamus and caudate nucleus.
- The floor of the inferior horn which is formed by the hippocampus, covered by the alveus, fimbria, and collateral eminence.
- The floor of the body of the lateral ventricle when traced backward becomes continuous with the roof of the inferior horn. Similarly, the choroid fissure in the body of the lateral ventricle lies between the fornix and thalamus, but in the inferior horn it lies above the fimbria and hippocampus.

Introduction

Each cerebral hemisphere contains a large C-shaped cavity known as the lateral ventricle. Each lateral ventricle consists of a body and three horns—anterior, posterior, and inferior. The anterior horn extends in the frontal lobe, posterior horn in the occipital lobe, and inferior horn is present in the temporal lobe. The cavity of the right and left ventricles communicates with the third ventricle through the interventricular foramen (**Fig. 34.1**).

The central part or body of the lateral ventricle extends anteroposteriorly between the interventricular foramen and splenium of the corpus callosum. In the cross-section, the central part is triangular and has three walls—a roof, a floor, and a medial wall. The anterior horn is present anterior to the interventricular foramen and extends forward in the frontal lobe. It has a roof, floor, medial, and anterior walls.

The inferior horn begins at the level of the splenium of the corpus callosum. It then passes downward behind the thalamus to run forward in the temporal lobe. The posterior horn is small and extends backward in the occipital lobe.

Surface Landmarks

1. See the location of the interventricular foramen in a midsagittal section of the cerebrum (**Fig. 34.2**).
2. Note the protruding choroid plexus between the superior surface of the thalamus and fornix.

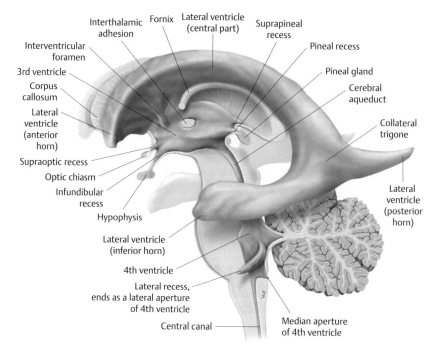

Fig. 34.1 Ventricles of the brain. Note the parts of the lateral ventricle: left lateral view. (From: Schuenke M, Schulte E, Schumacher U. THIEME Atlas of Anatomy. Head, Neck, and Neuroanatomy. Illustrations by Voll M and Wesker K. © Thieme 2020.)

3. In a midsagittal section, carefully remove the medial wall (septum pellucidum) of the anterior horn and central part of the lateral ventricle to see the superior surface of the thalamus and head and body of the caudate nucleus.

4. Trace the extent of the choroid fissure from the interventricular foramen to the anterior tip of the inferior horn. The choroid fissure is placed between the fornix and thalamus in the central part of the ventricle. It is placed between the fimbria and roof of the inferior horn in the inferior horn.

Dissection and Identification

Dissection of lateral ventricle (Video 34.1)

The dissection of the lateral ventricle is not easy. Students are suggested to take the help of their teacher for a successful dissection of the lateral ventricle. You should dissect the lateral ventricle in one complete half of the cerebral hemisphere belonging either to the right or left side. Follow the steps of dissection as listed below (**Figs. 34.2** and **34.3a, b**):

1. Give a vertical cut between the interventricular foramen and superior border of the cerebrum passing through the fornix, septum pellucidum, corpus callosum, and medial aspect of the cerebral hemisphere. Open the cut ends gently and take care that this incision does not

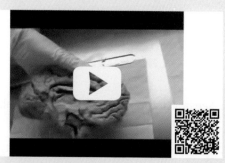

Video 34.1 Lateral ventricle.

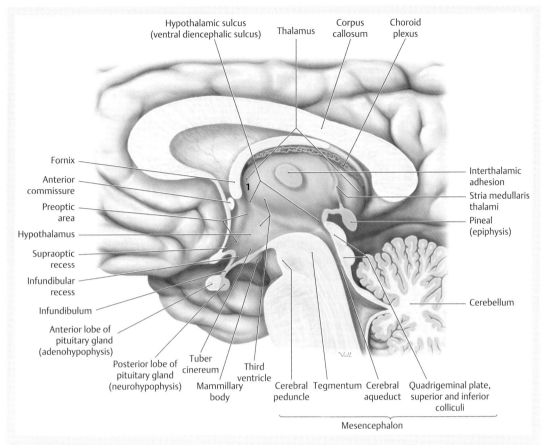

Fig. 34.2 Midsagittal section of the right hemisphere viewed from the medial side. 1, Interventricular foramen. (From: Schuenke M, Schulte E, Schumacher U. THIEME Atlas of Anatomy. Head, Neck, and Neuroanatomy. Illustrations by Voll M and Wesker K. © Thieme 2020.)

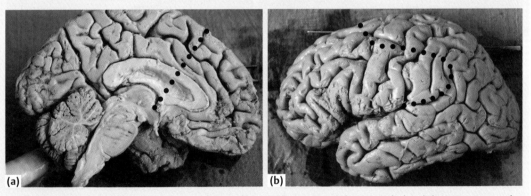

Fig. 34.3 **(a)** Medial surface of the cerebrum showing first incision from just behind the interventricular foramen to the superomedial border. **(b)** Incision on the superolateral surface to expose lateral ventricle. (Reproduced with permission from Pal, GP. Illustrated Textbook of Neuroanatomy. Lippincott Williams & Wilkins/Wolters Kluwer. 2013. Source: Prof. SD Joshi, SAIMS, Indore.)

go deep. The cut should extend only up to the lateral edge of the lateral ventricle, that is, at the junction of the undersurface of the roof (corpus callosum) and floor of the lateral ventricle (caudate nucleus).

2. Now turn the edge of the knife posteriorly and cut the hemisphere backward by keeping the point of the knife at the lateral edge of the lateral ventricle. You should observe the lateral edge of the lateral ventricle by carefully opening the cut ends of the hemisphere. Now the

incision will extend downward in a curved direction till the posterior ramus of the lateral sulcus is approached.

3. Now expose the insula by pulling the opercula and locate the circular sulcus at the inferior border of the insula. This sulcus separates the insula from the temporal lobe. Now extend the incision forward through the circular sulcus till it reaches the stem of the lateral sulcus. Take care that the tip of the knife is in the inferior horn of the lateral ventricle. You should keep on confirming this, from time to time, by opening the cut edges of the cerebral hemisphere.

4. By separating the cut edges gently, observe the choroid plexus in the inferior horn, which protrudes through the choroid fissure in its medial wall. Follow this choroid plexus backward and then in the body (stem) of the lateral sulcus, where it protrudes into the ventricle from its floor.

5. Now extend the cut in the stem of the lateral sulcus by separating the temporal lobe from the frontal lobe. The hemisphere is separated into two parts, that is, an anterior part and a posterior part. The anterior part containing the frontal lobe, anterior horn of the lateral ventricle, and brainstem and thalamus attached to it **(Fig. 34.4a)**. The posterior part contains the occipital and temporal lobes and encloses the body, posterior, and inferior horn of the lateral ventricle **(Fig. 34.4b)**. Gently separate the first part from the second part along the line of the choroid fissure (i.e., between the fornix and thalamus). Carefully cut the blood vessels entering the choroid fissure (internal cerebral veins and branches of the posterior choroidal artery). The choroid plexus will remain attached to the thalamus, while the arch of the fornix, fimbria, hippocampus, and the trunk and splenium of the corpus callosum will be separated along with the posterior part of the cerebrum.

6. The anterior and posterior parts may be fitted repeatedly to understand the parts and position of the ventricle and choroid fissure.

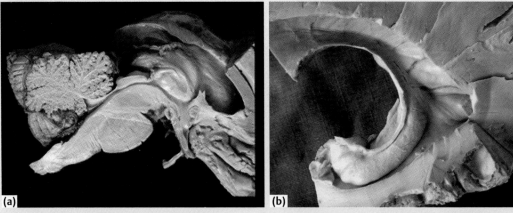

Fig. 34.4 **(a)** Anterior horn of the lateral ventricle, thalamus and brainstem seen after dissection containing the frontal lobe attached to it. **(b)** Dissection of occipital and temporal lobes containing posterior and inferior horns of the lateral ventricle. (Reproduced with permission from Pal, GP. Illustrated Textbook of Neuroanatomy. Lippincott Williams & Wilkins/Wolters Kluwer. 2013. Source: Prof. SD Joshi, SAIMS, Indore.)

Features of the Lateral Ventricle

The lateral ventricles are two in number and are present inside the right and left cerebral hemispheres. Each lateral ventricle consists of a body or central part located in the parietal lobe and three horns (i.e., anterior horn in the frontal lobe, posterior horn in the occipital lobe, and inferior horn in the temporal lobe). The central parts of the right and left lateral ventricles are separated from each other by the septum pellucidum (**Fig. 34.6**).

The anterior horn: The anterior end of the anterior horn is blind, while posteriorly it becomes continuous with the body of the lateral ventricle at the level of the interventricular foramen. Its anterior wall is formed by the genu of the corpus callosum, the roof by the body of the corpus callosum, floor by the rostrum of the corpus callosum, lateral wall by the head of the caudate nucleus, and medial wall by the septum pellucidum (**Fig. 34.5**).

The body or central part: The body extends anteriorly from the interventricular foramen to the level of splenium of the corpus callosum posteriorly. The medial wall of the central part of the lateral ventricle is formed by the septum pellucidum. The roof is formed by the trunk of the corpus callosum. The floor shows the following structures from the medial to the lateral sides: dorsal surface of the thalamus, thalamostriate vein, stria terminalis, and body of the caudate nucleus (**Fig. 34.6**).

The posterior horn: Two distinct ridges are seen in its medial wall, that is, the *bulb of the posterior horn* formed by the fibers of the forceps major. The lower ridge is formed by the calcarine sulcus and is known as the *calcar avis*. The roof, lateral wall, and floor of the posterior horn are formed by the tapetum.

The inferior horn: It presents a roof and a floor. The roof is formed by the tapetum of the corpus callosum laterally and tail of the caudate nucleus and stria terminalis medially. At the anterior end of the inferior horn, the tail becomes continuous with the amygdaloid body. The floor is formed by the collateral eminence laterally and hippocampus medially (refer to **Figs. 34.7–34.9**).

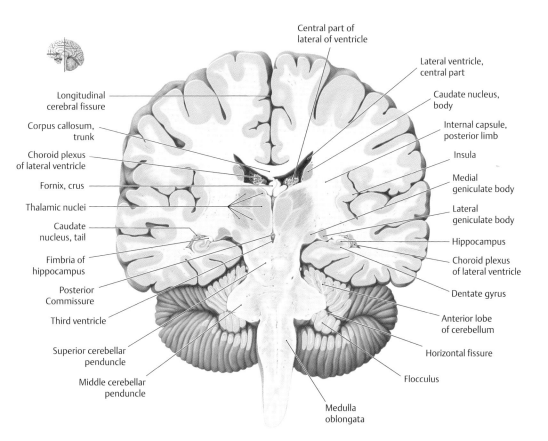

Fig. 34.5 Central part/body of lateral ventricle as seen in the coronal section of the cerebrum. (From: Schuenke M, Schulte E, Schumacher U. THIEME Atlas of Anatomy. Head, Neck, and Neuroanatomy. Illustrations by Voll M and Wesker K. © Thieme 2020.)

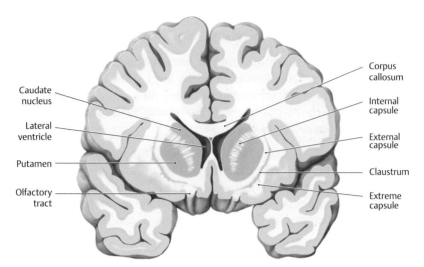

Fig. 34.6 Anterior horn of lateral ventricle as seen in the coronal section of the cerebrum. (From: Schuenke M, Schulte E, Schumacher U. THIEME Atlas of Anatomy. Head, Neck, and Neuroanatomy. Illustrations by Voll M and Wesker K. © Thieme 2020.)

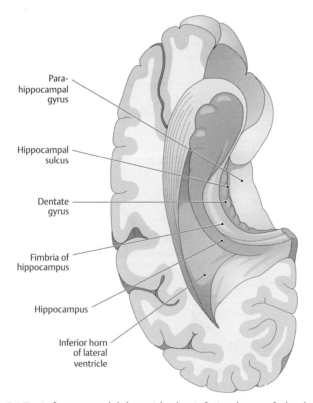

Fig. 34.7 Left temporal lobe with the inferior horn of the lateral ventricle exposed: transverse section, posterior view of the hippocampus on the floor of the inferior (temporal) horn. (From: Schuenke M, Schulte E, Schumacher U. THIEME Atlas of Anatomy. Head, Neck, and Neuroanatomy. Illustrations by Voll M and Wesker K. © Thieme 2020.)

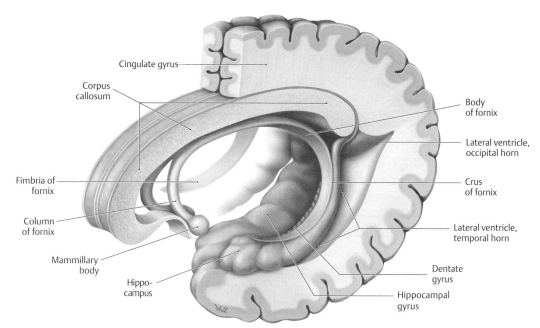

Fig. 34.8 Topography of the hippocampus, fornix, and corpus callosum (viewed from the upper left and other aspect). (From: Schuenke M, Schulte E, Schumacher U. THIEME Atlas of Anatomy. Head, Neck, and Neuroanatomy. Illustrations by Voll M and Wesker K. © Thieme 2020.)

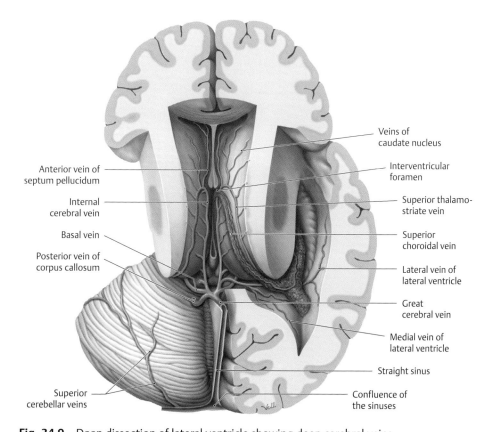

Fig. 34.9 Deep dissection of lateral ventricle showing deep cerebral veins.

▌ Clinical Notes

Ventriculography: The size, shape, and position of the ventricle can be visualized either by injecting air or radiopaque dye in the ventricular system. The ventricle may be distended as a result of obstruction in the circulation of the cerebrospinal fluid (CSF). The distortion and displacement of the ventricle may be due to the expanding tumor or intracranial hemorrhage.

1. However, these days the magnetic resonance imaging and computed tomographic scan of the brain are the investigation of choice.

2. *Hydrocephalus*: This condition results due to abnormal accumulation of the CSF in children. This leads to an abnormally large size of the head and degeneration of the brain tissue due to increased intracranial pressure. Hydrocephalus may result due to obstruction in the flow of CSF (obstructive hydrocephalus) or it may be due to overproduction or impaired absorption of CSF (communicating hydrocephalus).

The tumor of the choroid plexus may result in the overproduction of CSF. Obstruction in the flow of CSF may be due to the presence of tumor near the interventricular foramen leading to dilatation of the lateral ventricle on one side. The impaired absorption of CSF may be due to pathology in arachnoid granulation.

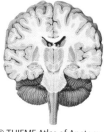
Learning Objectives

At the end of the dissection of the basal nuclei, you should be able to identify and understand the following:

- Parts of the caudate nucleus.
- Putamen and globus pallidus parts of the lentiform nucleus.
- Subthalamic nucleus.
- Substantia nigra.

Introduction

Basal nuclei are large masses of gray matter, which are located in the subcortical regions of the cerebrum. These nuclei belong to the motor system and play a major role in the voluntary movements. The motor functions of the basal nuclei are independent of the activity of the pyramidal system; therefore, these nuclei are considered a part of the extrapyramidal system.

Basal nuclei consist of the caudate nucleus, lentiform nucleus, subthalamic nucleus, and substantia nigra. Lentiform nucleus consists of two parts—putamen and globus pallidus (**Fig. 35.1a** and **b**). The putamen and caudate nucleus together form the corpus striatum. Substantia nigra is present in the midbrain (**Fig. 35.1a**), while the subthalamic nucleus is positioned between the thalamus and substantia nigra (**Fig. 35.2**).

Caudate nucleus and putamen (striatum) receive almost all the inputs of the basal nuclei. The axons of striatum terminate in the globus pallidus and substantia nigra, which in turn terminate in the thalamus and subthalamic nucleus.

Dissection and Identification

As such, no separate dissection of the basal nuclei is possible as these nuclei are deeply imbedded in the cerebrum (caudate, lentiform nuclei, and subthalamic nucleus) and midbrain (substantia nigra). The various parts of the caudate nucleus (head, body, and tail) can be seen during the dissection of the lateral ventricle. The substantia nigra can be seen in the midbrain. The putamen and globus pallidus parts of the lentiform nucleus are seen in both the coronal and horizontal (transverse) sections of the cerebral hemisphere.

Features of the Basal Nuclei

Caudate nucleus: The caudate nucleus is a C-shaped mass of gray matter that surrounds the thalamus and is present in the lateral ventricle (**Fig. 35.3**). It consists of head, body, and tail. The anterior end of the head is fused inferiorly with the lentiform nucleus (putamen). The body of the caudate nucleus is related to the thalamus on the medial side. The anterior end of the tail is in relation to the amygdaloid complex.

Lentiform nucleus: It is a convex mass of gray matter which is deeply situated in the cerebral hemisphere. Medially, it is related to the internal capsule while laterally it is separated from the claustrum by the fibers of the external capsule. The lentiform nucleus is divided into a lateral part (putamen) and a medial part (globus pallidus) (**Fig. 35.1b**).

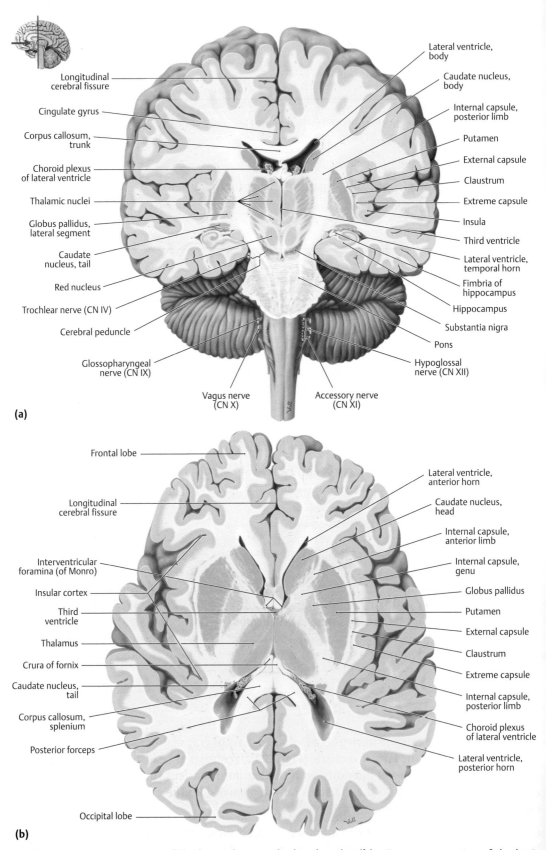

Fig. 35.1 (a) Coronal section of the brain showing the basal nuclei. **(b)** Transverse section of the brain showing the basal nuclei. (From: Schuenke M, Schulte E, Schumacher U. THIEME Atlas of Anatomy. Head, Neck, and Neuroanatomy. Illustrations by Voll M and Wesker K. © Thieme 2020.)

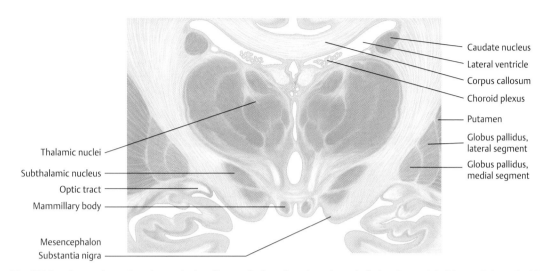

Fig. 35.2   Coronal section through the diencephalon showing the subthalamic nuclei. (From: Schuenke M, Schulte E, Schumacher U. THIEME Atlas of Anatomy. Head, Neck, and Neuroanatomy. Illustrations by Voll M and Wesker K. © Thieme 2020.)

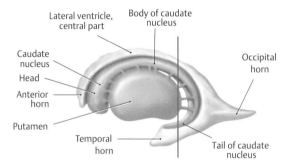

Fig. 35.3   Caudate nucleus and its relationship with the lateral ventricle and putamen. (From: Schuenke M, Schulte E, Schumacher U. THIEME Atlas of Anatomy. Head, Neck, and Neuroanatomy. Illustrations by Voll M and Wesker K. © Thieme 2020.)

Subthalamic nucleus: It is a small, biconvex mass of gray matter which lies below the thalamus and above the substantia nigra.

Substantia nigra: It is a large motor nucleus which is present in the midbrain (**Fig. 35.4**). It consists of two parts: pars reticulata and pars compacta. Cells of pars compacta contain neuromelanin, which gives a dark color to the substantia nigra. Substantia nigra synthesizes the neurotransmitter dopamine.

Connections of the substantia nigra: The caudate nucleus and putamen receive all inputs of the basal nuclei. Therefore, these nuclei are also known as input nuclei. The axons of the input nucleus project to the globus pallidus and substantia nigra. These are considered as major output nuclei. Fibers from the globus pallidus and substantia nigra terminate on the thalamus and subthalamic nucleus.

Dissection of basal ganglia is shown in **Figs. 35.1** and **35.2**.

Functions

The motor activity of basal nuclei is independent of the pyramidal motor system. Therefore, basal nuclei are included in the category of the extrapyramidal system.

Functions of the basal nuclei include programming of the normal voluntary movements and controlling of abnormal involuntary movements. Basal nuclei are also involved in cognitive and behavioral functions like reasoning, judgment, memory, and thought.

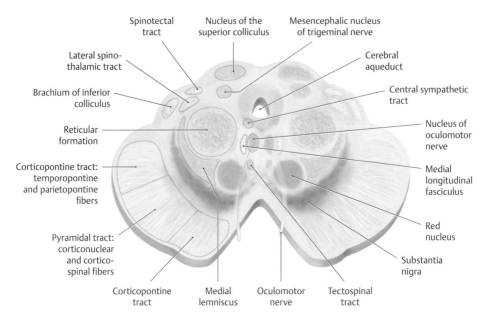

Fig. 35.4 Substantia nigra as seen in transverse section through the mesencephalon (midbrain): superior view. (From: Schuenke M, Schulte E, Schumacher U. THIEME Atlas of Anatomy. Head, Neck, and Neuroanatomy. Illustrations by Voll M and Wesker K. © Thieme 2020.)

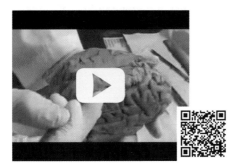

Video 35.1   Basal ganglia: Part I.

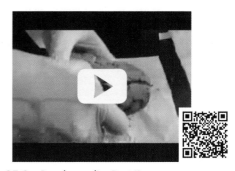

Video 35.2   Basal ganglia: Part II.

▌ Clinical Notes

1. *Parkinson disease*: It is a chronic progressive nervous disorder. This disease is characterized by tremors, muscular weakness, rigidity, and a peculiar gait. The disease is more common in males after the age of 60 years. The exact cause of the disease is unknown. It results due to the deficiency of neurotransmitter dopamine in the striatum. This deficiency occurs due to the degeneration of the dopaminergic neurons.

2. *Hemiballismus*: This condition results due to the small stroke lesion in the subthalamic nucleus. The hemiballismus is characterized by involuntary movements of the opposite limb. These movements resemble the movements of throwing; hence, it is called ballism.

3. *Huntington chorea*: It is a genetic disorder. The disease is characterized by chorea and dementia. The choreiform movements are involuntary movements of the limbs and twitching of the face. After some time, the patient becomes immobile and is unable to speak or swallow.

The disease is caused by the abnormal autosomal dominant gene, which causes the abnormal accumulation of *Huntington* protein in the neurons of the caudate nucleus and putamen.

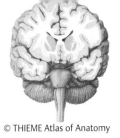

Learning Objectives

At the end of the study of the sections of the brain, you should be able to identify and understand the following:

Sections of Brain

- Interrelationship of various nuclei and their extent.
- Relationship of the white matter with the gray matter.
- Structure of various ventricles and their relations with the surrounding gray and white matter.

Introduction

The anatomy of the brain is complicated. For a comprehensive understanding of three-dimensional anatomy of the brain, it is necessary to study its sections in various planes, that is, the *coronal, transverse,* and *sagittal.* The sections of the brain should be learned after completing all other dissections of the brain as the knowledge of descriptive anatomy of the brain is necessary to understand these sections.

Sections of the brain in different planes give an idea about the position, extent, and shapes of various deeply situated collections of gray matter (nuclei) and their interrelationships. These sections also give an idea about the depth of a particular structure and ventricles from the surface. Knowledge of these sections is very important for understanding the images produced by the computed tomographic scan (CT scans) and magnetic resonance imaging (MRI). Some figures showing imaging of brain and images of cerebral angiography are included in this chapter.

Dissection and Identification

Sections of Brain

Under the supervision of your teacher, cut the sections of the brain with the help of a brain knife. If these sections are already present in the storage tank or museum cf your department, make use of them.

Coronal sections: Many coronal sections are selected. These sections are taken in a series, starting from the frontal lobe and gradually proceeding toward the occipital lobe. The representative site of the section is presented in a miniature figure at the left upper corner. The sections in this series are viewed from the anterior side (**Figs. 36.1–36.10**).

Transverse sections: In this series of horizontal sections, each section is viewed from above, thus the left side of the brain appears on the left side of the drawing. These sections are taken in a series, starting from the superior end of the brain and gradually proceeding toward the inferior end, that is, toward the brainstem (refer to **Fig. 35.1b**; **Figs. 36.11–36.15**).

Sagittal sections: The sagittal sections are taken in left cerebral hemisphere; thus, all these views are left lateral views. These sections are taken in a series, starting from the superficial aspect and gradually going toward the deeper aspect, till the section passes through the midline (**Figs. 36.16–36.23**).

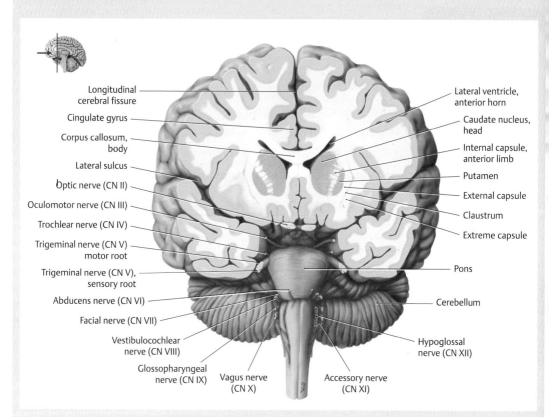

Fig. 36.1   Coronal section I. (Note: The representative site of the section is presented in a miniature figure at the left upper corner. This and other coronal sections are viewed from the anterior side.). (From: Schuenke M, Schulte E, Schumacher U. THIEME Atlas of Anatomy. Head, Neck, and Neuroanatomy. Illustrations by Voll M and Wesker K. © Thieme 2020.)

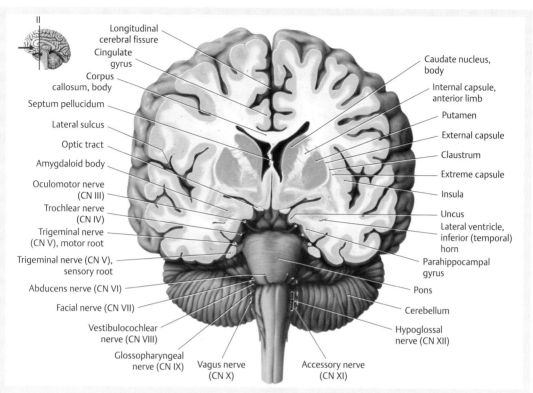

Fig. 36.2 Coronal section II. (From: Schuenke M, Schulte E, Schumacher U. THIEME Atlas of Anatomy. Head, Neck, and Neuroanatomy. Illustrations by Voll M and Wesker K. © Thieme 2020.)

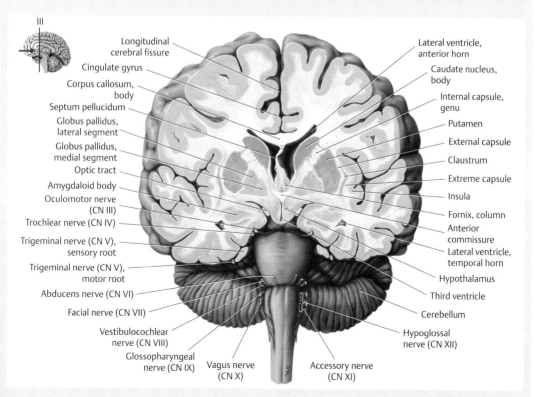

Fig. 36.3 Coronal section III. (From: Schuenke M, Schulte E, Schumacher U. THIEME Atlas of Anatomy. Head, Neck, and Neuroanatomy. Illustrations by Voll M and Wesker K. © Thieme 2020.)

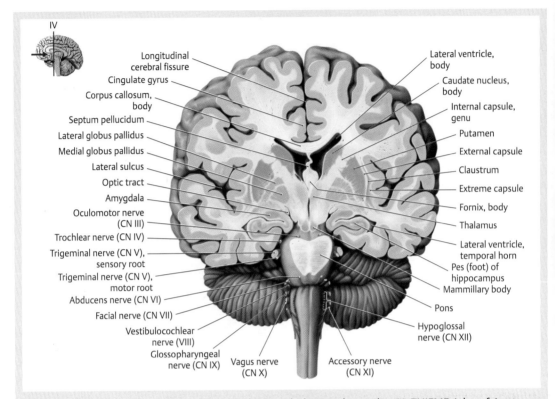

Fig. 36.4 Coronal section IV. (From: Schuenke M, Schulte E, Schumacher U. THIEME Atlas of Anatomy. Head, Neck, and Neuroanatomy. Illustrations by Voll M and Wesker K. © Thieme 2020.)

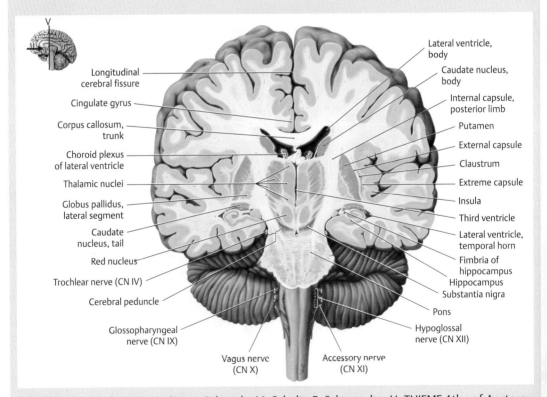

Fig. 36.5 Coronal section V. (From: Schuenke M, Schulte E, Schumacher U. THIEME Atlas of Anatomy. Head, Neck, and Neuroanatomy. Illustrations by Voll M and Wesker K. © Thieme 2020.)

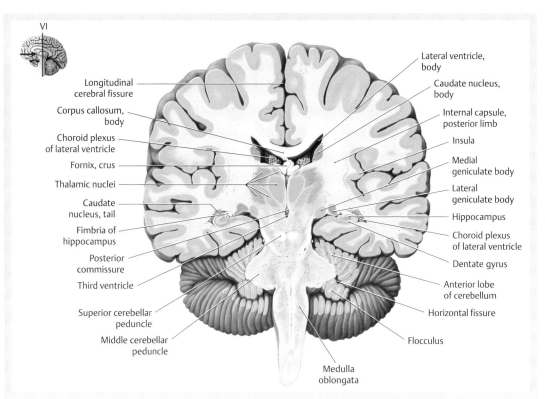

Fig. 36.6   Coronal section VI. (From: Schuenke M, Schulte E, Schumacher U. THIEME Atlas of Anatomy. Head, Neck, and Neuroanatomy. Illustrations by Voll M and Wesker K. © Thieme 2020.)

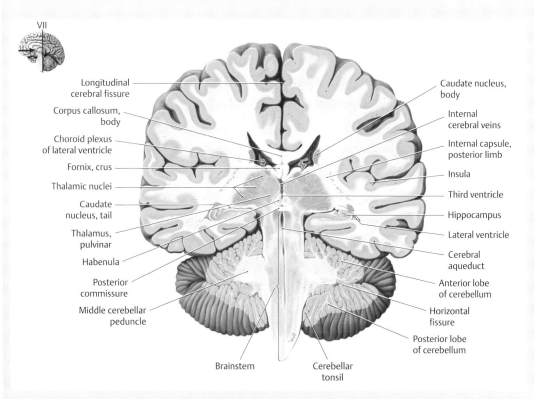

Fig. 36.7   Coronal section VII. (From: Schuenke M, Schulte E, Schumacher U. THIEME Atlas of Anatomy. Head, Neck, and Neuroanatomy. Illustrations by Voll M and Wesker K. © Thieme 2020.)

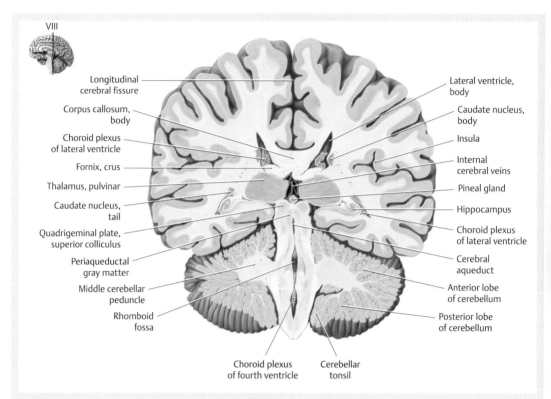

Fig. 36.8 Coronal section VIII. (From: Schuenke M, Schulte E, Schumacher U. THIEME Atlas of Anatomy. Head, Neck, and Neuroanatomy. Illustrations by Voll M and Wesker K. © Thieme 2020.)

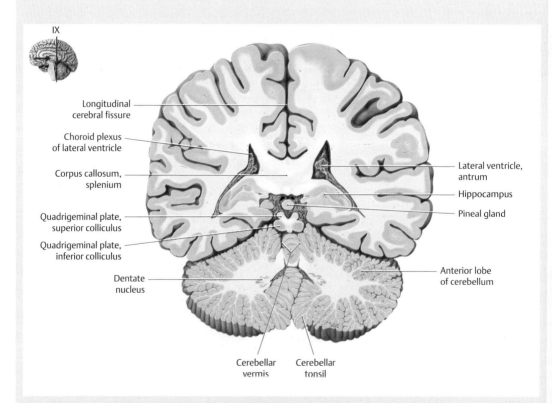

Fig. 36.9 Coronal section IX. (From: Schuenke M, Schulte E, Schumacher U. THIEME Atlas of Anatomy. Head, Neck, and Neuroanatomy. Illustrations by Voll M and Wesker K. © Thieme 2020.)

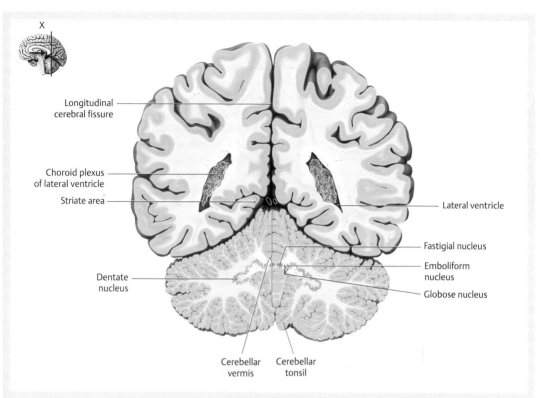

Fig. 36.10 Coronal section X. (From: Schuenke M, Schulte E, Schumacher U. THIEME Atlas of Anatomy. Head, Neck, and Neuroanatomy. Illustrations by Voll M and Wesker K. © Thieme 2020.)

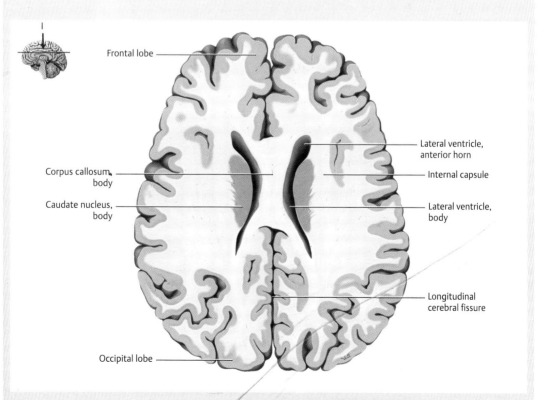

Fig. 36.11 Transverse (horizontal) section I. The transverse sections are viewed from above. (From: Schuenke M, Schulte E, Schumacher U. THIEME Atlas of Anatomy. Head, Neck, and Neuroanatomy. Illustrations by Voll M and Wesker K. © Thieme 2020.)

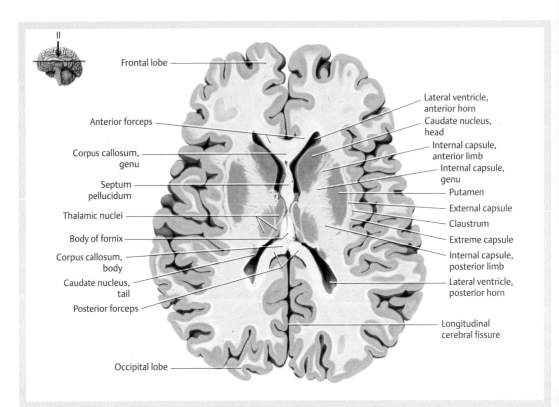

Fig. 36.12 Transverse section II. (From: Schuenke M, Schulte E, Schumacher U. THIEME Atlas of Anatomy. Head, Neck, and Neuroanatomy. Illustrations by Voll M and Wesker K. © Thieme 2020.)

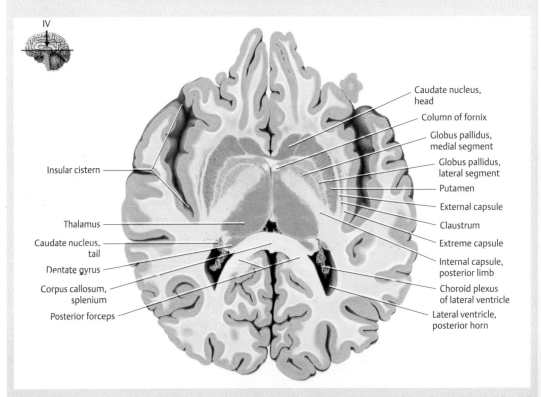

Fig. 36.13 Transverse section IV. (From: Schuenke M, Schulte E, Schumacher U. THIEME Atlas of Anatomy. Head, Neck, and Neuroanatomy. Illustrations by Voll M and Wesker K. © Thieme 2020.)

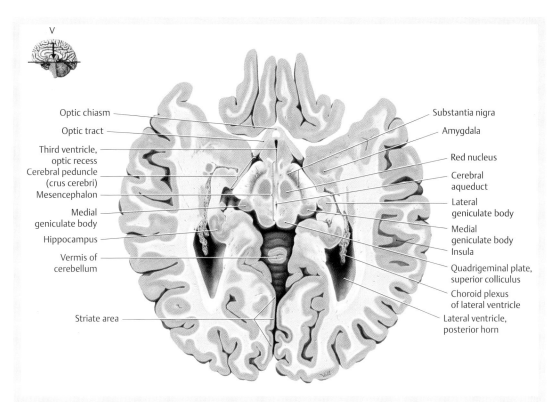

Fig. 36.14 Transverse section V. (From: Schuenke M, Schulte E, Schumacher U. THIEME Atlas of Anatomy. Head, Neck, and Neuroanatomy. Illustrations by Voll M and Wesker K. © Thieme 2020.)

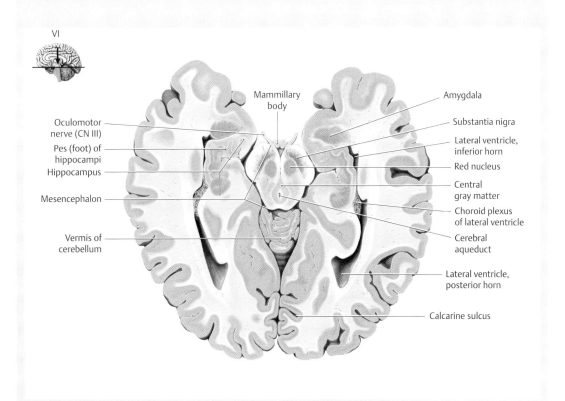

Fig. 36.15 Transverse section VI. (From: Schuenke M, Schulte E, Schumacher U. THIEME Atlas of Anatomy. Head, Neck, and Neuroanatomy. Illustrations by Voll M and Wesker K. © Thieme 2020.)

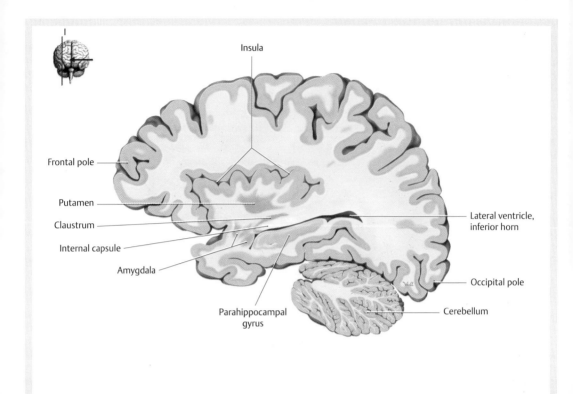

Fig. 36.16 Sagittal section I (left lateral view): Section through the insular cortex. (From: Schuenke M, Schulte E, Schumacher U. THIEME Atlas of Anatomy. Head, Neck, and Neuroanatomy. Illustrations by Voll M and Wesker K. © Thieme 2020.)

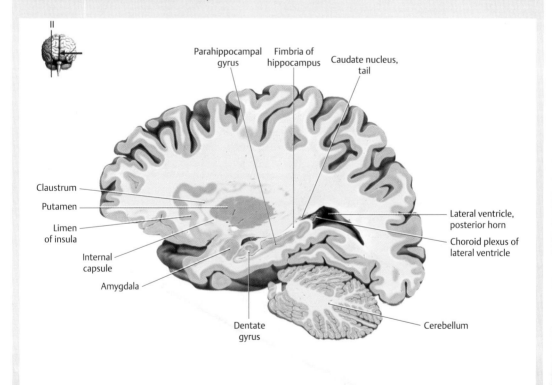

Fig. 36.17 Sagittal section II (left lateral view): Section through the amygdala. (From: Schuenke M, Schulte E, Schumacher U. THIEME Atlas of Anatomy. Head, Neck, and Neuroanatomy. Illustrations by Voll M and Wesker K. © Thieme 2020.)

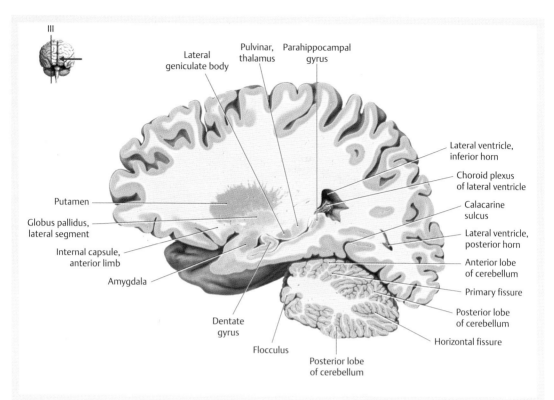

Fig. 36.18 Sagittal section III (left lateral view): Section through the geniculate body. (From: Schuenke M, Schulte E, Schumacher U. THIEME Atlas of Anatomy. Head, Neck, and Neuroanatomy. Illustrations by Voll M and Wesker K. © Thieme 2020.)

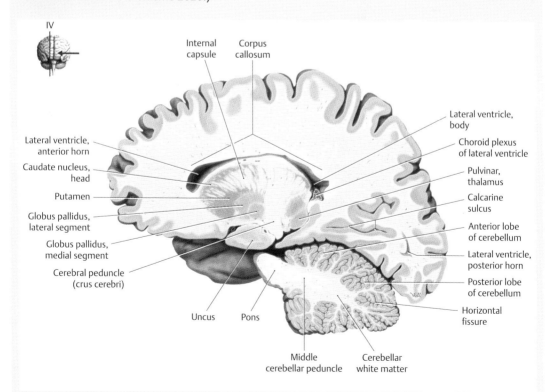

Fig. 36.19 Sagittal section IV (left lateral view): Section through the globus pallidus. (From: Schuenke M, Schulte E, Schumacher U. THIEME Atlas of Anatomy. Head, Neck, and Neuroanatomy. Illustrations by Voll M and Wesker K. © Thieme 2020.)

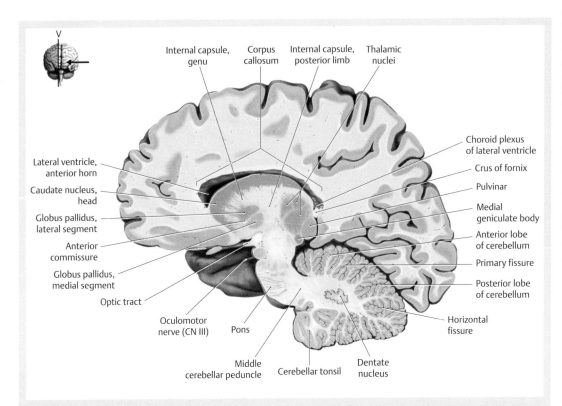

Fig. 36.20 Sagittal section V (left lateral view): Section through the caudate nucleus. (From: Schuenke M, Schulte E, Schumacher U. THIEME Atlas of Anatomy. Head, Neck, and Neuroanatomy. Illustrations by Voll M and Wesker K. © Thieme 2020.)

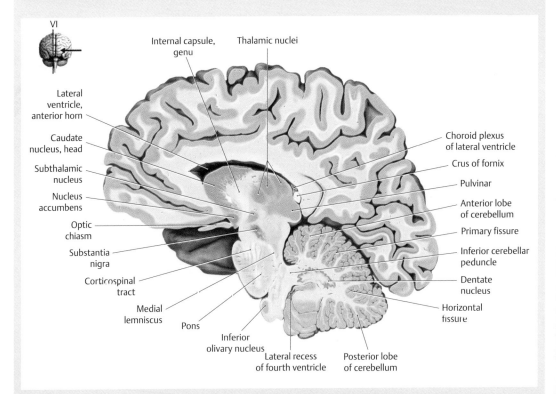

Fig. 36.21 Sagittal section VI (left lateral view): Section through the subthalamic nuclei. (From: Schuenke M, Schulte E, Schumacher U. THIEME Atlas of Anatomy. Head, Neck, and Neuroanatomy. Illustrations by Voll M and Wesker K. © Thieme 2020.)

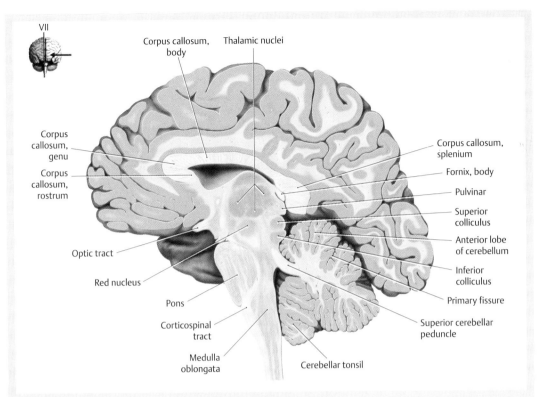

Fig. 36.22 Sagittal section VII (left lateral view): Section through the superior and inferior colliculi. (From: Schuenke M, Schulte E, Schumacher U. THIEME Atlas of Anatomy. Head, Neck, and Neuroanatomy. Illustrations by Voll M and Wesker K. © Thieme 2020.)

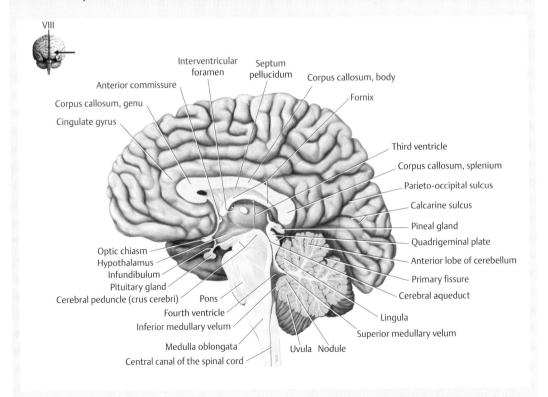

Fig. 36.23 Sagittal section VIII (left lateral view): Midsagittal section. (From: Schuenke M, Schulte E, Schumacher U. THIEME Atlas of Anatomy. Head, Neck, and Neuroanatomy. Illustrations by Voll M and Wesker K. © Thieme 2020.)

Index

A

Accessory nerve, 73
  branches of, 186
  dissection and identification of, 179
  injury to, 189
  nucleus and course of, 187f
Anesthetic block of inferior alveolar nerve, 94
Ansa cervicalis, 159–160, 162f
Anterior ciliary arteries, 247
Anterior commissure, 319
Anterior cranial fossae, 8, 9f
  dissection and identification of, 124
  location of, 123
  surface landmarks on, 123
Anterior spinal artery, 278
Anterior triangle of neck
  arteries of, 72, 72t
  dissection and identification of
    carotid triangle, 68, 68f, 70, 70f
    incision and reflection of skin, 66, 67f
    muscular triangle, 67, 68, 69f
    submental and digastric triangles, exposure of, 67
    superficial fascia, nerves and veins in, 67, 68f
  muscles related to, 71, 71t
  suprahyoid and infrahyoid regions of, 65, 66f
  surface landmarks on, 66
  veins of, 72–73, 73f
Arachnoid mater, 120, 277
Arachnoid villi and granulations, 121
Articular disc, exposure of, 96–97
Articular tubercle, 95, 96f
Arytenoid cartilages, 233
Ascending palatine artery, 206
Ascending pharyngeal artery, pharyngeal branches of, 206
Association fibers, 325
Atlanto-axial joint, 261, 266
Atlanto-occipital joint, 261, 263, 266
Atlas. *See* First cervical vertebrae
Auriculotemporal nerve, 81
Axis. *See* Second cervical vertebrae

B

Back of neck, 57
  dissection and identification of
    C1 spinal nerve, 60f, 61
    exposure and reflection of trapezius, 59–61, 60f
    greater occipital nerve, 60f, 61
    incision and reflection of skin, 58–59, 59f
    semispinalis capitis, 60f, 61
    suboccipital triangle, 60f, 61
    vertebral artery, 60f, 61
  muscles at, 62–63t
  spasm of muscles of, 63
  surface landmarks on, 58, 58f
Basal cerebral venous system, 275f
Basal nuclei, 338f
  composition of, 337
  dissection and identification of, 337
  features of, 337–338

functions of, 339–340
Basilar artery, 279
Basilar plexus of veins, 119
Bell's palsy, 40, 41
Benedikt syndrome, 294
Blood–brain barrier, 282
Brachial nerves, 175–176
Brachial plexus, 53–54
Brachiocephalic veins, 167f, 174
Brain, 308f
  anatomy of, 341
  arteries at base of, 276f
  arteries of, 278
    basilar, 279
    internal carotid, 279–280
  blood vessels of, 272–273
  dissection and identification of
    cerebral and cerebellar arteries, 275–277
    circle of Willis, 275–277
    cisterns and veins on cerebral hemisphere
      surface, 273–274
  and meninges in situ, 116f, 274f
  parts of, 269–272, 270f, 271f
  subarachnoid cisterns, 277–278, 277f
  superficial veins of, 274f, 275f, 278
  surface landmarks on, 273
Brain, midsagittal section of
  dissection and identification of, 317–318
  structures seen on, 318–320, 318f
    anterior commissure, 319
    circumventricular organs, 320
    corpus callosum, 318
    fornix, 318–319
    habenular commissure, 319
    hypothalamus, 319
    pineal gland, 319
    posterior commissure, 319
    septum pellucidum, 319
    thalamus, 319
    third ventricle, 320
Brain removal, from cranial cavity
  cranial meninges
    arachnoid mater, 120
    arachnoid villi and granulations, 121
    definition of, 118
    dura mater, 118–119
      dural folds, 119
      dural venous sinuses, 119
      paired sinuses, 120
      unpaired sinuses, 119–120
    pia mater, 121
  dissection and identification of
    arachnoid and pia maters, 117, 117f
    arachnoid mater, 115, 117
    dural venous sinuses and dural folds, 115
    middle meningeal vessels, 115
    removal of skull cap, 114–115, 114f
    subarachnoid space, 115, 117
  middle meningeal vessels, 118
  surface landmarks on, 113–114

Brain, sections of
    dissection and identification of, 341
        coronal sections, 342–347f
        sagittal sections, 342–347f, 350–353f
        transverse sections, 342, 347–349f
    functions of, 341
Brainstem, 283
    arteries of, 279f
    dissection to expose, 284–285
    external features of, 284f, 285f

C
Carotid body, 161
Carotid sheath, 159–161
Carotid sinus, 161
Caudate nucleus, 337, 339f
Cavernous petrosal sinus, 124f
Cavernous sinus, 132
    middle meningeal artery, 127–132
    relation of cranial nerves to, 130f
Central artery of retina, 247
Cerebellar cortex, 300
Cerebellar peduncles, 297, 298f
Cerebellomedullary cistern, 277
Cerebellum
    arteries of, 279f
    dissection and identification of
        cerebellar peduncles, 297, 298f
        choroid plexus, 298
        fissures and lobes, 295, 297
        inferior medullary velum, 298
        intracerebellar nuclei, 298
        median aperture of fourth ventricle, 298
    external features of, 296f, 297f, 299–300, 300f
    functions of, 295
    internal structure of, 300, 301f
    surface landmarks on, 295
Cerebral and cerebellar arteries, 275–277
Cerebral cortex, functional areas of, 313–314, 314f
Cerebral hemisphere, 329
    cisterns and veins on surface of, 273–274
    midsagittal section of brain to, 307–308
    poles, border, and sulci and gyri on superolateral
        surface of, 310f
    sulci and gyri on inferior surface of, 310f
    superficial veins of, 278
    sulci and gyri on medial surface of, 309
Cerebrum
    anterior part of, 332f
    composition of, 307
    dissection and identification of
        cerebral hemispheres, 307–309
        midsagittal section of brain, 308–309
    external features of
        gyri, 312–313
        limbic lobe and hippocampus, 313
        poles, surfaces, and borders, 312
        sulci, 312–313
    surface landmarks on, 307
Cervical groups of lymph nodes, 163
Cervical plexus, 162f
    branches of, 195–196
    dissection to roots and trunks of, 169, 171
    exposure of, 192, 193f
Cervical rib, 176
Cervical sympathetic trunk

branches of, 188
    ganglia of, 187
    injury to, 189
Cervical vertebrae, 15f
    constituents of, 15
    first, 16–17, 17f
    second, 18, 18f
    seventh, 19, 19f
Cervical vertebral joints. *See* Joints of neck region
Cervical viscera, 178f
Chalazion, 48
Chorda tympani nerve, 93, 216, 255
Choroid plexus, 298
Cingulum association fibers, 321–322
Circle of Willis, 275–277, 280–281, 280f
Circumvallate papillae, 216
Circumventricular organs, 320
Cisternal puncture, 63
Cisterna pontis, 277
Cistern of great cerebral vein, 278
Cistern of lateral sulcus, 278
Cochlear apparatus, 258–259
Commissural fibers, 325–326
Common carotid arteries, 172
Complete cleft palate, 208
Confluence of sinuses, 120
Conjunctiva, 46f, 47
Corneal grafts, 248
Corniculate cartilage, 233
Corona radiata, 323, 326
Corpus callosum, 319, 324–325
Cranial fossae
    anterior
        dissection and identification of, 124
        location of, 123
        surface landmarks on, 123
    middle
        dissection and identification of, 124–126
        location of, 123
        surface landmarks on, 123
    middle meningeal artery
        cavernous sinuses, 128–131
        course of, 127f
        frontal branch of, 127
        hypophysis cerebri, 127–128
        parietal branch of, 127
        sigmoid sinus, 132
        tentorium cerebelli, 131–132
        transverse sinus, 132
        trigeminal ganglion, 131
    posterior
        dissection and identification of, 126
        location of, 123
        surface landmarks on, 123
Cranial meninges
    arachnoid mater, 120
    arachnoid villi and granulations, 121
    definition of, 118
    dura mater, 118–119
        dural folds, 119
        dural venous sinuses, 119
        paired sinuses, 120
        unpaired sinuses, 119–120
    pia mater, 121
Cranial nerves and cavernous sinus, 130f
Cranial vault, 7

Cranial venous sinus, 124f
Craniovertebral joints, 264f, 265f
Cranium, interior of, 126f
Cricoarytenoid joints, 234
Cricoid cartilage, 232
Cricothyroid cartilage, 232–233
Cricothyroid joints, 233–234
Cricothyroid membrane, 232
Cricothyroid muscle, dissection of, 160, 234
Cricotracheal membrane, 233
Cuneiform cartilage, 233

D
Dacryocystitis, 48
Deep temporal fascia. *See* Temporal fascia
Diaphragma sellae, 119
Direction of enlargement of gland, 154
Dura mater
    dural folds, 119
    dural venous sinuses, 119
    paired sinuses, 120
    unpaired sinuses, 119–120

E
Ear
    dissection and identification of
        external acoustic meatus, 251
        internal ear, 253
        middle ear cavity, 251–252
        tympanic membrane, 251
    external (*See* External ear)
    internal (*See* Internal ear)
    middle (*See* Middle ear)
    parts of, 249, 250f
    surface landmarks on, 249
Enlargement of tubal tonsil, 208
Epicranial aponeurosis, 27
Epidural hemorrhage, 121
Epiglottic cartilage, 233
Epiphora, 48
Epistaxis, 229
Esophagus, 154
Esophagus, dissection of, 201
Ethmoidal air sinuses, 229
Eustachian tube, muscles of, 203f
External ear, 249
    auricle, 253
    dissection and identification of, 251
    external auditory meatus, 254
    surface landmarks on, 249
External laryngeal nerve, 160, 234, 240
Extraocular muscles
    of orbit, 139, 139t
    paralysis, 145–146
    of right eye, 137f
Eyeball, 241
    anterior segment of, 241, 244f, 246–247
    arterial supply of, 247
    blood supply of, 243f
    dissection and identification of, 241–243
    fibrous coat of, 245
    nerves of, 248
    nervous coat of, 245
    posterior segment of, 241, 247
    structure of, 242f
    surface landmarks on, 241

    vascular coat of, 245
    venous drainage of, 248
Eyelids
    dissection and identification of
        lacrimal gland and lacrimal sac, 45
        orbicularis oculi muscle, orbital septum, and
            nerves, 44–45
    functions of, 43
    layers of, 46–47, 46f
    margin of, 44f
    surface landmarks of, 43

F
Face
    arterial supply of, 38–39, 39f, 39t
    bleeding from, 41
    dangerous area of, 41, 41f
    dissection and identification of
        branches of facial nerve, 34, 35f
        cutaneous branches of trigeminal nerve, 34
        facial artery and vein, 34
        muscles of facial expression, 32, 33f, 34
        orbicularis oculi muscles, 34
        orbicularis oris, 34
        parotid duct, 34, 35f
        parotid gland, 34, 35f
        skin incision and reflection, 31–32, 32f
    muscles of, 37, 38t, 38t
    nerve supply of skin of, 36–37, 36f
    surface landmarks of, 31
    venous drainage of, 39, 40f
Facial artery
    in submandibular region, 108–109
    tonsillar branch of, 206
Facial nerve, 79, 80f
    branches of, 38
    dissection of branches of, 34, 35f
Falx cerebelli, 119
Falx cerebri, 119
First cervical vertebrae, 16–17, 17f
Fissures and lobes, 295, 297
Flocculonodular lobe, 299
Foramen magnum, structures passing through, 132
Forebrain, 272
Forehead skin
    blood vessels exposure beneath, 22–23
    muscles exposure beneath, 22–23
    nerve exposure beneath, 22–23
Fornix, 318–319
Fourth ventricle, 304f
    dissection and identification of
        floor of fourth ventricle, 303–304
        roof of fourth ventricle, 304, 305f
    features of, 306
    functions of, 303
    location of, 303
    median aperture of, 298
    surface landmarks on, 303
Foville syndrome, 291
Frontal air sinuses, 229

G
Glossopharyngeal nerve, 108, 184, 188
    branches of, 185
    course of, 185
    dissection and identification of, 179, 181f

Glottis, 231
Great auricular nerve, 81
Greater palatine artery, 206
Greater palatine nerve, 207

H

Habenular commissure, 319
Hard palate
    dissection of, 201
    neurovascular structures of, 203*f*
Head, 1
    dissection of, 201
    midsagittal section of, 199*f*
Hearing, mechanism of, 259
Hemiballismus, 340
Hindbrain, 272, 283, 283*f*
    cerebellum (*See* Cerebellum)
    medulla oblongata
        dissection and identification of, 284–285
        dorsal surface of, 286
        internal structure of, 286–287
        lesions of, 287
        surface landmarks on, 284
        transverse section of, 286*f,* 287*f*
        ventral surface of, 285
    pons, 289
        dissection and identification of, 288–289
        external features of, 289
        internal structure of, 290–291
        posterior surface of, 288
        surface landmarks on, 288
        ventral surface of, 288
Huntington chorea, 340
Hydrocephalus, 336
Hyoid bone, 15, 15*f*
Hypoglossal nerve, 73, 108, 162*f,* 216
    branches of, 187
    dissection and identification of, 179, 181*f*
    dissection of, 159–160
    injury, 217
    injury to, 189
Hypophysis cerebri, 132
Hypothalamus, 319

I

Incomplete cleft palate, 208
Inferior and middle cervical ganglia, dissection to, 169, 171
Inferior longitudinal bundle, dissection of, 323–324
Inferior medullary velum, 298
Inferior orbital fissure, 144–145
Inferior sagittal sinus, 119
Inferior thyroid artery, 149*f*
    dissection of, 234
    ligation of, 154
Infraorbital artery, 143–144
Infratemporal fossa, 85
    dissection to expose, 86–90, 89*f*
    lateral pterygoid muscle in, 92*f*
Infratemporal regions, 85
    arteries of, 93–94, 93*t*
    dissection and identification of
        infratemporal fossa, 86–90, 89*f*
        temporalis muscle, 86
    muscles related to, 89, 90*t*
    nerves of, 92–93, 92*t*

surface landmarks on, 85–86
veins of, 94, 94*f*
Insula, 311*f*
Internal capsule, 323, 326–327, 327*f*
Internal carotid artery, 279–280
    dissection and identification of, 180
    in upper part of neck, 177
Internal ear, 249, 256
    cochlear apparatus, 258–259
    dissection and identification of, 253
    schematic diagram of, 257*f*
    vestibular apparatus
        semicircular ducts, 258
        utricle and saccule, 257
Internal jugular vein, 180, 188
Internal laryngeal nerve, 239–240
Interpeduncular cistern, 277
Intervertebral joints, 261, 265–266
Intracerebellar nuclei, 298
Intracranial dural venous sinuses, 129*f*

J

Jaw, locking of, 101, 101*f*
Joints of larynx, 233–234
Joints of neck region, 266
    atlanto-axial joint, 261, 266
    atlanto-occipital joint, 261, 266
    dissection and identification of, 261
        atlanto-occipital joint, 263
        craniovertebral joints, 264*f,* 265*f*
        intervertebral joints, 265–266
        lateral atlantoaxial joint, 263
        medial atlantoaxial joint, 263
    intervertebral joints, 261
    ligaments of, 267*f*
    surface landmarks on, 261
    types of, 261
Jugulodigastric nodes, 163
Jugulo-omohyoid nodes, 163

L

Lacrimal apparatus, 47–48
Lacrimal canaliculus, 47
Lacrimal gland, 45, 47, 138–139
Lacrimal sac, 45, 47
Laryngeal and phrenic nerves, recurrent, 167–168
Laryngeal cartilages, 231*f*
    laryngeal mucosa covering, 236*f*
    and ligaments, anterolateral view of, 232*f*
    posterior view of, 233*f*
Laryngitis, 240
Laryngopharynx, 197
Larynx
    cavity of, 238
    dissection and identification of
        cricothyroid muscle, 234
        external laryngeal nerve, 234
        inferior thyroid artery, 234
        posterior cricoarytenoid muscle, 237
        recurrent laryngeal nerve, 234
        transverse and oblique arytenoid muscles, 237
        vocal and vestibular folds, 236
    dissection of, 201
    functions of, 231
    muscles of
        extrinsic, 231, 238–239

intrinsic, 231, 237*f*, 239, 239*t*
nerves of, 235*f*
    motor innervation, 240
    sensory innervation, 239–240
skeleton of, 231
surface landmarks on, 232–234
    arytenoid cartilages, 233
    corniculate cartilage, 233
    cricoid cartilage, 232
    cricothyroid cartilage, 232–233
    cricotracheal membrane, 233
    cuneiform cartilage, 233
    epiglottic cartilage, 233
    joints of larynx, 233–234
    quadrangular membrane, 233
    thyrohyoid membrane (ligament), 233
    thyroid cartilage, 232
vessels of, 235*f*, 240
Lateral atlantoaxial joint, dissection of, 263
Lateral nasal wall
    formation of, 224
    nerves and vessels of
        arteries and veins, 226, 226*f*
        autonomic supply, 226
        sensory nerve supply, 225–226
    vessels and nerves of, 223*f*
Lateral ventricle
    anterior horn of, 334*f*
    and caudate nucleus, 339*f*
    central part/body of, 333*f*
    dissection and identification of, 330–332
    features of, 332–335
        deep cerebral veins, 335*f*
    left temporal lobe with inferior horn of, 334*f*
    surface landmarks on, 329–330
Lentiform nucleus, 337
Lesser palatine arteries, 206
Lesser palatine nerve, 207
Ligation of superior thyroid artery, 154
Lingual artery, in submandibular region, 109
Lingual nerve, 108, 112, 216
Little area (Kiesselbach area), 229
Long ciliary nerves, 248
Long posterior ciliary arteries, 247
Ludwig's angina, 74
Lymphatic drainage, 208
Lymph nodes, 73
    cervical groups of, 163
    and lymph trunks, 176
    submandibular and submental groups of, 111–112, 112*f*
Lymphoid tissues of pharynx, 207

M
Mandible, 13–15, 14*f*, 88*f*
Mandibular fossa, 95, 96*f*
Mandibular nerve, 91*f*, 92, 92*t*
Maxillary artery, 93–94, 93*t*
Maxillary sinus
    arteries and veins, 229
    lymphatic drainage, 229
    nerves, 229
    shape of, 227
    walls and relations of, 227–228
Medial atlantoaxial joint, dissection of, 263
Medial nasal wall. *See* Nasal septum

Medial pterygoid muscle, 91*f*
Medulla oblongata
    dissection and identification of, 284–285
    dorsal surface of, 286
    internal structure of, 286–287
    lesions of, 287
    surface landmarks on, 284
    transverse section of, 286*f*, 287*f*
    ventral surface of, 285
Midbrain, 272
    dissection and identification of, 291–292
    dorsal surface of, 293
    internal structure of, 294*f*
        cerebral peduncles, 293–294
        at inferior colliculi level, 293
        at superior colliculi level, 294
        tectum, 294
    lateral surface of, 293
    lesions, 294
    parts of, 293*f*
    surface landmarks on, 291
    ventral surface of, 292
Middle cerebral artery, course and branches of, 276*f*
Middle cranial fossae, 8, 9*f*, 10
    dissection and identification of, 124–126
    location of, 123
    surface landmarks on, 123
Middle ear, 249
    anatomical relationships, 256*f*
    cavity of, 254
        arterial supply of, 256
        contents of, 255
        nerve supply of, 256
    dissection and identification of, 249, 251–252
    ear ossicles in, 252*f*
    infection of, 259
    lymphatic drainage of, 256
    muscles in, 255, 255*t*
    sagittal section through, 252*f*, 253*f*
    surface landmarks on, 249
    venous drainage of, 256
Middle meningeal artery, 132
    cavernous sinuses, 128–131
    course of, 127*f*
    frontal branch of, 127
    hypophysis cerebri, 127–128
    parietal branch of, 127
    sigmoid sinus, 132
    tentorium cerebelli, 131–132
    transverse sinus, 132
    trigeminal ganglion, 131
Millard–Gubler syndrome, 291
Mouth, floor of, 213*f*
Mumps, 83
Muscles of mastication, 89, 90*f*

N
Nasal cavity, 228*f*
    bones and cartilages forming, 219–220
    bony features of, 12
    dissection and identification of
        lateral wall of nose, 221
        nasal septum (medial nasal wall), 220–221
        pterygopalatine ganglion, 222–224
    lateral wall, 11*f*, 12
    lateral wall of, 224

medial wall, 10, 11*f*
right and left, 219
roof and floor, 12
surface landmarks on, 219–220
walls of, 219
Nasal septum
bones and cartilage of, 224
bones of, 12*f*
deviated, 230
dissection of, 220–221
formation of, 224
mucosa of, 222*f*
nerves and vessels of, 225
nerves of, 221*f*
vascular supply of, 222*f*
Nasolacrimal duct, 48
Nasopharynx, 197
Neck, midsagittal section of, 199*f*
Nose, sagittal section through, 223*f*

O
Occipital sinus, 119
Occipitofrontalis muscle and epicranial aponeurosis, 24, 24*f*
Occlusion of canal of Schlemm, 248
Ophthalmic artery, 142–142, 142*f*
Oral cavity, muscles of floor of, 211*f*
Orbicularis oculi muscle, 44–45
Orbit, 228*f*
arteries of
infraorbital, 143–144
ophthalmic, 142–142, 142*f*
dissection and identification of, 133, 134*f*
ciliary ganglion and common tendinous ring, 136–137
lacrimal gland, 137
nerves, vessels, and muscles, 135–136
optic nerves and structures, 136
periorbita, 134–135
removal of periosteum, 135–136
tendons of recti on sclera, 137
extraocular muscles of, 139, 139*t*
lacrimal gland, 138–139
nerves of
abducens, 142
ciliary ganglion, 142
frontal, 141
lacrimal, 141
nasociliary, 141
oculomotor, 141
optic, 140–141
trochlear, 142
surface landmarks on, 133
veins of, 144*f*
inferior orbital fissure and, 144–145
optic canal and, 145
superior orbital fissure and, 144, 145*f*
Orbital cavity, 10
Orbital septum, 44–45
Organ of corti, 258
Oropharynx, 197
Otic ganglion, 93

P
Palate, sagittal section through, 223*f*
Palatine branch of ascending pharyngeal artery, 206

Palatine tonsils, 204*f*, 207–208
Parahippocampal gyrus, 311*f*
Paranasal sinuses, 228*f*
Parapharyngeal space, 178*f*
Parathyroid glands, 151
dissection of, 149
preservation of, 155
Paratonsillar vein, 208
Parkinson disease, 340
Parotid abscess, 83
Parotid bed, 75
Parotid duct, 79
Parotid gland
lateral surface of, 76*f*, 77*f*
relations of, 79
shape of, 79
Parotid lymph nodes, 83, 83*f*
Parotid region, 75
arteries of, 81*f*, 82
dissection and identification of, 76–78
external carotid artery, 81, 81*f*
facial nerve, 79, 80*f*
muscles related to, 82
nerves of, 81
surface landmarks on, 75
veins of, 82, 82*f*
Parotid tumors, 83
Partial ptosis (drooping) of upper eyelid, 48
Pericranium, 24, 27, 29
Pharyngeal branches of ascending pharyngeal artery, 206
Pharyngeal mucosa, surface anatomy of, 202*f*
Pharyngeal muscles, 200*f*
Pharyngeal plexus
of nerves, 206–207
of veins, 206
Pharynx
arteries, 206
cavity of, 197
constrictors of, 201*f*
dissection and identification of, 198–199, 201
exposure of cavity of, 200–201
lymphoid tissues of, 207
muscles of, 204–205*t*
arrangement of, 204
dissection of, 202
subdivisions, 198*f*
surface landmarks on, 197–198
veins, 206
wall of, 197
Phrenic nerves, 53–54, 175
Pia mater, 121
Pineal gland, 319
Pituitary gland, subdivisions of, 128*f*
Pons, 289
dissection and identification of, 288–289
external features of, 289
internal structure of, 290–291
posterior surface of, 288
surface landmarks on, 288
ventral surface of, 288
Posterior commissure, 319
Posterior cranial fossae, 10
dissection and identification of, 126
location of, 123
surface landmarks on, 123

Posterior cricoarytenoid muscle, 237
Posterior inferior cerebellar artery, 278
Posterior spinal artery, 278
Posterior triangle
    description of, 55–56
    dissection and identification of
        boundaries of posterior triangle, 52, 52f
        brachial plexus, 53–54
        cutaneous nerves, 52, 52f
        floor of posterior triangle, 53, 54f
        incision and reflection of skin, 50–52, 51f
        occipital and subclavian triangles, 52–53
        phrenic nerve, 53–54
        subclavian vessels, 53–54
    floor of, 53, 54f
    nerves of, 56t
    roof of, 49
    subdivision of, 49
    surface landmarks of, 49–50, 50f
Prevertebral muscles, 191
    dissection and identification of, 191–192
    and intertransverse muscles, 194t
    and nerves, 195–196
    scalene and, 192f
    surface landmarks on, 191
    and veins, 195
    vertebral artery, 194–195
Projection fibers, 326–327
Pterygoid venous plexus, 94, 94f
Pterygopalatine ganglion, 227, 230
    branches of, 227
    exposure of, 222–224
Putamen and caudate nucleus, 339f

Q
Quadrangular membrane, 233

R
Raymond syndrome, 291
Recurrent laryngeal nerve, 148–149, 234, 240
Retina, layers of, 245f
Retinal detachment, 248
Retromandibular fossa. See Parotid bed
Retromandibular vein, 81–82
Right auricle, 250f
Right eye, extraocular muscle of, 137f, 138f
Right recurrent nerves, 175
Root of neck
    arteries of
        common carotid, 172
        subclavian, 172–173, 173–174t
    dissection and identification of, 166–171
    muscles of
        pre- and paravertebral, 172f
        scalene, 171, 171t
    nerves of
        brachial, 175–176
        lymph nodes and lymph trunks, 176
        phrenic, 175
        right recurrent, 175
    significance of, 165
    structures and their relationship at, 166f
    surface landmarks on, 165–166
    veins of, 174–175
Rotation of head, dizziness following, 63

S
Saccule, 257
Scala media, 258
Scala tympani, 258
Scala vestibuli, 258
Scalene muscles, 171, 171t, 192f
Scalene syndrome, 176
Scalenus anterior muscle, dissection to, 167–168
Scalp
    blood vessels of, 24–25, 24t
    clinical anatomy of, 27
    deeper dissection of, 26
    definition of, 21
    dissection and identification of, 22–23
    layers of, 23–24, 23f
    nerves of
        motor, 25, 25f
        sensory, 25, 26t
    surface landmarks, 21
Second cervical vertebrae, 18, 18f
Semicircular ducts, 258
Septum pellucidum, 319
Seventh cervical vertebrae, 19, 19f
Short ciliary nerves, 248
Short posterior ciliary arteries, 247
Sigmoid sinus, 120, 132
Sinusitis, 230
Skull
    anatomical position of, 1
    anterior aspect of, 2–3, 4f
    base of, 5, 6f
        anterior part of external aspect of, 5f, 6
        interior of, 7–10
        middle part of, 7
        posterior part of, 7
    bones of, 1, 1t
    internal aspect of, 7
    lateral aspect of, 4–5, 5f
    posterior aspect of, 2, 3f
    superior aspect of, 1–2, 2f
Soft palate, 197
    dissection of, 201
    muscles of, 203f, 205t
    surface landmarks on, 197–198
Sphenoidal air sinuses, 229
Sternomastoid and posterior belly of digastric muscle
    arteries of, 161
    carotid sheath, 160–161
    dissection and identification of, 158–160
    middle part of, 157
    nerves of
        ansa cervicalis, 161, 163
        lymph nodes, 163
    surface landmarks on, 158
    upper part of, 157
    veins of, 161
Straight sinus, 119
Stye, 48
Subclavian arteries, 167–168, 172–173, 173–174t
Subclavian vein, 174
Subclavian vessels, 53–54
Subdural hemorrhage, 121
Sublingual gland, 111
Submandibular/digastric triangle, 109f
Submandibular duct, 112
Submandibular gland, 103, 110–111

Submandibular lymph nodes and submandibular gland, 112
Submandibular parasympathetic ganglion, 103
Submandibular region, 103
 arteries of, 108–109
 dissection and identification of, 106f
  glossopharyngeal nerve, 105–106
  hyoglossus muscle, exposure of, 105, 106f
  lingual vessels, 105–106
  mylohyoid muscle, exposure of, 105
  styloid process, 105–106
  submandibular gland, exposure of, 105
  submental and digastric triangles, 104, 104f
 glands of, 110–111
 lymph nodes of, 103
 muscles of, 104, 104f, 107, 107f, 107t
 surface landmarks on, 103
 veins of, 109–110
 vessels of, 103
Submental triangle, enlargement of submental lymph node in, 74
Suboccipital triangle, 61–62
Substantia nigra, 339
Subthalamic nuclei, 339, 339f
Superficial fascia, 23, 27, 28–29
Superficial temporal region
 dissection and identification of, 28
 soft tissue layers of, 28–29, 28f
Superficial veins of cerebral hemisphere, 278
Superior laryngeal nerve, 148–149
Superior longitudinal bundle, dissection of, 322–323
Superior orbital fissure, 125f, 144, 145f
Superior sagittal sinus, 119
Superior thyroid artery, ligation of, 154
Supraclavicular nerves, 56f
Swelling of adenoids, 208
Sympathetic trunk
 dissection of, 160
 dissection to, 169, 171

T
Temple region. See Superficial temporal region
Temporal fascia, 29
Temporal fossa, 85
Temporalis muscle, 86
Temporal region, 85
 arteries of, 93–94, 93t
 dissection and identification of
  infratemporal fossa, 86–90, 89f
  temporalis muscle, 86
 muscles related to, 89, 90t
 nerves of, 92–93, 92t
 surface landmarks on, 85–86
 veins of, 94, 94f
Temporomandibular (TM) joint, 91f
 description of, 97–98
 dissection and identification of, 96–97, 97f
 interior of, 97f
 ligaments of, 100f
 movements of, 98–101
  chewing, 101
  depression, 98, 99f
  elevation, 101
  protraction, 98, 98f
  retraction, 98, 98f

surface landmarks on, 95, 96f
Tentorium cerebelli, 119, 131–132
Thalamus, 319
Third ventricle, 320
Thoracic duct, 148–149, 174
Thoracic outlet, 165
Thoracic pleura, 175
Thrombosis of dural venous sinuses, 121
Thymus, 149
Thyroglossal cyst or sinus, 154
Thyrohyoid membrane (ligament), 233
Thyroid cartilage, 232
Thyroidectomy, 155
Thyroid gland
 arteries of, 151, 152f
 blood vessels of, 148–149
 dissection and identification of, 147–149
 false capsule of, 150
 location of, 147
 lymphatic drainage of, 151
 nerves of, 151
 neurovasculature, 153f
 parts/lobes of, 150, 150f
 surface landmarks on, 147
 veins of, 151, 152f
Thyroid surgery, anatomical considerations during, 154
Tongue
 artery of, 215
 dissection and identification of
  hyoglossus muscle, 212–214
  on midsagittal section of head, 210–211
  sublingual gland and submandibular duct, 212, 212f
 dorsum of, 209, 210f
 functions of, 209
 lymphatic drainage of, 216–217, 216f
 midsagittal section of, 211f
 muscles of
  extrinsic, 214, 215t
  intrinsic, 212–214, 214f, 215f
 nerves of, 213f, 216
 root, body, and tip of, 209
 substance of, 209
 surface landmarks on, 209
 veins of, 216
 ventral aspect of, 209, 210f
 vessels of, 213f
Tonsillar branch of facial artery, 206
Trachea, 153–154, 201
Tracheotomy, 155
Transverse and oblique arytenoid muscles, 237
Transverse sinus, 120, 132
Trigeminal ganglion, 131
Trigeminal neuralgia, 40
Tympanic cavity. See Middle ear
Tympanic membrane, 254–255

U
Uncinate fasciculus, dissection of, 323
Uncus, 311f
Upper part of cervical vessels and nerves
 accessory nerve, 186
 cervical part of internal carotid artery, 182–183
 cervical part of sympathetic trunk, 187–188
 cervical part of vagus nerve, 185–186

dissection and identification of, 178–180
  accessory nerve, 179
  cervical viscera and parapharyngeal space, 178*f*
  glossopharyngeal nerve, 179, 181*f*
  hypoglossal nerve, 179, 181*f*
  internal carotid artery and internal jugular vein, 180
  parapharyngeal space, 180, 182*f*
  sympathetic trunk, 179
  vagus nerve, 179, 180*f*, 181*f*
  glossopharyngeal nerve, 184–185
  hypoglossal nerve, 186–187
  internal jugular vein, 183–184
  surface landmarks on, 177
Utricle, 257

V
Vagus nerve, 73, 188
  branches of, 185–186
  dissection and identification of, 179, 180*f*, 181*f*
  dissection to, 167–168
Ventral rami of cervical nerves, exposure of, 192
Ventriculography, 320, 336
Vertebral artery
  branches of, 195
  exposure of, 192
  intracranial branches of, 278
  origin, course, and parts of, 193*f*

parts of, 194–195
second part of, 196
Vertebral vein, 195
Vestibular apparatus
  semicircular ducts, 258
  utricle and saccule, 257
Vocal and vestibular folds, 236

W
Weber syndrome, 294
Wharton duct. *See* Submandibular duct
White matter of cerebellum, 300
White matter of cerebrum
  association fibers, 325
  commissural fibers, 325–326
  dissection and identification of
    cingulum association fibers, 321–322
    corona radiata, 323
    corpus callosum, 324–325
    inferior longitudinal bundle, 323–324
    internal capsule, 323
    superior longitudinal bundle, 322–323
    uncinate fasciculus, 323
  internal capsule, 326–327, 327*f*
  projection fibers, 326–327

Z
Zygomatic arch, 87*f*

oin our Student Ambassador Program

e you a medical student with a strong
ssion for improving education in your field?

ecome a Thieme Student's Champion!

**Scan the QR Code
to Sign Up Today!**

https://bit.ly/3qJr2la

About the Student's Champion Program

As a Student's Champion, you will be part of a select group of individuals who act as ambassadors for Thieme. You will have the opportunity to promote our mission of enhancing medical education, while gaining valuable skills and experiences along the way.

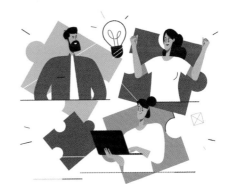

© rikkyal/stock.adobe.com

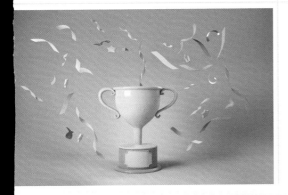

Program benefits and opportunities

- Solve real-world problems of students
- Develop leadership and management skills
- Expand your professional network
- Collaborate with a leading international publisher

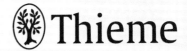

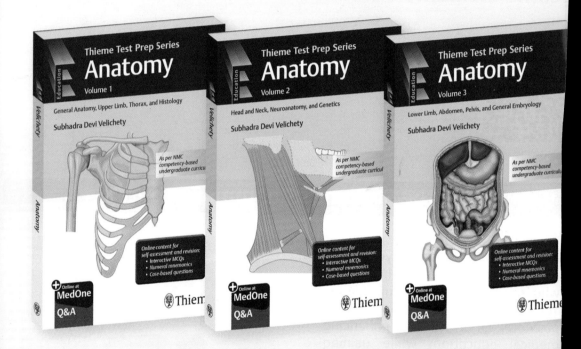

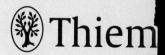